T0263635

Hepatitis C Direct Acting Antivirals: The New Standard of Care

Guest Editor

FRED POORDAD, MD

CLINICS IN LIVER DISEASE

www.liver.theclinics.com

Consulting Editor
NORMAN GITLIN, MD

August 2011 • Volume 15 • Number 3

SAUNDERS an imprint of ELSEVIER, Inc.

W.B. SAUNDERS COMPANY

A Division of Elsevier Inc.

1600 John F. Kennedy Boulevard, Suite 1800 • Philadelphia, PA 19103-2899

http://www.theclinics.com

CLINICS IN LIVER DISEASE Volume 15, Number 3
August 2011 ISSN 1089-3261, ISBN-13: 978-1-4557-1107-9

Editor: Kerry Holland

Clinics in Liver Disease (ISSN 1089-3261) is published quarterly by Elsevier Inc., 360 Park Avenue South, New York, NY 10010-1710. Months of issue are February, May, August, and November. Business and Editorial Offices: 1600 John F. Kennedy Blvd., Ste. 1800, Philadelphia, PA 19103-2899. Customer Service Office: 3251 Riverport Lane, Maryland Heights, MO 63043. Periodicals postage paid at New York, NY and additional mailing offices. Subscription prices are $251.00 per year (U.S. individuals), $124.00 per year (U.S. student/resident), $343.00 per year (U.S. institutions), $333.00 per year (foreign individuals), $171.00 per year (foreign student/resident), $413.00 per year (foreign instituitions), $290.00 per year (Canadian individuals), $171.00 per year (Canadian student/resident), and $413.00 per year (Canadian institutions). Foreign air speed delivery is included in all *Clinics* subscription prices. All prices are subject to change without notice. **POSTMASTER:** Send address changes to *Clinics in Liver Disease*, Elsevier Health Sciences Division, Subscription Customer Service, 3251 Riverport Lane, Maryland Heights, MO 63043. **Customer Service: Telephone: 1-800-654-2452 (U.S. and Canada); 314-447-8871 (outside U.S. and Canada). Fax: 314-447-8029. E-mail: journalscustomerservice-usa@elsevier.com (for print support); journalsonlinesupport-usa@elsevier.com (for online support).**

Reprints. For copies of 100 or more of articles in this publication, please contact the Commercial Reprints Department, Elsevier Inc., 360 Park Avenue South, New York, NY 10010-1710. Tel.: 212-633-3812; Fax: 212-462-1935; E-mail: reprints@elsevier.com.

Clinics in Liver Disease is covered in *MEDLINE/PubMed (Index Medicus)*, Science Citation Index Expanded, Journal Citation Reports/Science Edition, and Current Contents/Clinical Medicine.

Printed and bound by CPI Group (UK) Ltd, Croydon, CR0 4YY

Transferred to Digital Print 2011

Contributors

CONSULTING EDITOR

NORMAN GITLIN, MD, FRCP(LONDON), FRCPE(EDINBURGH), FACG, FACP
Formerly, Professor of Medicine, Chief of Hepatology, Emory University; Currently, Consultant, Atlanta Gastroenterology Associates, Atlanta, Georgia

GUEST EDITOR

FRED POORDAD, MD
Chief, Hepatology, Cedars-Sinai Medical Center; Associate Professor of Medicine, Hepatology Department, David Geffen School of Medicine at University of California Los Angeles, Los Angeles, California

AUTHORS

JOSEPH AHN, MD, MS
Assistant Professor of Medicine, Loyola University Medical Center, Maywood, Illinois

BRUCE R. BACON, MD
James F. King MD Endowed Chair in Gastroenterology; Professor of Internal Medicine, Division of Gastroenterology and Hepatology, St Louis University School of Medicine, St Louis, Missouri

MARIA BUTI, MD
Professor of Medicine, Liver Unit, Hospital General Universitario Valle Hebron; CIBERHED del Instituto Carlos III, Barcelona, Spain

SANDRA CIESEK, MD
Klinik für Gastroenterologie, Hepatologie und Endokrinologie, Medizinische Hochschule Hannover; Abteilung für Experimentelle Virologie, Twincore, Zentrum für Experimentelle und Klinische Infektionsforschung GmbH, Hannover, Germany

ARCHITA P. DESAI, MD
Fellow, Section of Gastroenterology, Hepatology and Nutrition, Department of Medicine, University of Chicago Medical Center, Chicago, Illinois

PAUL V. DESMOND, MBBS, FRACP
Associate Professor, Department of Gastroenterology and Hepatology, St Vincent's Hospital, Fitzroy, Victoria, Australia

DOUGLAS T. DIETERICH, MD
Professor of Medicine, Division of Liver Diseases, Mount Sinai School of Medicine, New York, New York

RAFAEL ESTEBAN, MD
Professor of Medicine, Liver Unit, Hospital General Universitario Valle Hebron; CIBERHED del Instituto Carlos III, Barcelona, Spain

STEVEN L. FLAMM, MD
Professor of Medicine, Northwestern Feinberg School of Medicine, Chicago, Illinois

ROBERT G. GISH, MD
Division of Gastroenterology, University of California at San Diego, San Diego, California

JACINTA A. HOLMES, MBBS
Hepatology Fellow, Department of Gastroenterology and Hepatology, St Vincent's Hospital, Fitzroy, Victoria, Australia

JAWAD A. ILYAS, MD, MS
Liver Center, St Luke's Episcopal Hospital; Departments of Medicine and Surgery, Baylor College of Medicine, Houston, Texas

IRA JACOBSON, MD
Chief of the Division of Gastroenterology and Hepatology; Vincent Astor Distinguished Professor of Clinical Medicine, The Joan Sanford I. Weill Cornell Medical College; Attending Physician, New York-Presbyterian Hospital Cornell Campus, New York, New York

OMER KHALID, MD
Division of Gastroenterology and Hepatology, St Louis University School of Medicine, St Louis, Missouri

PAUL Y. KWO, MD
Professor of Medicine; Medical Director, Liver Transplantation, Gastroenterology/Hepatology Division, Indiana University School of Medicine, Indianapolis, Indiana

ERIC J. LAWITZ, MD, CPI
Alamo Medical Research, San Antonio, Texas

ANNMARIE LIAPAKIS, MD
Fellow Division of Gastroenterology and Hepatology, Weill Cornell Medical College, New York, New York

MICHAEL P. MANNS, MD
Klinik für Gastroenterologie, Hepatologie und Endokrinologie, Medizinische Hochschule Hannover, Hannover, Germany

NICHOLAS A. MEANWELL, PhD
Department of Medicinal Chemistry, Bristol-Myers Squibb Research and Development, Wallingford, Connecticut

FERNANDO E. MEMBRENO, MD, MSc
Alamo Medical Research, San Antonio, Texas

NANCY REAU, MD
Associate Professor, Section of Gastroenterology, Hepatology and Nutrition, Department of Medicine, Center for Liver Diseases, University of Chicago Medical Center, Chicago, Illinois

MITCHELL L. SHIFFMAN, MD
Director, Liver Institute of Virginia, Bon Secours Health System, Richmond and Newport News, Virginia

ALEXANDER J. THOMPSON, MBBS, FRACP, PhD
Director of Hepatology Research, Department of Gastroenterology and Hepatology, St Vincent's Hospital, Fitzroy, Victoria, Australia; Duke Clinical Research Institute, Duke University Medical Center, Durham, North Carolina

MARIE-LOUISE C. VACHON, MD, MSc
Fellow, Divisions of Infectious Diseases; Division of Liver Diseases, Mount Sinai School of Medicine, New York, New York

JOHN M. VIERLING, MD
Professor of Medicine and Surgery; Chief of Hepatology; Director of Advanced Liver Therapies, Liver Center, St Luke's Episcopal Hospital; Departments of Medicine and Surgery, Baylor College of Medicine, Houston, Texas

THOMAS VON HAHN, MD
Klinik für Gastroenterologie, Hepatologie und Endokrinologie, Medizinische Hochschule Hannover, Hannover, Germany

TANIA M. WELZEL, MD
Department of Medicine 1, JW Goethe University Hospital, Frankfurt, Germany

STEFAN ZEUZEM, MD
Chairman, Department of Medicine 1, JW Goethe University Hospital, Frankfurt, Germany

RONG ZHAO, MD, PhD
Department of Medicine, Indiana University School of Medicine, Indianapolis, Indiana

Contents

pegylated interferon (Peg-IFN) and ribavirin therapy achieve curative responses in 40% to 80% of patients, depending on genotype. Recognition of new therapeutic targets for HCV therapy has led to development of novel therapies. The purpose of this review is to summarize the status of novel therapeutics for CHC that promise to increase the safety and efficacy of therapy.

Boceprevir: A User's Guide **537**

Paul Y. Kwo and Rong Zhao

Given its essential role in the process of hepatitis C virus (HCV) replication, the viral NS3/4A serine protease is arguably the most thoroughly characterized HCV enzyme and the most intensively pursued anti-HCV target for drug development thus far. Recent data have demonstrated promise for the NS3 protease inhibitor boceprevir, which, when added to the standard of care peginterferon and ribavirin, improves sustained virological response while shortening duration of therapy in genotype-1–infected individuals. This review discusses the mechanism of action of boceprevir, its effects on HCV, and its viral resistance.

Telaprevir User's Guide **555**

AnnMarie Liapakis and Ira Jacobson

For a decade, standard therapy for patients with genotype 1 chronic HCV (HCV G1) consisted of pegylated interferon (Peg-IFN) alfa-2a or Peg-IFN alfa-2b, combined with ribavirin. Despite the improved efficacy of this therapy over others, the overall sustained virologic response rate in patients with HCV G1 was still low. This article discusses phase I, II, and III trials examining telaprevir's role in treating patients with HCV. We have now entered an era of combination therapy utilizing direct acting anti-virals, the start of which was marked by the FDA approval of HCV protease inhibitors.

Management of the Treatment-Experienced Patient Infected with Hepatitis C Virus Genotype 1: Options and Considerations **573**

Omer Khalid and Bruce R. Bacon

Individuals infected with hepatitis C virus (HCV) are at risk for cirrhosis and/or hepatocellular carcinoma. Treatment of HCV infection has undergone several revisions over the past 15 years and continues to evolve. The current major advance is with the protease inhibitors in addition to pegylated interferon and ribavirin. The emergence of resistance needs to be monitored carefully as newer and more potent drugs are added to the interferon and ribavirin backbone drugs. In addition, adverse events will be more frequent and some novel ones will require special attention.

The HIV/HCV-Coinfected Patient and New Treatment Options **585**

Marie-Louise C. Vachon and Douglas T. Dieterich

Hepatitis C (HCV) treatment is on the cusp of change with the approval of the first direct-acting antivirals: telaprevir and boceprevir. Drug–drug interactions with HIV antiretrovirals, increased toxicity, and rapid selection of HCV-resistant mutants are among the treatment complexities expected

FORTHCOMING ISSUES

November 2011

Orthotopic Liver Transplantation

Paul Martin, MD and
Cynthia Levy, MD,
Guest Editors

February 2012

Hepatic Encephalopathy

Kevin Mullen, MD, *Guest Editor*

May 2012

Key Consultations in Hepatology

Steven L. Flamm, MD, *Guest Editor*

RECENT ISSUES

May 2011

Diagnosis and Therapy of Hepatocellular Carcinoma: Status Quo and a Glimpse at the Future

Adrian Reuben, BSc, MBBS, FRCP, FACG,
Guest Editor

February 2011

Hepatobiliary Manifestations of Diseases Involving Other Organ Systems

Ke-Qin Hu, MD, *Guest Editor*

November 2010

Diagnostic Challenges in Liver Pathology

Jay H. Lefkowitch, MD, *Guest Editor*

RELATED INTEREST

Gastroenterology Clinics of North America, September 2010 (Vol. 39, No. 3)
Clinical Pharmacology of Gastrointestinal and Liver Disease
Richard H. Hunt, FRCP, FRCPEd, FRCPC, FACG, AGAF, *Guest Editor*

Preface

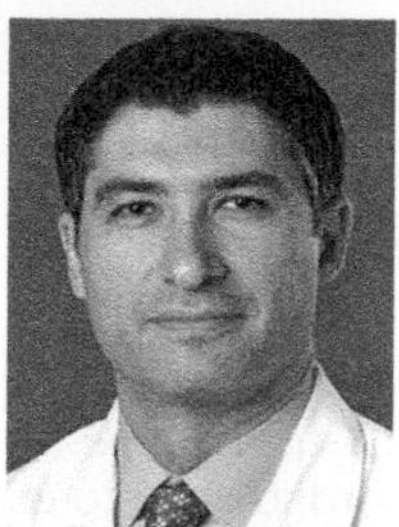

Fred Poordad, MD
Guest Editor

The field of hepatitis C saw a historic year in 2011 with the approval of the first two direct-acting antiviral agents targeting a nonstructural protein of the virus. This advance has been heralded as revolutionary in its potential impact on the care of the hepatitis C patient and the direction of future research.

While these two new compounds, boceprevir and telaprevir, offer a significant improvement in sustained response rates, they are still used with a backbone of interferon and ribavirin. The adverse event profile remains problematic and not all patients are eligible to receive these agents. The field is now quickly progressing toward less toxic regimens, including some with no interferon.

This issue of *Clinics in Liver Disease* begins with Drs Esteban and Buti looking back at the career of interferon, and its ongoing utility in the treatment of hepatitis. Dr Reau then assesses the treatment landscape to tell us who is left to treat. Dr Thompson reviews the exciting emerging field of genetic variability and its impact on treatment decision-making. Drs Kwo and Jacobson then give us a very in-depth overview of the two new protease inhibitors, followed by Dr Manns' assessment of the next wave of this class of drug. Dr Lawitz and Gish explore the polymerase inhibitors and NS5A inhibitors, which are likely to be major players in the combination therapy arena, while Dr Flamm gives a review and insight into other compounds we have heard less about but may have a future impact. The excitement of having so many new compounds to experiment with is tempered by the realization that mixing and matching drugs may not be so straightforward. Dr Zeuzem tells us what makes sense in this regard, while Drs Vierling and Bacon gives us some practical considerations on how to treat patients today with what we currently have available. There are many subgroups of special interest when treating hepatitis C, and Drs Dieterich and Vachon discuss one of these important groups, the HIV co-infected patient. Finally, Dr Shiffman peers into the future and speculates on what the treatment of hepatitis C will look like without interferon, and when that may happen.

I think this issue will spark interest in observing where the field of hepatitis C therapy is going, and I would like to thank all of the authors for their hard work and excellent

Clin Liver Dis 15 (2011) xiii–xiv
doi:10.1016/j.cld.2011.06.001

contributions. I would like to thank Dr Norman Gitlin for giving me the honor of guest editing this issue and particularly Kerry Holland for her patience and support.

Fred Poordad, MD
Hepatology Department
Cedars-Sinai Medical Center
8635 West 3rd Street
Suite 1060
Los Angeles, CA 90048, USA

E-mail address:
Fred.poordad@cshs.org

1990–2010: Two Decades of Interferon-Based Therapy

Maria Buti, MD[a,b,*], Rafael Esteban, MD[a,b]

KEYWORDS

• Hepatitis C • Interferon • Ribavirin

The currently recommended therapy for chronic hepatitis C infection is a combination of pegylated interferon (peginterferon) and ribavirin, which results in sustained clearance of hepatitis C virus (HCV) in at least half of patients. Nonetheless, getting to this point has been a long trip.[1] The history of interferon for the treatment of chronic hepatitis C began almost 25 years ago when hepatitis C was called non-A, non-B hepatitis and the only marker of treatment success was normalization of transaminase values. The year 1989 witnessed an important step forward when Michael Houghton identified the HCV, enabling the development of the first assays to determine HCV RNA and assess the virologic response to therapy.[2] The next step was the introduction of ribavirin, a drug whose mechanism of action is still poorly understood, which increased the response rate and decreased relapses.[3] Then came the development of pegylated interferon, a long-lasting interferon taken once a week that reaches greater, and more maintained serum levels, thereby increasing the sustained virologic response (SVR).[4] However, the story of interferon is a still a work in progress. New types of interferon, such as interferon-λ, which has a different mechanism of action and probably a better safety profile, are under investigation in phase 3 studies. The results of these trials could change the treatment approach to HCV.

INTERFERON FOR NON-A, NON-B HEPATITIS

Interferons are host-derived proteins produced by nucleated cells in response to viruses. These agents represent the early, preantibody response to viral infection.

The authors are consultants for Merck, Gilead, Novartis, BMS, and Janseen.

[a] Liver Unit, Hospital General, Universitario Valle Hebron, Paseo Valle Hebron 119, Barcelona 08035, Spain

[b] CIBERHED del Instituto Carlos III, Barcelona, Spain

* Corresponding author. Liver Unit, Hospital General, Universitario Valle Hebron, Paseo Valle Hebron 119, Barcelona 08035, Spain.

E-mail address: Mbuti@vhebron.net

Clin Liver Dis 15 (2011) 473–482

doi:10.1016/j.cld.2011.05.007

liver.theclinics.com

Three types of interferon produced by different cell populations have been described.[5,6] Alpha interferon is produced by B lymphocytes and monocytes, beta interferon by fibroblasts, and gamma or immune interferon by the helper-inducer subset of T lymphocytes. Interferons elicit an antiviral response in cells by binding to specific cell receptors and activating intracellular enzymes, such as 2′,5′-oligoadenylate synthetase, which activates ribonucleases that can destroy viral mRNAs within the infected cells. In addition, interferons have other properties such as immunomodulatory actions, amplifying HLA class I antigen expression on membranes of virus-infected cells, and augmenting natural killer cell activity.[6–9]

The first study with interferon for the treatment of chronic non-A, non-B hepatitis was a small trial of recombinant human interferon-α2b performed in 1983 by Hoofnagle and colleagues.[10] The investigators treated 10 patients who had chronic non-A, non-B hepatitis with doses of 0.5 to 5 μg of recombinant human interferon-α. Elevated serum aminotransferase levels decreased rapidly during therapy and eventually fell to normal or near normal in 8 of the 10 patients. Prolonged treatment was associated with a sustained improvement in aminotransferase levels and a marked improvement in hepatic histology, even though low doses of interferon-α had been used. These findings suggested that long-term, low-dose interferon-α therapy could be effective in controlling the disease activity in some patients with chronic non-A, non-B hepatitis, and provided proof that interferon, with its broad antiviral activity, was effective against the still undiscovered agent of non-A, non-B hepatitis.

Six years later, in 1989, Davis and colleagues[11] published the first prospective, randomized, controlled trial assessing the role of interferon therapy in naïve patients with chronic hepatitis C. One hundred and sixty-six patients with chronic hepatitis C were randomly assigned to receive either 3 million or 1 million units of recombinant interferon-α 3 times weekly for 24 weeks, or to receive no treatment. The probability of normalization or near normalization of serum alanine aminotransferase (ALT) levels after 6 months of interferon therapy was 46% in patients treated with 3 million units (P<.001) and 28% in those treated with 1 million units (P<.02), but only 8% in untreated patients. Patients who received 3 million units of interferon showed histologic improvement, with regression of lobular and periportal inflammation. Relapse within 6 months after completion of treatment occurred in 51% of patients treated with 3 million units of interferon and 44% of those treated with 1 million units. This study was the first to show that a 24-week course of interferon therapy was effective in controlling disease activity in many patients with hepatitis C, although relapse after stopping treatment was common.

Both studies were performed before HCV had been identified and included patients with chronic non-A, non-B hepatitis, and the criteria used to assess treatment response were normalization of ALT levels and/or improved liver histology. Following these studies, other trials confirmed the initial results in larger numbers of patients and identified certain variables, such as young age, short duration of infection, and elevated ALT levels, associated with a greater response to therapy.

A major milestone in the interferon story occurred in 1989, when Michel Houghton identified and characterized the HCV.[2] After nearly 6 years of intensive investigation at Chiron Laboratories Corporation, in which numerous molecular biology methods were used to determine the viral etiology of parenterally transmitted non-A, non-B viral hepatitis, a single cDNA clone was isolated, shown to be derived from a new flavi-like virus, and named hepatitis C virus. The HCV clone was isolated using a novel, blind immunoscreening method with antibodies derived from a clinically diagnosed non-A, non-B patient, and was found to encode an immunodominant epitope within the HCV nonstructural protein 4. Its viral origin was demonstrated by its specific hybridization to a large single-stranded RNA molecule of about 10,000 nucleotides found only in non-A, non-B hepatitis–infected samples, and which shared distant sequence identity with flaviviruses. Subsequent work demonstrated that HCV was the principal cause of parenterally transmitted non-A, non-B hepatitis around the world, with an estimated 170 million global carriers.[12,13]

Identification of HCV enabled the development of serologic markers such as anti-HCV antibodies and, even more important, the detection of HCV RNA, the best marker of active HCV infection. In 1990, Shindo and colleagues[14] published the first clinical observation evaluating the effect of interferon on HCV RNA, and reported an association between undetectable HCV RNA and normalization of ALT values. Thus, HCV RNA determination was found to be a valuable virologic marker of therapy response.

At that time, 3 types of interferon-α were under development: recombinant interferon-α2b and interferon-α2a, and a monoclonal antibody–purified lymphoblastoid alpha interferon named interferon lymphoblastoid, as well as a type of beta interferon.[15,16] Lymphoblastoid interferon-α is a mixture of different interferons, and is produced by stimulation of a human cell line with Sendai virus.

A randomized study was performed to compare the short-term and long-term efficacy and safety of interferon-α2b with that of lymphoblastoid interferon in a 24-week treatment course. One thousand and seventy-one patients with chronic hepatitis C were randomized to receive either lymphoblastoid interferon or interferon-α2b. The efficacy results of the two interferons were similar, but interferon lymphoblastoid seemed to have a better safety profile.[17] Following this multicenter study, interferon lymphoblastoid was retired because of limitations in its development. Interferon-β was used mainly in Japan, and was reported to have a better safety profile but with a lower efficacy.[18–20] Later, a second interferon-α2 was developed and named α2a. The efficacy of this interferon was similar to that obtained with α2b, and both were approved for the treatment of chronic hepatitis C.[21]

Interferon-α was approved as hepatitis C therapy in 1991. However, the overall rate of SVR, defined as the absence of HCV RNA in serum at least 6 months after the discontinuation of therapy, was low (generally <20%) with interferon-α monotherapy.[1]

Most patients relapsed after short courses (6 months) of therapy, and sustained viral-negative response occurred in only 21% of treated patients.[1] One way to increase the SVR rates was by prolonging interferon treatment for up to 12 to 24 months. This method increased the durability of the initial response, resulting in a mean sustained response rate of 35%.[1] It also significantly increased the cost and inconvenience of the treatment, and relapse remained common. The main pitfalls of this therapy were that interferon required parenteral injections, had multiple adverse effects, and resulted in a poor overall response rate.

INTERFERON AND RIBAVIRIN

The second important advance in hepatitis C therapy came with the use of ribavirin. Ribavirin is a nucleoside analogue with known activity against several flaviviruses. When HCV was identified as a flavivirus, ribavirin was an obvious treatment choice. Ribavirin had little effect on serum HCV RNA levels, but led to improvements in aminotransferase levels and histologic activity of the liver.[22–24] More importantly, when it was combined with interferon, ribavirin increased the rate of SVR. Two pivotal studies with either interferon-α2b or interferon-α2a given in combination with ribavirin for 48 weeks yielded SVR rates of 40% to 50%; that is, 2 to 3 times those obtained with interferon alone. The SVR rate ranged from 16% to 28% in patients with genotype 1, and 66% to 69% in those with genotypes 2 or 3.[25,26] Ribavirin was approved for use as an adjunct to interferon therapy for hepatitis C in 1998.

PEGYLATED INTERFERONS

A third advance in hepatitis C therapy came soon after, with the development of pegylated forms of interferon that allow once-weekly rather than thrice-weekly injections. This long-acting interferon, pegylated interferon (peginterferon), is produced by the covalent attachment of polyethylene glycol (PEG) to the interferon molecule. With its increased half-life, peginterferon can be given as a weekly dose.[4,27] Two peginterferon formulations are currently approved for the treatment of hepatitis C: α2a (Pegasys, Roche) and α2b (Peg-Intron, Schering-Plough). In two large trials of these agents, the rates of sustained virologic response to a 48-week course of peginterferon and ribavirin were 54% and 56%, as compared with 44% and 47% with standard interferon and ribavirin, and only 29% with peginterferon alone.[28,29] Response rates were higher among patients with genotype 2 or 3 than among those with genotype 1. A subsequent trial of different regimens of peginterferon-α2a and ribavirin showed that patients with genotype 2 or 3 could be treated with a lower dose of ribavirin (800 mg rather than 1000–1200 mg daily), and that SVR rates after 24 weeks of therapy (81% and 84%) were similar to the rates after 48 weeks of therapy (79% and 80%).[28–30]

Treatment of chronic hepatitis C involves a combination of weekly subcutaneous injections of peginterferon and twice-daily oral doses of ribavirin.[28,29] The recommended dose of peginterferon-α2a is 180 μg per week[29] and that of peginterferon-α2b is 1.5 μg/kg body weight per week.[28] The optimal duration of therapy and the ribavirin dose vary according to the HCV genotype. Patients with genotype 1 should receive ribavirin for 48 weeks at a daily dose of 1000 mg (if their body weight is 75 kg or less) or 1200 mg (if their weight exceeds 75 kg).[28–31] Patients with genotype 2 or 3 infection should receive 24 weeks of combination therapy with a ribavirin dose of 800 mg daily.[30,32–34] There is little information on the treatment of hepatitis C in patients with genotypes 4, 5, or 6,[35] and the regimen for genotype 1 is usually recommended for these cases.

In the United States, peginterferon-α2b was approved in 2001 and peginterferon-α2a in 2002. The cost of a 48-week course of peginterferon and ribavirin ranges from $30,000 to $40,000, depending on local charges and the dose and brand of drugs used. The expenditure associated with monitoring and physician visits should also be considered in weighing the costs of therapy.

Three general patterns of response occur with treatment: an SVR, a transient virologic response and relapse or breakthrough, and nonresponse. In patients with an SVR, HCV RNA levels usually decrease rapidly with the start of therapy, become undetectable within 4 to 24 weeks, and remain undetectable throughout the course of treatment and follow-up. ALT levels decrease within a few weeks after the decline in HCV RNA levels, usually become normal during treatment, and remain normal during follow-up. With the use of current regimens, overall SVR rates are 75% to 80% among patients with HCV genotype 2 or 3 infection and 40% to 50% among those with genotype 1.[28–36] Among patients with genotype 1, the SVR rates are lower in blacks (28%) than in whites (52%).[36] Other factors associated with a lower response rate are higher initial levels of HCV RNA (>600,000 IU/mL), male sex, higher body weight, and more advanced liver fibrosis.

Not all patients with HCV RNA that becomes undetectable during treatment have an SVR. In 10% of patients, HCV RNA reappears in serum later, during the course of treatment (as a breakthrough), and in 20% it reappears when therapy is stopped (as a relapse). In patients with a relapse, HCV RNA usually reappears within a few weeks after discontinuation of therapy, and ALT levels increase toward pretreatment levels thereafter.

In some patients with chronic hepatitis C, HCV RNA remains detectable during treatment (nonresponse) and treatment provides little clinical benefit. Nonresponse is uncommon among patients with genotype 2 or 3, but it occurs in at least 30% of patients with genotype 1. In this situation, the recommendation is to stop treatment at week 12 if the drop in HCV RNA levels is less than 2 logs or at week 24 if HCV RNA remains detectable.[37] Individualization of therapy offers the possibility of tailoring treatment to particular patients and selecting the treatment duration that ensures the best chance of achieving SVR while avoiding overtreatment.[28–42]

Side effects of peginterferon and ribavirin affect most patients under treatment.[43] The most common adverse effects of peginterferon are myalgias, fatigue, and hematologic effects. In addition, psychological side effects such as depression, anxiety, irritability, sleep disturbance, and difficulty concentrating can occur.

Two peginterferon-α molecules are commercially available for the treatment of chronic hepatitis C, and these differ in the size and nature of the covalently attached PEG moiety, with resulting differences in pharmacokinetics and dosing regimens. Peginterferon-α2b has a linear 12-kDa PEG chain covalently attached primarily to histidine-34 of interferon-α2b, releasing native interferon-α2b. The branched, 40-kDa PEG chain of peginterferon-α2a is covalently attached via stable amide bonds to lysine residues of interferon-α2a, and circulates as an intact molecule. Consequently, peginterferon-α2a has a longer half-life and reduced clearance compared with native interferon-α2a, and can be given once weekly regardless of body weight.[44] Peginterferon-α2b has a shorter half-life in serum than peginterferon-α2a and requires dosing based on body weight (**Table 1**). The majority of head-to-head randomized controlled trials, including the large, randomized IDEAL (Individualized Dosing Efficacy vs Flat Dosing to Assess Optimal Pegylated Interferon Therapy) trial (N = 3070),[36] have demonstrated similar SVR rates for peginterferon-α2a and peginterferon-α2b in combination with ribavirin (41% vs 39%, respectively). Nonetheless, two randomized controlled trials (N = 431 and N = 320)[45,46] have shown a statistically significant benefit for peginterferon-α2a (66% vs 54% and 69% vs 54%). Furthermore, two large retrospective studies and one prospective observational study in real-life settings

Table 1
Characteristics of the pegylated interferons

Parameter	Pegylated Interferon-α2a	Pegylated Interferon-α2b
Structural		
Molecular weight (kDa)	40	12
Polyethylene glycol structure	Branched	Linear
Pharmacokinetics		
Absorption half-life (h)	50	50
Time to T_{max} (h)	45–70	15–44
Mean C_{max} (μg/L)	14–26	20–32
Elimination half-life (h)	65	22–60
Volume of distribution (L)	8–12	31–73
Clearance (mL/h)	60–100	725
Posology/Administration		
Registration name	Pegasys	Peg-Intron
Route of administration	Subcutaneous	Subcutaneous
Dosage	180 μg weekly	1.5 μg/kg weekly

have shown a significant benefit for peginterferon-α2a versus peginterferon-α2b, although the SVR rates were generally lower than those seen in controlled trials.[47] Peginterferon plus ribavirin, as the standard of care for patients with chronic hepatitis C, may in the future form the basis of improved treatment regimens that include new, targeted anti-HCV agents to increase SVR rates even further.

OTHER INTERFERONS AND NEW INTERFERONS

Interferon alphacon-1 or consensus interferon (CIFN) was approved for the treatment of chronic hepatitis C in 1997, before combination treatment with peginterferon-α and ribavirin became available in the United States. It is a synthetic, recombinant type I interferon derived by aligning the most commonly observed amino acid in each position of several alpha-interferon nonallelic subtypes to generate a consensus sequence (**Table 2**).[48] At present, the use of this drug is restricted to a subgroup of patients who have failed a previous course of treatment.[49] This drug is not approved in Europe and its use in the United States is limited. Albumin–IFN-α2b (AlbIFN-α) is an 85.7-kDa molecule resulting from the genetic fusion of human albumin and interferon-α2b, designed to increase drug exposure and improve patient compliance through less frequent dosing (see **Table 2**). AlbIFN-α has a half-life of approximately 6 days, supporting dosing at 2- to 4-week intervals. AlbIFN-α induces the interferon-specific OAS1 gene, with a mechanism of action similar of that of peginterferon-α.[50] Nevertheless, two recent parallel phase 3 studies in genotype 1 (ACHIEVE 1 including 1331 patients)[51] and in genotype 2 or 3 (ACHIEVE 2/3 including 933 patients)[52] failed to demonstrate better tolerability and efficacy of Alb-IFNα compared with pegylated interferon and ribavirin. Conversely, side effects were more common in the AlbIFN-α group than in the peginterferon-α2a groups, particularly a larger number of pulmonary adverse effects. These safety concerns prompted the US Food and Drug Administration and European Health Care Agency to ask for additional data, which was not provided in the time allotted; hence, the drug was not approved.[53]

Another interferon is currently under development. Interferon-λ (IFN-λ1), also known as IL-29, is a type III interferon that suppresses HCV replication in vitro through mechanisms similar to type I interferons (see **Table 2**). These drugs are cytokines with interferon type I–like antiviral activities. However, IFN-λ1 shows more rapid activation of STAT and a delayed yet prolonged effect on the expression of various interferon-stimulated genes. Of importance is that expression of IFN-λ1 receptors is restricted to B lymphocytes and epithelium-derived cells, including hepatocytes, providing the rationale for reduced adverse events, especially hematological toxicity, compared with interferon-α, which exerts its actions through widely distributed interferon-α tissue receptors.[54,55] Pegylated IFN-λ1 (PegIFN-λ1) developed as a recombinant form of human IFN-λ1 conjugated with a 20-kDa linear PEG chain, is now under evaluation

Table 2
New interferon (IFN) molecules

	Consensus IFN	AlbIFN-α2b	IFN-λ
Type of Interferon	I	I	III
Phase	Licensed in USA	Withdrawn	Phase 2
Advantages	None	Longer half-life	Fewer AEs
Disadvantages	Daily dosing	More AEs	Unknown

Abbreviation: AEs, adverse events.

in phase 2b studies. Much of the scientific popularity of PegIFN-λ1 derives from the recent discovery, by 3 independent genome-wide association studies, that single-nucleotide polymorphisms located near the IL-28B encoding region on chromosome 19 are strongly associated with HCV patients' response to peginterferon-α and ribavirin[56–58]; the results of trials with PegIFN-λ1 are expected in 2012.

In conclusion, over the 25 years of interferon use for the treatment of chronic hepatitis C, this drug has been continuously adapted to provide better formulations, a longer half-life, and fewer side effects. Thus it will remain as the backbone of new protease inhibitor regimens (telaprevir-based and boceprevir-based therapies)[59] for the treatment of patients with chronic hepatitis C infected by genotype 1.

REFERENCES

1. Ghany MG, Strader DB, Thomas DL, et al. Diagnosis, management, and treatment of hepatitis C: an update. Hepatology 2009;49:1335–74.
2. Choo QL, Kuo G, Weiner AJ, et al. Isolation of a cDNA clone derived from a blood-borne non-A, non-B viral hepatitis genome. Science 1989;21(244):359–62.
3. Di Bisceglie AM, Shindo M, Fong TL, et al. A pilot study of ribavirin therapy for chronic hepatitis C. Hepatology 1992;16:649–54.
4. Glue P, Fang JW, Rouzier-Panis R, et al. Pegylated interferon-α2b: pharmacokinetics, pharmacodynamics, safety and preliminary efficacy data. Clin Pharmacol Ther 2000;68:556–67.
5. Liang TJ, Rehermann B, Seeff LB, et al. Pathogenesis, natural history, treatment, and prevention of hepatitis C. Ann Intern Med 2000;132:296–305.
6. Sen GC. Viruses and interferons. Annu Rev Microbiol 2001;55:255–81.
7. Tilg H. New insights into the mechanisms of interferon α: an immunoregulatory and anti-inflammatory cytokine. Gastroenterology 1997;112:1017–21.
8. Mogensen KE, Lewerenz M, Reboul J. The type I interferon receptor: structure, function, and evolution of a family business. J Interferon Cytokine Res 1999;19:1069–98.
9. Peters M. Actions of cytokines on the immune response and viral interactions: an overview. Hepatology 1996;23:909–16.
10. Hoofnagle JH, Mullen KD, Jones DB. Treatment of chronic non-A, non-B hepatitis with recombinant human alpha interferon. A preliminary report. N Engl J Med 1986;315:1575–8.
11. Davis GL, Balart LA, Schiff ER, et al. Treatment of chronic hepatitis C with recombinant interferon alfa. A multicenter randomized, controlled trial. Hepatitis Interventional Therapy Group. N Engl J Med 1989;321(22):1501–6.
12. Lavanchy D. The global burden of hepatitis C. Liver Int 2009;29(Suppl 1):74–81.
13. Kim WR. The burden of hepatitis C in the United States. Hepatology 2002;36(Suppl):S30–4.
14. Shindo M, Di Bisceglie AM, Cheung L, et al. Decrease in serum hepatitis C viral RNA during alpha-interferon therapy for chronic hepatitis C. Ann Intern Med 1991;1(115):700–4.
15. Jacyna MR, Brooks MG, Loke RH, et al. Randomised controlled trial of interferon alfa (lymphoblastoid interferon) in chronic non-A non-B hepatitis. BMJ 1989;14(298):80–6.
16. Kakumu S, Yoshioka K, Wakita T, et al. A pilot study of ribavirin and interferon beta for the treatment of chronic hepatitis C. Gastroenterology 1993;105:507–12.
17. Farrell GC, Bacon BR, Goldin RD. Lymphoblastoid interferon alfa-n1 improves the long-term response to a 6-month course of treatment in chronic hepatitis C

compared with recombinant interferon alfa-2b: results of an international randomized. Hepatology 1998;27:1121–7.
18. Kakizaki S, Takagi H, Yamada T, et al. Evaluation of twice-daily administration of interferon-beta for chronic hepatitis C. J Viral Hepat 1999;6:315–9.
19. Yoshioka K, Yano M, Hirofuji H, et al. Randomized controlled trial of twice-a-day administration of natural interferon beta for chronic hepatitis C. Hepatol Res 2000;18:310–9.
20. Shiratori Y, Nakata R, Shimizu N, et al. High viral eradication with a daily 12-week natural interferon-beta treatment regimen in chronic hepatitis C patients with low viral load. IFN-beta Research Group. Dig Dis Sci 2000;45:2414–21.
21. Ouzan D, Babany G, Valla D, et al. Comparison of high initial and fixed-dose regimens of interferon-alpha2a in chronic hepatitis C: a randomized controlled trial. French Multicenter Interferon Study Group. J Viral Hepat 1998;5:53–9.
22. Reichard O, Andersson J, Schvarcz R, et al. Ribavirin treatment for chronic hepatitis C. Lancet 1991;337:1058–61.
23. Lau JY, Tam RC, Liang TJ, et al. Mechanism of action of ribavirin in the combination treatment of chronic HCV infection. Hepatology 2002;35:1002–9.
24. Feld JJ, Hoofnagle JH. Mechanism of action of interferon and ribavirin in treatment of hepatitis C. Nature 2005;436:967–72.
25. Poynard T, Marcellin P, Lee SS, et al. Randomised trial of interferon alpha2b plus ribavirin for 48 weeks or for 24 weeks versus interferon alpha2b plus placebo for 48 weeks for treatment of chronic infection with hepatitis C virus. International Hepatitis Interventional Therapy Group (IHIT). Lancet 1998;352:1426–32.
26. McHutchison JG, Gordon SC, Schiff ER. Interferon alfa-2b alone or in combination with ribavirin as initial treatment for chronic hepatitis C. Hepatitis Interventional Therapy Group. N Engl J Med 1998;339:1485–92.
27. Harris JM, Martin NE, Modi M. Pegylation: a novel process for modifying pharmacokinetics. Clin Pharmacokinet 2001;40:539–51.
28. Manns MP, McHutchison JG, Gordon SC, et al. Peginterferon alfa-2b plus ribavirin compared with interferon alfa-2b plus ribavirin for initial treatment of chronic hepatitis C: a randomised trial. Lancet 2001;358:958–65.
29. Fried MW, Shiffman ML, Reddy KR, et al. Peginterferon alfa-2a plus ribavirin for chronic hepatitis C virus infection. N Engl J Med 2002;347:975–82.
30. Hadziyannis SJ, Sette H Jr, Morgan TR, et al. Peginterferon alfa-2a and ribavirin combination therapy in chronic hepatitis C: randomized study of treatment duration and ribavirin dose. Ann Intern Med 2004;140:346–55.
31. Zeuzem S, Buti M, Ferenci P, et al. Efficacy of 24 weeks treatment with peginterferon alfa-2b plus ribavirin in patients with chronic hepatitis C infected with genotype 1 and low pretreatment viremia. J Hepatol 2006;44:97–103.
32. Dalgard O, Bjoro K, Hellum KB, et al. Treatment with pegylated interferon and ribavirin in HCV infection with genotype 2 or 3 for 14 weeks: a pilot study. Hepatology 2004;40:1260–5.
33. Mangia A, Santoro R, Minerva N, et al. Peginterferon alfa-2b and ribavirin for 12 vs. 24 weeks in HCV genotype 2 or 3. N Engl J Med 2005;352:2609–17.
34. von Wagner M, Huber M, Berg T, et al. Peginterferon-alpha-2a (40KD) and ribavirin for 16 or 24 weeks in patients with genotype 2 or 3 chronic hepatitis C. Gastroenterology 2005;129:522–7.
35. Kamal SM. Hepatitis C virus genotype 4 therapy: progress and challenges. Liver Int 2011;31(Suppl 1):45–52.
36. McHutchison JG, Lawitz EJ, Shiffman ML. Peginterferon alfa-2b or alfa-2a with ribavirin for treatment of hepatitis C infection. N Engl J Med 2009;361:580–93.

37. Davis GL, Wong JB, McHutchison JG. Early virologic response to treatment with peginterferon alfa-2b plus ribavirin in patients with chronic hepatitis C. Hepatology 2003;38:645–52.
38. Ferenci P, Fried MW, Shiffman ML. Predicting sustained virological responses in chronic hepatitis C patients treated with peginterferon alfa-2a (40 KD)/ribavirin. J Hepatol 2005;43:425–33.
39. Kamal SM, El Kamary SS, Shardell MD. Pegylated interferon alpha-2b plus ribavirin in patients with genotype 4 chronic hepatitis C: the role of rapid and early virologic response. Hepatology 2007;46:1732–40.
40. Pearlman BL, Ehleben C, Saifee S. Treatment extension to 72 weeks of peginterferon and ribavirin in hepatitis C genotype 1-infected slow responders. Hepatology 2007;46:1688–94.
41. Berg T, von Wagner M, Nasser S. Extended treatment duration for hepatitis C virus type 1: comparing 48 versus 72 weeks of peginterferon-alfa-2a plus ribavirin. Gastroenterology 2006;130:1086–97.
42. Buti M, Lurie Y, Zakharova NG, et al. Randomized trial of peginterferon alfa-2b and ribavirin for 48 or 72 weeks in patients with hepatitis C virus genotype 1 and slow virologic response. Hepatology 2010;52:1201–7.
43. Fried MW. Side effects of therapy of hepatitis C and their management. Hepatology 2002;36(Suppl 1):S237–44.
44. Foster GR. Review article: pegylated interferons: chemical and clinical differences. Aliment Pharmacol Ther 2004;20:825–30.
45. Rumi MG, Aghemo A, Prati GM. Randomized study of peginterferon-alpha2a plus ribavirin vs peginterferon-alpha2b plus ribavirin in chronic hepatitis C. Gastroenterology 2010;138:108–15.
46. Ascione A, De Luca M, Tartaglione MT. Peginterferon alfa-2a plus ribavirin is more effective than peginterferon alfa-2b plus ribavirin for treating chronic hepatitis C virus infection. Gastroenterology 2010;138(1):116–22.
47. Aghemo A, Colombo M. Peginterferon alfa-2B versus peginterferon alfa-2A with ribavirin for the treatment of chronic hepatitis C: the pursuit of an ideal. Gastroenterology 2010;138:386–9.
48. Blatt LM, Davis JM, Klein SB, et al. The biologic activity and molecular characterization of a novel synthetic interferon-alpha species, consensus interferon. J Interferon Cytokine Res 1996;16:489–99.
49. Bacon BR, Shiffman ML, Mendes F. Retreating chronic hepatitis C with daily interferon alfacon-1/ribavirin after nonresponse to pegylated interferon/ribavirin: DIRECT results. Hepatology 2009;49:1838–46.
50. Balan V, Nelson DR, Sulkowski MS. A phase I/II study evaluating escalating doses of recombinant human albumin-interferon-alpha fusion protein in chronic hepatitis C patients who have failed previous interferon-alpha-based therapy. Antivir Ther 2006;11:35–45.
51. Zeuzem S, Sulkowski MS, Lawitz EJ. ACHIEVE-1 Study Team. Albinterferon alfa-2b was not inferior to pegylated interferon-alpha in a randomized trial of patients with chronic hepatitis C virus genotype 1. Gastroenterology 2010;139:1257–66.
52. Nelson DR, Benhamou Y, Chuang WL. ACHIEVE-2/3 Study Team. Albinterferon alfa-2b was not inferior to pegylated interferon-alpha in a randomized trial of patients with chronic hepatitis C virus genotype 2 or 3. Gastroenterology 2010;139:1267–76.
53. Human Genome Sciences announces preliminary feedback from FDA on Zalbin BLA for chronic hepatitis C [press release]. Rockville (MD): Human Genome

Sciences, Inc.; June 14, 2010. Available at: http://www.hgsi.com/latest/human-genome-sciences-announces-preliminary-feedback-from-fda-on-zalbin-bla-for-chronic-hepati-7.html. Accessed January 6, 2011.

54. Miller DM, Klucher KM, Freeman JA. Interferon lambda as a potential new therapeutic for hepatitis C. Ann N Y Acad Sci 2009;1182:80–7.
55. Muir AJ, Shiffman ML, Zaman A. Phase 1b study of pegylated interferon lambda 1 with or without ribavirin in patients with chronic genotype 1 hepatitis C virus infection. Hepatology 2010;52:822–32.
56. Ge D, Fellay J, Thompson AJ. Genetic variation in IL-28B predicts hepatitis C treatment-induced viral clearance. Nature 2009;461:399–401.
57. Tanaka Y, Nishida N, Sugiyama M. Genome-wide association of IL28B with response to pegylated interferon-alpha and ribavirin therapy for chronic hepatitis C. Nat Genet 2009;41:1105–9.
58. Thomas DL, Thio CL, Martin MP. Genetic variation in IL28B and spontaneous clearance of hepatitis C virus. Nature 2009;461:798–801.
59. Pawlotsky JM. The results of phase III clinical trial with telaprevir and boceprevir presented at the liver meeting 2010: a new standard of care for hepatitis C virus genotype 1 infection, but with issues still pending. Gastroenterology 2011;140(3):746–54.

Naives, Nonresponders, Relapsers: Who Is There Left to Treat?

Archita P. Desai, MD[a], Nancy Reau, MD[b,*]

KEYWORDS

• Hepatitis C • Epidemiology • Pegylated interferon • Ribavirin
• Non-responders • Relapse

Hepatitis C, previously known as non-A, non-B hepatitis, became a reportable disease in 1982. After intense investigation, the causative agent, the hepatitis C virus, was first isolated and characterized in 1989. Since that time, hepatitis C virus (HCV) infection has been recognized as a staggering problem both in the United States and worldwide. It is now well documented that HCV is the most common chronic bloodborne infection in the United States and is the leading cause of liver transplantation.[1–3]

INCIDENCE

The true incidence of HCV is difficult to assess, as most patients with new infection are asymptomatic, with clinical signs of acute hepatitis C apparent in only 30% to 40% of infections.[4] It is also believed that there is underreporting by health care providers of diagnosed cases.[2] Most importantly, individuals at highest risk of infection, such as injection drug users, may not have access to or seek health care, decreasing the likelihood of timely diagnosis of newly acquired HCV infection. Therefore, although only 878 cases of confirmed acute hepatitis C were reported in the United States in 2008, the Centers for Disease Control and Prevention (CDC) estimates that approximately 18,000 new HCV infections occurred that year, after adjusting for asymptomatic infection and underreporting.[5] Fortunately, our understanding of HCV and its

The authors have nothing to disclose.
Financial Support and conflicts: none.

[a] Section of Gastroenterology, Hepatology and Nutrition, Department of Medicine, University of Chicago Medical Center, 5841 South Maryland Avenue, MC 4076, Chicago, IL 60637, USA
[b] Section of Gastroenterology, Hepatology and Nutrition, Department of Medicine, Center for Liver Diseases, University of Chicago Medical Center, 5841 South Maryland Avenue, MC 4076, Chicago, IL 60637, USA
* Corresponding author.
E-mail address: nreau@medicine.bsd.uchicago.edu

Clin Liver Dis 15 (2011) 483–495
doi:10.1016/j.cld.2011.05.011

transmission has greatly lowered rates of newly acquired HCV infection over the past 2 decades through education, needle-exchange programs, and screening of blood products. As a result, most infected individuals acquired their disease during the 1980s and early 1990s. Specifically, a 5-fold to 10-fold decrease in incidence of acute hepatitis C was observed in the early 1990s.[6,7] Since then, the incidence of acute HCV infection has been steady and estimated at a rate of 0.3 cases per 100,000.[5] These incidence estimates for hepatitis C are derived by adjusting rates from the Sentinel Counties Study of Viral Hepatitis (1982–2006), an active surveillance program put into place by the CDC (1982–2006) to monitor new cases of HCV infection.

PREVALENCE

Because 85% of patients with HCV infection progress to chronic hepatitis, prevalence rates of HCV are staggering. The most recent National Health and Nutrition Examination Survey (NHANES) found that 1.3% of the US population, or more than 3 million people, have chronic hepatitis C.[3] Furthermore, this number is likely to be an underestimate as several high-risk groups were excluded from this analysis, such as those who are incarcerated, homeless, or institutionalized. In a study looking at the prevalence of HCV infection in users of the Department of Veterans Affairs (VA) medical centers, the prevalence of HCV antibody positivity was 4%, and 75% of these patients were positive for HCV RNA.[8] Even higher rates of HCV infection were reported by Briggs and colleagues[9] when studying the users of the San Francisco VA Medical Center with about 18% of patients being positive for anti-HCV, of which 78.6% were viremic. Rates of HCV infection are even higher in the incarcerated population. Among US prison inmates, approximately 12% to 35% had evidence of chronic HCV infection.[10] Different rates of HCV infection are documented in these and other epidemiologic studies because the prevalence varies by several key patient characteristics that are not represented uniformly in the groups of individuals captured by these studies. Those at highest risk for HCV infection are injection drug users, persons who received a blood transfusion or other blood products before 1992, persons who received a bone marrow or solid organ transplant before 1992, those with multiple sexual partners, human immunodeficiency virus (HIV)-infected individuals, those with a history of military service, those who are incarcerated and institutionalized, and those who are homeless or of low socioeconomic status.[2,9,11,12]

In addition, two important demographic features of individuals infected with HCV are also shifting with time: age and race. First, the average age of patients with HCV infection is increasing. Because of the significant decline in annual incidence of HCV infection over the past 2 decades, the prevalence is driven by a cohort of patients infected when rates of new infection were high. As this cohort ages, the peak prevalence shifts to an older age group. To illustrate this point, about 10 years ago, the third NHANES showed a peak prevalence of 3.9% in those aged 30 to 39.[1] Based on the current NHANES data, the prevalence of anti-HCV increased with age from 1.0% in those 20 to 29 years of age to a peak of 4.3% in those 40 to 49 years of age. It then decreased to 1.6% in those 50 to 59 years of age and 0.9% in persons aged 60 years or older. Based on these data, we expect that the prevalence of HCV in younger age groups will continue to decline as the proportion of individuals with newly acquired HCV declines or stays at low levels. In contrast, the prevalence of chronic hepatitis from HCV will increase in the older population and it is projected that without effective interventions, a decline in prevalence will only begin to occur by 2040 because of aging and natural deaths among the cohort of patients infected in the 1980s to 1990s.[13]

The prevalence of HCV also varies in different racial groups over time. African American patients are more likely to have evidence of HCV infection. According the current NHANES data, non-Hispanic black individuals were twice as likely at non-Hispanic white and Mexican American individuals to have antibodies to HCV, 3.0% versus 1.5% versus 1.3% respectively. Interestingly, when broken down by age group, they found that this difference was largely driven by the differences in prevalence in older persons. A striking 9.4% of non-Hispanic black participants 40 to 49 years of age were positive for anti-HCV compared with 3.8% of non-Hispanic white persons (P<.0001). When looking at participants younger than 40, the prevalence between the 2 groups was similar (1.2% vs 1.1%, P = .73).[3] These data indicate that the incidence of HCV infection is equalizing between African American and white individuals; however, clinicians will continue to see a racial difference in those with HCV infection as they manage patients infected during an era when non-Hispanic black persons were more likely to be infected than white persons.

Finally, when considering the prevalence of HCV, it is important to consider prevalence of the different genotypes of the hepatitis C virus. The hepatitis C virus has significant genetic heterogeneity, with 6 different genotypes and several subtypes. Most individuals in the United States with chronic hepatitis C are infected with HCV genotype 1a or 1b with rates as high as 71.5% in tertiary care referral centers.[14] Similar rates of genotype 1 infections were seen in the third NHANES Survey, with 56.7% of patients positive for HCV RNA having genotype 1a and 17% having genotype 1b.[1] Approximately 15% are infected with genotype 2a or 2b and 5% to 7% with 3a, 1% with genotype 4, and 3% with genotype 6.[1] The impact of HCV genotype on clinical behavior is debated in the literature but it is clear that genotype greatly affects response to current standard therapy regimens, with patients infected with genotypes 2 and 3 experiencing much higher rates of sustained virologic response than those infected with genotype 1. Extrapolating from these treatment outcomes, one can safely assume that the proportion of patients infected with genotype 1 HCV will increase: because patients with genotype 2 or 3 disease are more frequently encouraged to consider therapy, treatment typically results in cure and thus without viremia they subsequently are less likely to transmit their infection to others.

DISEASE BURDEN OF HCV INFECTION

The enormous burden of disease related to hepatitis C is fueled by the prevalence of disease combined with the high rates of cirrhosis and its ensuing complications in certain groups of individuals. Currently, HCV is thought to account for 40% of all chronic liver disease. Similarly, 30% to 40% of patients who have received or are waiting for a liver transplant are infected with HCV.[2] It is predicted that without more effective therapy, the disease burden and mortality from HCV infection will increase twofold to threefold over the next 2 decades in the United States as the number of persons with long duration of infection grows (**Fig. 1**).[15,16] Most HCV-infected persons are only now reaching an age when complications of liver disease, such as hepatic decompensation, hepatocellular carcinoma, and death, may start to develop, and multiple studies have predicted a rise in future HCV-related morbidity and mortality rates.[3,13,17,18] Using a complex model looking at multiple cohorts and the natural history of HCV infection, Davis and colleagues[18] project that the proportion of all HCV cases with cirrhosis will increase to 25% in 2010, 37% in 2020, and 45% in 2030, and the number of patients with hepatic decompensation will continue to increase dramatically over the next 30 years as more patients develop cirrhosis. It is also projected that the number of liver-related deaths will increase through 2022.

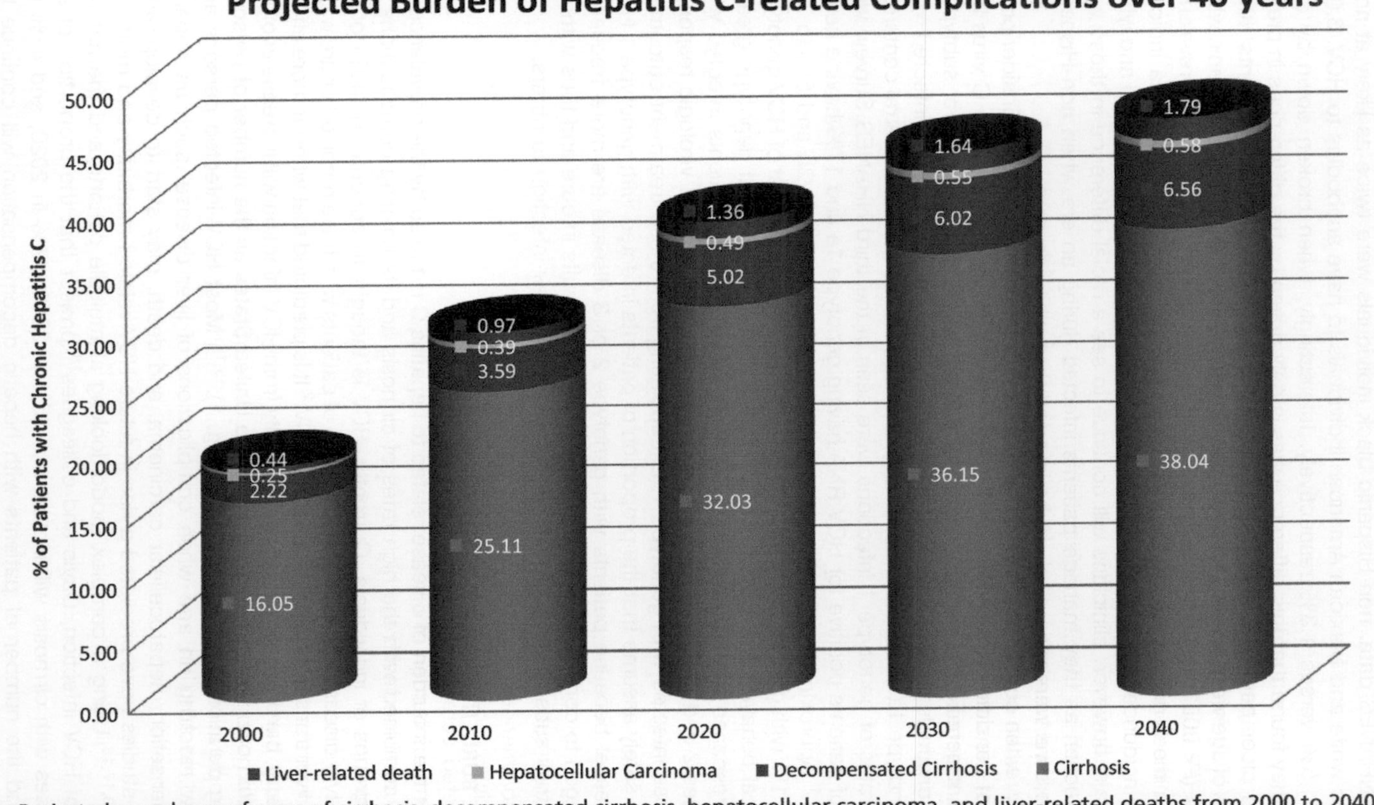

Fig. 1. Projected prevalence of cases of cirrhosis, decompensated cirrhosis, hepatocellular carcinoma, and liver-related deaths from 2000 to 2040 in 10-year intervals (numbers reported are percentage of all individuals with chronic hepatitis C). (*Data from* Davis GL, Albright JE, Cook SF, et al. Projecting future complications of chronic hepatitis C in the United States. Liver Transpl 2003;9[12682882]:331–8.)

Although fewer than 7500 deaths were attributed to HCV in 2004,[19] this is projected to increase each decade through 2030.[18]

It is important to consider that treatment will reduce the number of cases of decompensated cirrhosis in nearly direct proportion to the proportion of patients who are treated. Specifically, treating 25%, 50%, or 100% of all patients with HCV in 2010 would decrease rates of cirrhosis in 2020 by 1.0%, 7.8%, and 15.6%, respectively. In addition, if better sustained virological response (SVR) rates are achieved, treatment of 50% of HCV-infected individuals would reduce rates of cirrhosis by 15.2% in just 10 years.[18] SVR is almost always used as a surrogate for virological cure, as there is a clear link between achieving SVR and substantial improved long-term outcomes including a reduction in the risk of progression to cirrhosis and the development of its associated complications, as well as a lower overall mortality rate. In addition, in those patients with high-grade fibrosis and cirrhosis who achieve SVR with therapy, there is a lower rate of progression to need for liver transplantation.[20]

Therefore, the current burden placed on the health care system by HCV infection is significant considering the prevalence of infection. However, as the large cohort of currently infected patients ages, complications of liver disease and the burden on the health care system will increase dramatically until a significant majority is treated successfully. If SVR can be achieved for the large majority of persons with chronic hepatitis C, we will see a dramatic decline in the prevalence of cirrhosis, hepatocellular carcinoma, and the number of patients needing liver transplantation.

WHO IS LEFT TO TREAT?

Patients Naïve to Therapy

There are many patients yet naïve to therapy for their chronic HCV infection, but this number is unknown. This, in a large part, is because of the asymptomatic nature of chronic hepatitis from HCV infection. It is unknown what proportion of HCV-positive persons in the United States are aware of their infection, but it is likely a substantial proportion of individuals with chronic HCV infection. Universal screening for HCV would allow better identification of all patients with chronic HCV, but this has not been recommended. Currently, the most cost-effective approach to detecting HCV infection is to screen individuals who have an identifiable risk factor.[11,21–23] Although this targeted screening approach leads to identification of those at high risk for acquiring the infection, there are many individuals infected with HCV who do not have any of these features in their history. In their analysis of the current NHANES data, Armstrong and colleagues[3] found that using the screening criteria, such as history of injection drug use, blood transfusion before 1992, or abnormal alanine aminotransferase levels (ALT), would identify 85% of persons 20 to 59 years of age and 87% of persons 60 or older. Therefore, about 15% of patients with chronic HCV would not be identified and given our conservative estimate of prevalence of 3 million people in the United States, 450,000 individuals with chronic hepatitis would be missed. In addition, our current screening criteria identify many patients who may be more difficult to treat, that is, older patients who received a blood transfusion before 1992, older patients with more comorbid conditions, those actively using injection drugs, individuals infected with HIV, patients with end-stage renal disease on hemodialysis, and organ transplant recipients, but misses those who might have better rates of viral eradication, that is, younger patients with minimal histologic changes and few comorbid conditions.

Importantly, Singer and Younossi[21] found that universal screening can be cost effective if half of the patients who test positive are treated. However, treatment rates are currently much lower than this threshold. In addition, current recommendations for selection of patients for treatment are biased toward treating patients with more advance disease (METAVIR stage 3 or 4) disease,[11] as they have the most to benefit from successful therapy. Yet, this population has also been proven as one of the most difficult to treat, both because of complications from cirrhosis and a substantially lower rate of SVR in those with advanced disease. In addition, some clinicians are hesitant to treat patient subsets that were not well represented in the large registration trials, which were restrictive in their exclusion criteria. For example, patients with normal ALT values were excluded, which can be up to 40% of those with chronic HCV in the community.[3] Because of these and other factors, recent data show that antiviral treatment rates are lower than 30% and as low as 6% in a report looking at HCV treatment in injection drug users in Baltimore.[24–26] When looking at reasons for low treatment uptake in the community, Falck-Ytter and colleagues[27] found that 37% of individuals considered for treatment did not adhere to an appointment for evaluation and education, 34% had a medical contraindication, 13% had ongoing substance abuse, 11% of patients chose to defer treatment, and 5% had normal ALT levels.

As we acquire data from studies evaluating the efficacy of treatment in patients who were excluded in the registration trials who potentially have a good risk-benefit ratio as well as with improved SVR rates, some of the barriers to HCV treatment in the community will no longer play a major role. Primary care providers may refer patients more often when more successful treatment options are available, patients are more likely to attend this initial evaluation with a specialist and accept therapy when the risk-benefit ratio of therapy is improved, and specialists will be more likely to treat special patient groups that previously had been deemed inappropriate candidates for treatment when higher rates of success are expected.

Given our limited efforts to identify individuals with chronic HCV and the currently low treatment rates of individuals with HCV in the community, it can safely be inferred that the number of patients naïve to therapy is large. With improvements in our ability to achieve SVR with new therapies, universal screening may become cost effective. If instituted, universal screening would undoubtedly increase the number of individuals aware of their chronic hepatitis C infection and accordingly add to the group of treatment-naïve individuals. In addition, with studies documenting the feasibility, benefits, and safety of treatment on specialized populations in whom treatment was thought to be contraindicated, the pool of treatment-naïve patients eligible and willing to consider therapy will continue to grow.

Treatment-Experienced Patients

The ultimate goal of therapy for chronic hepatitis C is to prevent cirrhosis, liver disease–related complications, and death from HCV infection. However, the slow progression to these end points in patients with chronic hepatitis C makes it difficult to demonstrate efficacy of therapeutic options if only these clinical end points are used. Therefore, treatment responses are most often defined by a surrogate virological parameter rather than a clinical end point.

After initiating treatment, several types of virological responses may occur and are delineated according to their timing relative to the course of treatment. SVR, defined as the absence of HCV RNA from serum 24 weeks following discontinuation of therapy, is generally regarded as "virological cure." On the other hand, treatment-experienced patients are a heterogeneous group, including those who fail to clear their sera of HCV RNA after 24 weeks of therapy, as well as those whose virus returns either after treatment is discontinued or while on therapy. Nonresponders to anti-HCV therapy are broken down into null responders, who fail to decrease their HCV RNA by 2 logs after 12 weeks of therapy; partial responders, those who decrease their HCV RNA by 2 logs but are still HCV RNA–positive at week 24 of therapy; and those patients who experience breakthrough (those who initially cleared virus with therapy but have replication resume despite continued treatment). During follow-up, relapsers are patients who experience a reappearance of HCV RNA in serum after therapy is discontinued despite having cleared their sera at the end of treatment (**Table 1**).

Standard interferon was first approved for HCV therapy in 1991; however, SVR rates were only 10% to 15%.[28,29] The success of therapy has markedly improved with the addition of ribavirin and pegylating interferon, yet SVR rates still remain suboptimal at less than 50% in most genotype 1 subgroups.[30–33] Based on data from the 3 large registration trials, approximately, 35% of patients infected with HCV genotype 1 and 7% of those with HCV genotype 2 or 3 are nonresponders, whereas 23% with HCV genotype 1 and 13% with HCV genotype 2 or 3 relapse to standard therapy.[30–32,34] Thus, there is a rapidly growing pool of patients who have failed attempts at prior therapy.

Baseline characteristics help predict those who are likely to have a favorable response with therapy. Individuals with genotypes 2 and 3 infection have a higher SVR rate than those with genotypes 1 and 4.[11,34] Similarly, those with a low viral load are more likely to achieve SVR.[11,32,34] More recently, polymorphisms of the interleukin 28B (IL28B) gene are found to predict higher SVR rates in those with CC versus CT and TT genotypes.[35] Other less consistently reported patient characteristics associated with a greater likelihood of response to therapy include nonmodifiable baseline factors such as female gender, age younger than 40 years, non-African American race, elevated ALT levels, and the absence of bridging fibrosis or cirrhosis on liver biopsy.[11,33,34]

Modifiable factors associated with favorable outcomes include higher doses of peginterferon and ribavirin, longer duration of therapy for those with genotypes 1and 4 infection, lower body weight (<75 kg), and the absence of insulin resistance.[11,33,34] In addition, there are fewer data to guide therapy for patients with HIV, those with compensated and decompensated cirrhosis, those with advanced kidney disease, those following solid organ transplantation including liver transplantation, those with acute hepatitis C, those actively using injection drugs, and those with psychiatric illness. In these patients, although there are limited data to guide the decision to start therapy and how to treat these groups of patients, the risk-benefit ratio of therapy must be evaluated for each individual patient.[11,34]

Viral kinetics in response to therapy are also useful in predicting successful response to therapy or failure of therapy in patients, especially those infected with genotype 1 (see **Table 1**). An early virological response (EVR) is defined as a more than 2 log reduction of serum HCV RNA at week 12 of therapy compared with the baseline level. Currently, in patients with genotype 1 infection, the strongest negative predictor of achieving SVR is the failure to achieve an EVR. Ninety-seven percent to 100% of treatment-naive patients with HCV genotype 1 infection who did not reach an EVR failed to achieve SVR.[31,36] In these patients, treatment may be discontinued as likelihood of SVR is very low.[11]

Rapid virological response (RVR), defined as undetectable HCV RNA at week 4 of treatment, was also found to predict a high likelihood of achieving an SVR.[36,37] In addition, using RVR is helpful in deciding length of therapy in patients with genotype 1. Specifically, the SVR rate was 89% in patients who achieved an RVR and 19% in those treated for 24 weeks who did not achieve an RVR, and these rates did not change significantly for those treated for 48 weeks.[37] Therefore, using RVR has the advantage

Table 1
Virological responses during therapy: definitions and clinical significance

Virological Response	Definition	Clinical Implication
Rapid virological response (RVR)	HCV RNA negative at treatment week 4 by a sensitive PCR-based quantitative assay	Predicts high likelihood of SVR (85%–90%)[36,37]
Early virological response (EVR)	≥2 log reduction in HCV RNA level compared with baseline HCV RNA level (partial EVR) or HCV RNA negative at treatment week 12 (complete EVR)	Failure to achieve EVR predicts failure to achieve SVR (97%–100%) Therapy can be stopped if EVR not achieved[11,29,36]
End-of-treatment response (ETR)	HCV RNA negative by a sensitive PCR-based quantitative assay at the end of 24 or 48 weeks of treatment	Required for SVR by definition
Sustained virological response (SVR)	HCV RNA–negative 24 weeks after cessation of treatment	Considered virological cure Best predictor of long-term response with relapse rate 1%–3%[20]
Partial response or breakthrough	Decrease in HCV RNA by >2 logs from baseline but still HCV RNA–positive at week 24 or reappearance of HCV RNA in serum while still on therapy	Response to retreatment with peginterferon and ribavirin (40 %)[41] Response to retreatment with telaprevir in combination with peginterferon and ribavirin (57%–62%)[41]
Relapse	Reappearance of HCV RNA in serum after therapy is discontinued	Response to retreatment with peginterferon and ribavirin (20%–29%)[41,43] Response to retreatment with telaprevir in combination with peginterferon and ribavirin (69%–76%)[41] Response to retreatment with Boceprevir in combination with peginterferon and ribavirin (69%–75%)[43]
Nonresponse	Failure to clear HCV RNA from serum after 24 weeks of therapy	Response to retreatment with peginterferon and ribavirin (7%–9%)[41,43] Response to retreatment with telaprevir in combination with peginterferon and ribavirin(38%–39%)[41] Response to retreatment with boceprevir in combination with peginterferon and ribavirin (40%–52%)[43]
Null response	Failure to decrease HCV RNA by <2 logs after 24 weeks of therapy <1 log at 4 weeks of therapy (eNR)	Response to retreatment with telaprevir in combination with peginterferon and ribavirin (31%)[8] Response to retreatment with boceprevir in combination with peginterferon and ribavirin (33%–34%)[5] For eNR: Response to retreatment with peginterferon and ribavirin (0%)[43,45]

Abbreviations: HCV, hepatitis C virus; PCR, polymerase chain reaction.

of limiting exposure to and the side effects of therapy in patients who are as likely to achieve SVR with shorter lengths of therapy. It is important to note that only 10% to 24% of patients with genotype 1 infection achieved RVR.[11,36,37]

The management of treatment-experienced patients is even more challenging than treatment-naïve subjects, as various management strategies have not shown good outcomes for these patients. The HALT-C trial evaluated the role of long-term antiviral therapy with the goal of preventing progressive liver disease. Although serum ALT levels, HCV RNA, and hepatic necroinflammation were significantly reduced in the treated arm, long-term therapy did not decrease their primary outcome of long-term complications, including death, hepatic decompensation, hepatocellular carcinoma, or progression to cirrhosis.[38] Re-treating subjects with combination peginterferon and ribavirin is also not an effective strategy, as only 5% to 16% are successful in attaining SVR.[39,40] Based on studies looking at retreatment of patients who experienced treatment failure, our current practice guidelines actually discourage retreatment unless the first course was suboptimal.[11] Yet, the management of treatment-experienced individuals requires individual consideration, as not all subsets behave identically. In the REPEAT trial, those who had relapsed from prior therapy actually attained SVR at much higher rates that those with nonresponse.[40] This will also be true when considering retreatment with triple therapy once the first direct-acting antivirals (DAAs) become approved.

Although there are fewer nonresponders and relapsers as standard of care has moved to peginterferon alfa-2a or alfa-2b with weight-based ribavirin, still 30% to 40% of patients do not respond to peginterferon with ribavirin and up to 20% of patients relapse after completing therapy.[31] Considering several pivotal trials, although 40% to 60% do not attain SVR, approximately 15% to 30% relapsed after therapy was discontinued, and therapy was discontinued for 30% at treatment week 12 because of defined stopping rules based on futility.[21,29,34] Nonresponders will be more difficult to manage than relapsers, whereas the most difficult subset to manage will be null-responders (see **Table 1**). In the telaprevir studies of treatment failures (PROVE-3 and REALIZE [preliminary data]), retreatment with 12 to 24 weeks of triple therapy followed by 12 to 24 weeks of peginterferon and ribavirin resulted in SVR in only 38% to 39% for nonresponders versus 69% to 86% for relapsers versus 31% of null-responders.[41,42] In the boceprevir study (RESPOND-2), preliminary results indicate that 40% to 52% of nonresponders to peginterferon and ribavirin will achieve SVR compared with 69% to 75% of relapsers versus only 33% or 34% of early null-responders.[43] These initial data confirm that null-responders will remain a clinical challenge for several years to come.

How Many Are Left to Treat?

Based on our knowledge of the prevalence of chronic hepatitis C, and current treatment initiation and success rates, we can begin to estimate the number of patients with chronic hepatitis C who are still left to be treated (**Fig. 2**). Specifically, based on the 2010 US Census, there were 281.4 million US residents. From the most current NHANES data, we can estimate that 1.3%, or 3.7 million, of the US population has chronic hepatitis C. It is projected that 60% to 70% of those with chronic hepatitis C will go on to develop chronic liver disease.[13,23,44] Although all of these individuals should receive therapy, at best only about 30% of patients in the community are evaluated for therapy.[24–26] Of this small population, an estimated 25% of patients will initiate treatment because of contraindications to combination pegylated interferon and ribavirin therapy or patient refusal of therapy.[28–30,34] Therefore, of the 2.6 million people who will likely progress in their liver disease from chronic hepatitis C in the

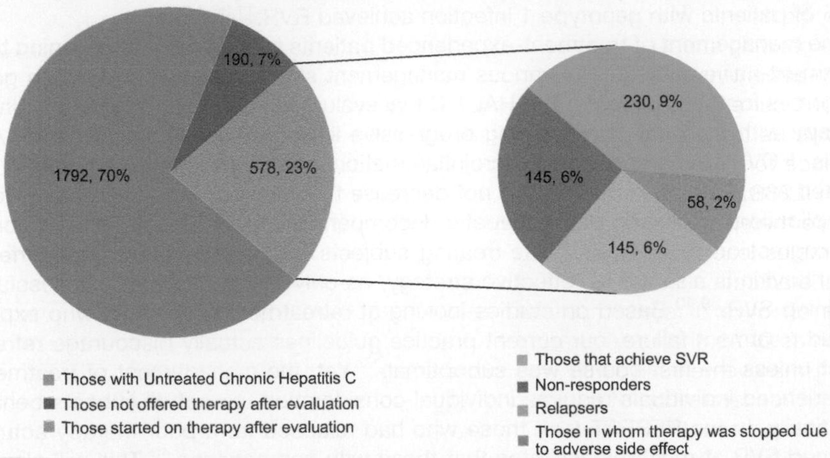

Fig. 2. Based on 2010 US Census Data, 3.7 million residents have chronic hepatitis C and of these 2.6 million will go on to develop significant liver disease. Of these, only an estimated 30% will be evaluated for therapy and only 23% will begin therapy. A minority will achieve SVR whereas others will be nonresponders, relapsers, or have therapy discontinued because of adverse side effects. (Numbers are reported in hundred-thousands, percentage of total number of individuals with chronic hepatitis predicted to develop significant liver disease.)

United States, only about 580,000 patients will be offered therapy. Of the patients offered therapy with pegylated interferon and ribavirin, about 40%, or 230,000 patients, will achieve SVR, whereas 25%, or 145,000 patients, will not respond, another 25%, or 145,000 patients, will relapse, and 10%, or 58,000 patients, will have to discontinue therapy because of an adverse event.[34] All in all, of all patients with chronic hepatitis C who should be treated, only about 10% of patients will be cured of their infection with current standard of care therapy using pegylated interferon and ribavirin. With the addition of DAAs to this therapy regimen, preliminary data suggest that we will be able to recapture about 40% to 50% of nonresponders and 70% to 80% of relapsers.[41–43]

SUMMARY

Hepatitis C has a high prevalence in the United States, driven currently by high rates of chronic infection. The disease burden of HCV will only continue to increase over the next 20 to 30 years by many estimates unless an effective therapy is both approved and broadly used. Although it is difficult to predict who will progress to develop more significant liver disease, cirrhosis, and its complications, it is clear that the peak prevalence of HCV is moving to older age groups. As these individuals progress in age, they are also more likely to develop other comorbid conditions that are negative factors for consideration for or response to current therapy. In addition, our current treatment uptake rates are low in many groups of patients, as many patients are unaware of their infection, chose not to undergo treatment, are not candidates for treatment, or are unable to complete the course of treatment. This is compounded by limited success rates for many subgroups of patients and the significant adverse side effects associated with pegylated interferon and ribavirin–based regimens.

Although the current key management questions clinicians must answer while evaluating patients with chronic hepatitis C include who should be treated, when should they be treated, and with what regimen, these clinical questions will be compounded by a growing subset of treatment-experienced patients in addition to the large number of treatment-naïve individuals.

Our currently available pegylated interferon and ribavirin combination therapy allows us to successfully treat a small subset of patients with a greater than 70% chance for SVR: those with genotype 2 or 3, those with low viral load, and those with IL28B genotype CC. In this subset of patients, treatment should be initiated, as future therapy will offer little to no improvement in SVR rates, and waiting for future therapies leads to the possibility of missing a window of opportunity for successful viral eradication with currently available therapy. For those where current therapy is less effective or contraindicated, there is great expectation that newer therapies, such as DAAs, including telaprevir and boceprevir, will improve viral clearance rates. With improvements in ability to achieve SVR with agents such as telaprevir and boceprevir, reexamination of the utility of universal screening or more inclusive screening for chronic hepatitis C is warranted. In addition, trials to evaluate new therapies and optimize the use of triple drug therapies are needed if HCV is to be successfully controlled and its incumbent morbidity and mortality drastically lowered for all groups of patients.

REFERENCES

1. Alter MJ, Kruszon-Moran D, Nainan OV, et al. The prevalence of hepatitis C virus infection in the United States, 1988 through 1994. N Engl J Med 1999;341(10451460): 556–62.
2. Kim WR. The burden of hepatitis C in the United States. Hepatology 2002; 36(5 Suppl 1):S30–4.
3. Armstrong GL, Wasley A, Simard EP, et al. The prevalence of hepatitis C virus infection in the United States, 1999 through 2002. Ann Intern Med 2006;144(10):705–14.
4. Koretz RL, Abbey H, Coleman E, et al. Non-A, non-B post-transfusion hepatitis. Looking back in the second decade. Ann Intern Med 1993;119(2):110–5.
5. CDC.gov. Viral hepatitis statistics & surveillance. 2010. Available at: http://www.cdc.gov/hepatitis/Statistics/index.htm. Accessed January 20, 2011.
6. Armstrong GL, Alter MJ, McQuillan GM, et al. The past incidence of hepatitis C virus infection: implications for the future burden of chronic liver disease in the United States. Hepatology 2000;31(10706572):777–82.
7. CDC.gov. Viral hepatitis statistics & surveillance table 1a. 2010. Available at: http://www.cdc.gov/hepatitis/Statistics/2008Surveillance/Table1a.htm. Accessed January 20, 2011.
8. Dominitz JA, Boyko EJ, Koepsell TD, et al. Elevated prevalence of hepatitis C infection in users of United States veterans medical centers. Hepatology 2005; 41(1):88–96.
9. Briggs ME, Baker C, Hall R, et al. Prevalence and risk factors for hepatitis C virus infection at an urban Veterans Administration medical center. Hepatology 2001; 34(6):1200–5.
10. Weinbaum CM, Sabin KM, Santibanez SS. Hepatitis B, hepatitis C, and HIV in correctional populations: a review of epidemiology and prevention. AIDS 2005; 19(Suppl 3):S41–6.
11. Ghany MG, Strader DB, Thomas DL, et al. Diagnosis, management, and treatment of hepatitis C: an update. Hepatology 2009;49(4):1335–74.

12. Gough E, Kempf MC, Graham L, et al. HIV and hepatitis B and C incidence rates in US correctional populations and high risk groups: a systematic review and meta-analysis. BMC Public Health 2010;10:777.
13. Davis GL, Albright JE, Cook SF, et al. Projecting future complications of chronic hepatitis C in the United States. Liver Transpl 2003;9(12682882):331–8.
14. Lau JY, Davis GL, Prescott LE, et al. Distribution of hepatitis C virus genotypes determined by line probe assay in patients with chronic hepatitis C seen at tertiary referral centers in the United States. Hepatitis Interventional Therapy Group. Ann Intern Med 1996;124(10):868–76.
15. Recommendations for prevention and control of hepatitis C virus (HCV) infection and HCV-related chronic disease. Centers for Disease Control and Prevention. MMWR Recomm Rep 1998;47(RR–19):1–39.
16. Wong JB, McQuillan GM, McHutchison JG, et al. Estimating future hepatitis C morbidity, mortality, and costs in the United States. Am J Public Health 2000; 90(11029989):1562–9.
17. El-Serag HB, Davila JA, Petersen NJ, et al. The continuing increase in the incidence of hepatocellular carcinoma in the United States: an update. Ann Intern Med 2003;139(14623619):817–23.
18. Davis GL, Alter MJ, El-Serag H, et al. Aging of hepatitis C virus (HCV)-infected persons in the United States: a multiple cohort model of HCV prevalence and disease progression. Gastroenterology 2010;138(2):513–21, 521 e1–6.
19. Wise M, Bialek S, Finelli L, et al. Changing trends in hepatitis C-related mortality in the United States, 1995–2004. Hepatology 2008;47(4):1128–35.
20. Aronsohn A, Reau N. Long-term outcomes after treatment with interferon and ribavirin in HCV patients. J Clin Gastroenterol 2009;43(7):661–71.
21. Singer ME, Younossi ZM. Cost effectiveness of screening for hepatitis C virus in asymptomatic, average-risk adults. Am J Med 2001;111(8):614–21.
22. Alter MJ, Seeff LB, Bacon BR, et al. Testing for hepatitis C virus infection should be routine for persons at increased risk for infection. Ann Intern Med 2004; 141(15520428):715–7.
23. CDC.gov. Hepatitis C FAQs for health professionals. 2010. Available at: http://www.cdc.gov/hepatitis/HCV/HCVfaq.htm#c1. Accessed January 20, 2011.
24. Shatin D, Schech SD, Patel K, et al. Population-based hepatitis C surveillance and treatment in a national managed care organization. Am J Manag Care 2004;10(4):250–6.
25. Mehta SH, Genberg BL, Astemborski J, et al. Limited uptake of hepatitis C treatment among injection drug users. J Community Health 2008;33(3):126–33.
26. Kanwal F, Hoang T, Kramer JR, et al. Increasing prevalence of HCC and cirrhosis in patients with chronic hepatitis C virus infection. Gastroenterology 2011;140(4): 1182, e1–1188.
27. Falck-Ytter Y, Kale H, Mullen KD, et al. Surprisingly small effect of antiviral treatment in patients with hepatitis C. Ann Intern Med 2002;136(4):288–92.
28. Carithers RL Jr, Emerson SS. Therapy of hepatitis C: meta-analysis of interferon alfa-2b trials. Hepatology 1997;26(3 Suppl 1):83S–8S.
29. McHutchison J. Hepatitis C therapy in treatment-naive patients. Am J Med 1999; 107(6B):56S–61S.
30. Manns MP, McHutchison JG, Gordon SC, et al. Peginterferon alfa-2b plus ribavirin compared with interferon alfa-2b plus ribavirin for initial treatment of chronic hepatitis C: a randomised trial. Lancet 2001;358(9286):958–65.
31. Fried MW, Shiffman ML, Reddy KR, et al. Peginterferon alfa-2a plus ribavirin for chronic hepatitis C virus infection. N Engl J Med 2002;347(13):975–82.

32. Hadziyannis SJ, Sette H Jr, Morgan TR, et al. Peginterferon-alpha2a and ribavirin combination therapy in chronic hepatitis C: a randomized study of treatment duration and ribavirin dose. Ann Intern Med 2004;140(5):346–55.
33. McHutchison JG, Lawitz EJ, Shiffman ML, et al. Peginterferon alfa-2b or alfa-2a with ribavirin for treatment of hepatitis C infection. N Engl J Med 2009;361(6): 580–93.
34. Seeff LB, Ghany MG. Management of untreated and nonresponder patients with chronic hepatitis C. Semin Liver Dis 2010;30(4):348–60.
35. Thompson AJ, Muir AJ, Sulkowski MS, et al. Interleukin-28B polymorphism improves viral kinetics and is the strongest pretreatment predictor of sustained virologic response in genotype 1 hepatitis C virus. Gastroenterology 2010; 139(1):120, e118–129.
36. Ferenci P, Fried MW, Shiffman ML, et al. Predicting sustained virological responses in chronic hepatitis C patients treated with peginterferon alfa-2a (40 KD)/ribavirin. J Hepatol 2005;43(3):425–33.
37. Jensen DM, Morgan TR, Marcellin P, et al. Early identification of HCV genotype 1 patients responding to 24 weeks peginterferon alpha-2a (40 kd)/ribavirin therapy. Hepatology 2006;43(5):954–60.
38. Di Bisceglie AM, Shiffman ML, Everson GT, et al. Prolonged therapy of advanced chronic hepatitis C with low-dose peginterferon. N Engl J Med 2008;359(23): 2429–41.
39. Cheruvattath R, Rosati MJ, Gautam M, et al. Pegylated interferon and ribavirin failures: is retreatment an option? Dig Dis Sci 2007;52(3):732–6.
40. Jensen DM, Marcellin P, Freilich B, et al. Re-treatment of patients with chronic hepatitis C who do not respond to peginterferon-alpha2b: a randomized trial. Ann Intern Med 2009;150(8):528–40.
41. McHutchison JG, Manns MP, Muir AJ, et al. Telaprevir for previously treated chronic HCV infection. N Engl J Med 2010;362(14):1292–303.
42. Foster GR, Zeuzem S, Andreone P, et al. Telaprevir-based therapy in G1 HCV-infected patients with prior null response, partial response or relapse to peginterferon/ribavirin: REALIZE trial final results. Hepatology International 2011;5(1): PS02–4.
43. Bacon BR, Gordon SC, Lawitz E, et al. Boceprevir for previously treated chronic HCV genotype 1 infection. N Engl J Med 2011;364(13):1207–17.
44. Poynard T, Ratziu V, Charlotte F, et al. Rates and risk factors of liver fibrosis progression in patients with chronic hepatitis c. J Hepatol 2001;34(5):730–9.
45. Reau N, Satoskar R, Te H, et al. Evaluation of early null response to pegylated interferon and ribavirin as a predictor of therapeutic nonresponse in patients undergoing treatment for chronic hepatitis C. Am J Gastroenterol 2011;106(3): 452–8.

Redefining Baseline Demographics: The Role of Genetic Testing in Hepatitis C Virus Infection

Jacinta A. Holmes, MBBS[a], Paul V. Desmond, MBBS, FRACP[a], Alexander J. Thompson, MBBS, FRACP, PhD[a,b,*]

KEYWORDS

- Hepatitis C virus infection • Peginterferon/ribavirin
- Predictors of treatment outcome • Genetic testing • *IL28B*
- Interferon-λ • *ITPA* • Ribavirin-induced anemia

It is estimated that 3% of the world's population (130–170 million people) are chronically infected with the hepatitis C virus (HCV).[1] Progression to cirrhosis occurs in more than 20% over time, and these patients are subsequently at risk of developing end-stage liver disease and hepatocellular carcinoma.[2] HCV infection is now the leading indication for liver transplantation.[1] Viral eradication has been shown to improve survival and reduce the risk of hepatocellular carcinoma.[3] The current standard of care (SOC) for chronic hepatitis C (CHC) infection consists of pegylated interferon (Peg-IFN) combined with ribavirin (RBV). Overall success rates are disappointing, with a sustained virological response (SVR), defined as undetectable HCV RNA level 6 months post therapy, achieved by only 54% to 56% of patients.[4–6] Treatment is also costly and may be associated with significant toxicity. It would therefore be clinically useful to be able to accurately predict at baseline which patients are most likely to achieve SVR, both to prioritize their treatment and spare unnecessary morbidity for those with very low probability of clearance.

Disclosures: AJ Thompson is a coapplicant of 2 patents related to the *IL28B* and ITPA discoveries.

[a] Department of Gastroenterology and Hepatology, St Vincent's Hospital, 41 Victoria Parade, Fitzroy 3065, Victoria, Australia

[b] Duke Clinical Research Institute, Duke University Medical Center, PO Box 17969, Durham, NC 27710, USA

* Corresponding author. Department of Gastroenterology and Hepatology, St Vincent's Hospital, 41 Victoria Parade, Fitzroy 3065, Victoria, Australia.

E-mail address: alexander.THOMPSON@svhm.org.au

Clin Liver Dis 15 (2011) 497–513
doi:10.1016/j.cld.2011.05.009

Several baseline factors have been identified as associated with response to SOC treatment, including both viral and host factors. The most important viral factor has been HCV genotype, the strongest baseline predictor of treatment response, with genotype 2/3 HCV (HCV-2/3) patients achieving SVR rates of approximately 70% to 80% with 24 weeks duration of treatment, compared with 40% to 50% for genotype 1 HCV (HCV-1) patients treated for 48 weeks.[4–7] Low baseline viral load (<400,000–800,000 IU/mL) was also an important predictor of response.[4–7] Amino acid mutations in the HCV core protein (arginine 70 and/or leucine 91) and the HCV nonstructural (NS) 5A protein (interferon sensitivity-determining region [ISDR], IFN/RBV resistance-determining region) have been associated with IFN response in Japanese patients infected with genotype 1b HCV, although this has not been replicated in Western populations.[8–14]

Host factors that have been associated with poor treatment response include male gender, older age, high body mass index, advanced liver fibrosis stage, hepatic steatosis, insulin resistance, and low serum lipid levels.[4–6,15–19] Ethnicity has also been strongly associated with treatment outcome, with reported response rates in African American patients approximately half that seen in Caucasians.[20,21] By contrast, response rates in Asian populations were higher than those reported in Caucasian studies.[22–24] This result strongly suggested that genetic factors might play an important role in determining sensitivity to IFN-based antiviral therapy.

Genetic variation in the region of the *interleukin (IL)28B* gene on chromosome 19 has recently been identified to be strongly associated with treatment outcome in HCV-1 patients treated with Peg-IFN and RBV.[25–28] Patients carrying the good-response variant had 2- to 3-fold higher rates of SVR. Differences in allele frequency between patients of different racial groups explained much of the recognized ethnic disparity in SVR rates. Subsequently, *IL28B* polymorphism was also found to be associated with spontaneous clearance of acute HCV infection.[28,29] More recently, genetic association studies have also investigated determinants of treatment-related toxicity and have identified 2 functional variants in the *inosine triphosphatase* (*ITPA*) gene on chromosome 20 that protect against RBV-induced hemolytic anemia.[30,31] These genetic discoveries will enhance clinicians' ability to personalize treatment decisions for patients, informing both the likelihood of success as well as the probability of hematologic morbidity. This review article addresses the recent advances made in our understanding of genetic predictors of HCV treatment outcome, and how they might be used in current clinical practice.

GENETIC TESTING

Discovery of IL28B

Genome-wide association studies

Genome-wide association studies (GWAS) have recently identified single-nucleotide polymorphisms (SNPs) in the region of the *IL28B* gene on chromosome 19 that strongly predict treatment response in patients infected with HCV-1. This discovery was reported simultaneously by 3 independent groups in North America, Australia/Northern Europe, and Japan (**Fig. 1**).[25–28]

Ge and colleagues[25] studied 1137 North American HCV-1 patients of European American (n = 871), African American (n = 191), and Hispanic (n = 75) ancestry from the IDEAL study cohort.[32] The primary analysis was for genetic determinants of SVR; nonresponder patients were excluded if they were less than 80% adherent to therapy. The genotyping platform used was the Illumina Human610-quad BeadChip. Seven SNPs were significantly associated with SVR ($P<10^{-8}$). The top-discovery SNP was

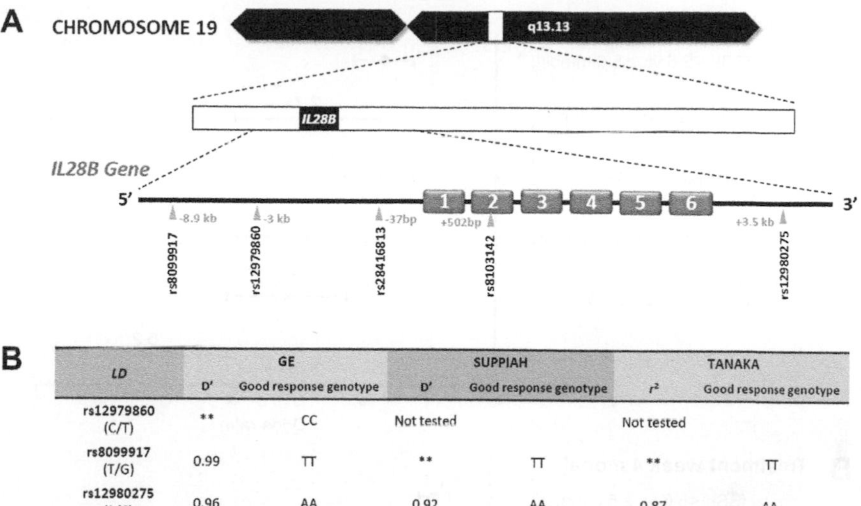

LD	GE		SUPPIAH		TANAKA	
	D'	Good response genotype	D'	Good response genotype	r^2	Good response genotype
rs12979860 (C/T)	**	CC	Not tested		Not tested	
rs8099917 (T/G)	0.99	TT	**	TT	**	TT
rs12980275 (A/G)	0.96	AA	0.92	AA	0.87	AA

Fig. 1. (*A*) Chromosome 19 with *IL28B* region with the location and linkage of the top 3 association SNPs associated with SVR and 2 proposed functional variants across the 3 GWAS studies. (*B*) The Tag SNPs are listed with their linkage disequilibrium score (r^2/D'), and the good-response genotype. (*Data from* Refs.[25–27])

rs12979860 ($P = 1.37 \times 10^{-28}$), which is located 3 kilobases (kb) upstream of the *IL28B* gene. The 6 other SNPs were all in the same genetic region, and included rs8099917 and rs12980275. All 7 SNPs were in high linkage disequilibrium (LD, SNPs that are inherited together), and adjustment for rs12979860 largely attenuated the association of the other SNPs with SVR, suggesting that all 7 SNPs were tagging a common genetic signal. The top-association SNP, rs12979860, is a biallelic polymorphism, with 3 possible genotypes: CC, CT, and TT. The CC (good-response) genotype had a 2- to 3-fold higher rate of SVR in all 3 ethnic groups as compared with CT and TT genotypes. In addition, the good-response C allele was more common in the European American population (39%) than in the African American population (16%), explaining more than 50% of the difference in treatment response seen between these racial populations. In a separate multiethnic population with unknown HCV status, the C allele frequency was even higher in East Asians, which mirrors the high SVR rates that have been reported in Asian populations.[22–24] On multivariate analysis, *IL28B* genotype was independently associated with SVR, and had the highest odds ratio (OR) favoring SVR compared with conventional predictors of treatment response (**Fig. 2**A). Resequencing (fine mapping) of the *IL28B* region identified two potential causative SNPs: rs28416813 (37 base pairs upstream of the *IL28B* translation initiation codon) and rs8103142 (nonsynonymous SNP in exon 2, arginine at position 70 to lysine, K70R). Both are in such high LD with the top-association SNP, rs12979860, that it was not possible to statistically differentiate a causal SNP. Two other interesting observations were made. In patients with CHC, the frequency of the good-response C allele was lower than in an ethnically matched non-HCV control population, suggesting that the C allele might favor spontaneous clearance. The second observation was that the rs12979860 was the only common genetic variant associated with viral load set-point at baseline. Paradoxically, the good-response CC genotype patients had a higher baseline viral load (6.35 vs 6.16 $\log_{10}$ IU/mL).

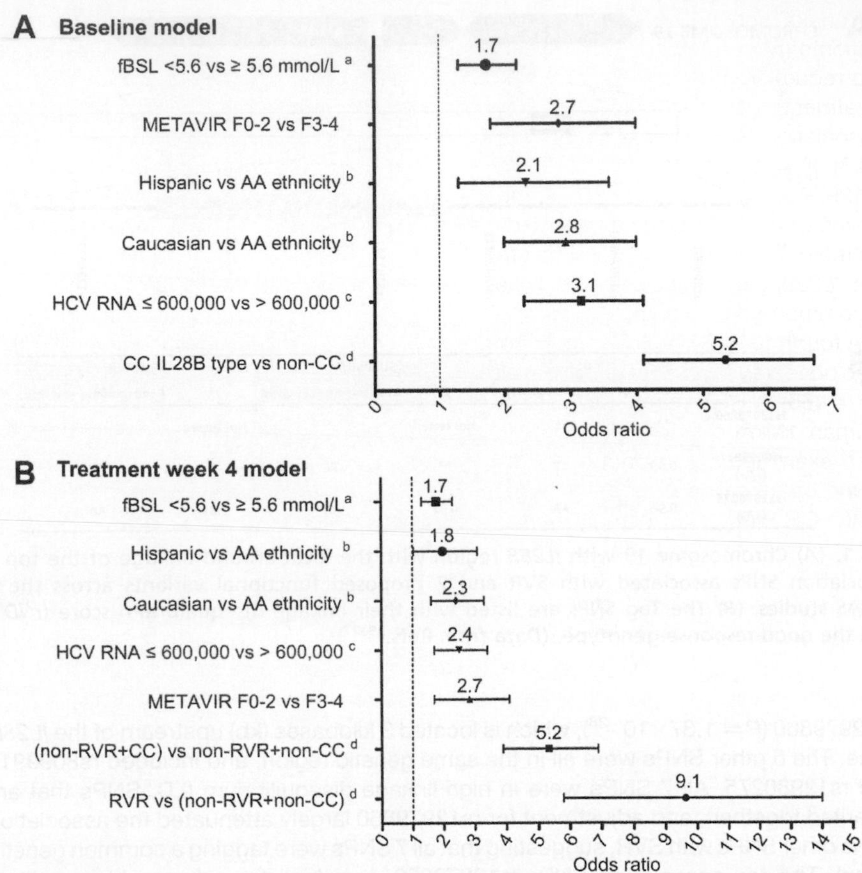

Fig. 2. Multivariate logistic regression odds ratios for conventional pretreatment predictors of SVR. (*A*) *IL28B* is included in the baseline multivariate model. (*B*) Week-4 treatment response (RVR vs non-RVR). [a] fBSL, fasting blood sugar level; [b] AA, African American; [c] IU/mL; [d] rs12979860 *IL28B* genotype. (*Data from* Thompson AJ, Muir AJ, Sulkowski MS, et al. Interleukin-28B polymorphism improves viral kinetics and is the strongest pre-treatment predictor of sustained virological response in genotype 1 hepatitis C virus. Gastroenterology 2010;139:120–9.)

The results of a second GWAS were reported by Suppiah and colleagues.[26] This study investigated determinants of SVR in Caucasian HCV-1 patients from Australia and Europe (N = 848). Their top-association SNP was rs8099917 located 8.9 kb upstream of the *IL28B* gene. The good-response (TT) genotype was associated with a twofold increase in SVR (OR for SVR =1.98, $P = 9.25 \times 10^{-9}$). A second SNP, rs12980275, was identified on haplotype analysis of tag SNPs in the *IL28B* region to be associated with SVR ($P = 7.74 \times 10^{-10}$). Several other SNPs of genome-wide significance were also identified as part of a common 6-allele haplotype block associated with treatment response. It must be noted that the top-discovery SNP tested in the Ge study (rs12979860)[25] was not included on the Illumina Infinium Human Hap300/CNV370-Quad BeadChip used in this GWAS. In Caucasian patients enrolled in the study by Ge, rs12979860 and rs8099917 were in linkage disequilibrium ($D' = 0.99$), and the good-response CC genotype (rs12979860) corresponded to the TT genotype of rs8099917.

Tanaka and colleagues[27] performed a GWAS in a Japanese cohort of HCV-1 patients (N = 314). Null virological response (NVR, defined as failure to attain a 2-log reduction in HCV RNA at week 12 and detectable HCV viremia 24 weeks post treatment) was the clinical phenotype defined for the primary analysis. Their top-association SNP in this study was rs8099917 (overall OR for NVR = 27.1 [14.6–50.3], $P = 2.68 \times 10^{-32}$). rs8099917 was also strongly associated with SVR. Again, rs12979860 was not included on the Affymetrix SNP 6.0 Array chip used in this study. Seven other SNPs were associated beyond the genome-wide threshold, found either on the basis of LD and haplotype structure or by fine resequencing studies. All were in the *IL28B* gene region and in linkage disequilibrium with rs8099917, representing a common genetic signal.

A fourth GWAS published later from the Swiss Hepatitis C and HIV cohort studies[28] also observed an association between *IL28B* polymorphisms and treatment outcomes (N = 465) in HCV genotypes 1 to 4 (rs12979860 was not genotyped on the Illumina Human 1M-Duo Human Hap550/Human610W-Quad BeadChips). In addition, they also examined the impact of rs8099917 on spontaneous clearance (N = 347) and found that the poor-response allele was associated with a significantly higher risk of CHC; OR was 6.02 and 2.2 for homozygotes and heterozygotes, respectively (see *IL28B* and spontaneous clearance in acute hepatitis C infection).

IL28B genotype and viral kinetics

A separate intention-to-treat analysis was performed on the IDEAL pharmacogenetics cohort, including all patients regardless of the level of adherence.[33] Viral kinetics early in treatment were significantly improved in patients carrying the good-response *IL28B* genotype. At week 2 of treatment, the earliest time point sampled, the median reduction of serum HCV RNA in Caucasian good-response patients was 2.6 $\log_{10}$ IU/mL, compared with 0.9 $\log_{10}$ IU/mL and 0.6 $\log_{10}$ IU/mL for CT and TT patients, respectively. These patients subsequently had higher rates of rapid virological response (RVR, defined as negative HCV RNA at week 4 of treatment), and complete early virological response (cEVR, defined as negative HCV RNA level at week 12 of treatment). A 2-$\log_{10}$ IU/mL reduction in serum HCV RNA was almost universal in these Caucasian good-response patients at week 12 (97%). Subsequently, relapse rates were lower. A similar pattern of HCV RNA reduction by *IL28B* genotype was observed in African American patients, although the magnitude of HCV RNA decline was less marked. The association between *IL28B* polymorphism and on-treatment viral kinetics has subsequently been shown to be mainly due to an effect on phase 1 kinetics.[34,35]

IL28B genotype and week 4 RVR

IL28B genotype has been shown to be strongly predictive of week 4 viral clearance. In the IDEAL pharmacogenetics study, 28% of Caucasian good-response (CC) patients attained RVR versus 5% in both CT and TT patients (rs12979860).[33] The majority of patients who attained RVR carried the CC genotype (77%). Of interest, once RVR was attained all patients did well, regardless of *IL28B* genotype (SVR = 85%, 76%, and 100% for CC, CT, and TT patients). In patients who did not attain RVR, *IL28B* genotype was important: subsequent SVR rate was 66% if CC genotype, but only 31% and 24% in CT and TT genotypes (see **Fig. 2**B).[33] The sensitivity of *IL28B* genotype for SVR was 56% and the positive predictive value (PPV) of *IL28B* genotype for SVR was 69%. In comparison, the sensitivity of RVR for SVR was 25% but the PPV was 84%.[33] Therefore it seems likely that *IL28B* genotype at baseline, and RVR at week 4, will have complementary use in the clinic, where *IL28B* genotyping can identify approximately 40% of patients who will have a good response to IFN-based treatment, even in non-RVR patients, and RVR identifies a smaller number of patients who will do well regardless of genetic background.

IL28B and HCV genotype 2/3

Several retrospective studies have investigated the association between *IL28B* genotype and treatment outcome in HCV-2/3.[36–41] The heterogeneous study designs, and disparity between the ratio of HCV-2:HCV-3 and *IL28B* allele frequencies among study populations makes direct comparison difficult. The high rate of SVR in these IFN-sensitive genotypes also complicates analysis, as a similar relative effect size (in terms of OR) will dictate that large cohorts will be required to show statistical differences between relative rates of SVR. A well-characterized cohort of Caucasian HCV-2/3 patients from Italy treated with variable-duration Peg-IFN and RBV demonstrated that rs12979860 genotype was an independent predictor of SVR, with SVR rates of 82%, 75%, and 58% in CC, CT, and TT patients, respectively.[42] In RVR patients, *IL28B* genotype had no effect on SVR; however, in non-RVR patients *IL28B* genotype strongly predicted subsequent SVR; 87% in CC patients versus 29% in TT patients ($P<.0002$). *IL28B* was also associated with SVR in cohorts from Germany and Japan.[37,38] In a study by Rauch and colleagues,[28] HCV genotype (HCV-2/3 vs HCV-1/4) and *IL28B* genotype (rs8099917) were both independently associated with SVR. However, in a subanalysis limited to the HCV-2/3 patients (n = 230) the association was suggestive but did not reach statistical significance (OR = 1.62 [0.80–3.31], $P = .18$). No analysis according to week 4 response was presented. *IL28B* polymorphism has been associated with early viral kinetics but not overall SVR in other European and Taiwanese cohorts.[36,39–41,43] Thus, the role of *IL28B* genotype in HCV-2/3 treatment outcomes is less clear. The authors believe that there is likely to be a relationship between *IL28B* polymorphism and IFN sensitivity, but that clinical utility will be less than in HCV-1, given the high overall response rates. More prospective studies, stratifying for *IL28B* genotype and week 4 virological response, are required.

IL28B genotype in other clinical situations

***IL28B* genotype in HCV/human immunodeficiency virus coinfection** In HCV and human immunodeficiency virus (HIV) coinfected patients, *IL28B* genotype remains a strong predictor of SVR.[44–47] As seen in HCV monoinfection, the association is strongest in the setting of HCV-1 (75% in CC patients vs 38% in non-CC patients, OR 3.7, $P<.0001$), and weaker in HCV-3. *IL28B* has also been shown to be associated with treatment outcome in HCV-4–infected patients.[44]

***IL28B* genotype and liver transplantation** HCV recurrence after liver transplant is universal, and HCV infection can be aggressive and lead to rapid progression to cirrhosis.[48–51] Unfortunately, treatment response rates have been disappointing and there is a risk that IFN may precipitate rejection.[50–53] Patients must be carefully selected for treatment, which remains controversial. In this context, *IL28B* genotype has recently been investigated as a predictor of treatment response for posttransplant HCV in 3 retrospective case series. The first study evaluated the relationship between *IL28B* genotype, both donor and recipient, and IFN-based treatment outcome in a Japanese cohort.[54] Carriage of the rs8099917 good-response genotype by the recipient, or the donor liver, was associated with higher rates of SVR. The benefit was additive in patients in whom both recipient and donor liver carried the good-response genotype. No patients who carried the poor-response *IL28B* genotype, and who also received a poor-response genotype donor liver, attained an SVR. A second study of 189 liver transplant patients from North America found that rs12979860 was independently associated with SVR in both donor and recipients.[55]

Again, the effect of the good-response genotype in the donor *and* recipient was additive and strongly predictive of SVR, and high rates of treatment failure were observed if neither the recipient nor the donor was good-response genotype. A third cohort from Germany confirmed a key role for *IL28B* genotype in posttransplant HCV outcomes.[56] Although more studies are required, these early data suggest a potential role for *IL28B* genotyping in organ allocation protocols.

***IL28B* genotype and direct-acting antivirals** The influence of *IL28B* polymorphisms in the setting of direct-acting antivirals (DAAs) is not yet known. The most advanced DAAs in clinical development are the protease inhibitors boceprevir and telaprevir.[57–59] There is only one article in the literature that has examined *IL28B* genotype and treatment outcomes with triple therapy (SOC plus telaprevir).[60] In a small heterogeneous cohort of Japanese HCV-1 patients, representing a mix of prior nonresponders and treatment-naïve patients, and who were treated with variable-duration triple therapy, good-response *IL28B* genotype was strongly associated with SVR (SVR rate of 84% in good-response genotype vs 28% and 32% in poor-response genotypes for rs12979860 and rs8099917, respectively). More recent interim analyses of phase 2 DAA studies suggest that the addition of a DAA to SOC attenuates the association between *IL28B* genotype and early virological responses, although *IL28B* genotype did remain relevant.[61] Further studies are required.

***IL28B* and spontaneous clearance in acute hepatitis C infection** *IL28B* polymorphisms have been associated with spontaneous clearance of HCV. Thomas and colleagues[29] observed that *IL28B* genotype (candidate polymorphism rs12979860) was strongly associated with spontaneous clearance in an injecting drug user population: the good-response CC genotype was associated with an approximately threefold increase in spontaneous clearance. Similar findings were noted in a subsequent GWAS.[28] In this study from the Swiss HIV/HCV cohort several SNPs in the region of the *IL28B* gene exceeded the threshold for genome-wide significance, and the top-discovery SNP was rs8099917, OR 2.31, $P = 6.07 \times 10^{-9}$ (again, data for rs12979860 were not included in the final analysis). Of note, no association with common variants in any other genetic region was noted.

The association between rs12979860 and spontaneous clearance was investigated in 190 patients from the German anti-D cohort, a unique group of women exposed to anti-D contaminated with a single strain of HCV-1.[62] Spontaneous viral clearance was significantly higher in the good-response rs12979860 genotype (64% in CC vs 24% in CT and 6% in TT). The good-response genotype was also associated with a higher rate of jaundice (33% vs 16% in CT/TT patients), perhaps suggesting that historical studies of treatment response in acute HCV may have enrolled a disproportionate number of good-responder patients. Patients with the poor-response *IL28B* genotype and who were not jaundiced at presentation did particularly poorly (clearance rate of 13.7%). *IL28B* polymorphism was also associated with acute clearance and jaundice in patients from the ATAHC study.[63] The data suggest that anicteric poor-responder *IL28B* genotype patients might benefit from early antiviral therapy, rather than waiting 12 to 24 weeks from exposure, as recommended by most guidelines.

***IL28B* mechanisms**

IL28B is located on chromosome 19 and encodes IFN-λ3, a type 3 interferon (see **Fig. 1**A). There are 3 members of the family: *IL29* (IFN-λ1), *IL28A* (IFN-λ2), and *IL28B* (IFN-λ3).[64,65] IFN-λ is induced by stimuli that also induces type I IFNs, such as viral infection (through the viral pattern recognition receptors RIG-I and Toll-like receptors 3, 7, and 9). IFN-λ1, -λ2, and -λ3 signal through the common IFN-λ receptor

(IFNLR). Expression of the IFNLR is restricted compared with the ubiquitous type I IFN receptor; it is known to be expressed by epithelial cells (including hepatocytes) and plasmacytoid dendritic cells, but not by most hematopoietic cell lines. Activation leads to induction of IFN-stimulated genes (ISGs) via the Jak-STAT pathway, also used by the type I IFN receptor.[64,65] IFN-λ has in vitro and in vivo antiviral efficacy.[66,67] Pegylated IL-29 is currently in clinical development for HCV as a less toxic alternative to IFN-α; it is hoped that the restricted expression of the IFNLR will be associated with less hematological toxicity and flu-like symptoms.[65] Although the association between *IL28B* polymorphism and viral clearance is biologically plausible, the exact mechanism for its effect is not understood. There are two key issues: identification of the causal variant, and definition of the immunologic consequences of *IL28B* genotype.

Causal variant

GWAS test for association between clinical phenotype and common genetic variants (frequency 1%–5% in the population), also known as SNPs. Common genetic variants may be inherited together in haplotype blocks (such variants are said to be in LD). Therefore the genetic variation in a haplotype block can be captured by testing one representative SNP (a "tag" SNP). Genotyping chips therefore include tag SNPs chosen to cover the expression of all genes. There is some redundancy in the tag SNPs chosen, which differ according to chip and manufacturer. For example, rs12979860 and rs8099917 are both tag SNPs for a common haplotype block in Caucasians. The causal variant for the *IL28B*-SVR association is likely to be within this tagged haplotype block, but the polymorphism itself is not yet known. Putative functional SNPs have been identified in the region, including rs8103142, a nonsynonymous SNP in exon 2 of *IL28B* (K70R) (**Fig. 3**) and rs28416813, a guanosine to cytosine substitution 37 base pairs upstream of the translation initiation codon, in a recognized promoter region. Due to the high LD between the SNPs (r^2>0.85 for both SNPs), it has not been possible to differentiate which, if either, was the causal SNP in studies to date.

Beyond identification of the causal variant, there is little yet known about the biological mechanism underlying this genetic association. One possibility is that polymorphism affects gene expression; however, the relationship between *IL28B* genotype and expression of *IL28B* mRNA remains controversial.[25–27,66,67] *IL28B* genotype has been associated with intrahepatic ISG expression in several studies wherein the poor-response genotypes have been associated with increased expression, consistent with previous data linking ISG expression to IFN treatment response.[68,69] This association with liver ISG expression was not seen in healthy controls, suggesting that the correlation is specific to HCV infection.[70] Further functional studies investigating the immunology associated with *IL28B* genotype and treatment response are required.

Inosine Triphosphatase Polymorphisms and Ribavirin-Associated Anemia

Inosine triphosphatase polymorphisms and anemia

RBV is an essential part of therapy for HCV, increasing on-treatment antiviral potency[71,72] and reducing relapse rates.[73] Dose reduction or cessation is associated with lower SVR rates.[74,75] Unfortunately, RBV-induced hemolytic anemia is a common dose-limiting side effect of treatment, reported in approximately 15% of the patients enrolled in the phase 3 registration studies.[71]

A GWAS of RBV-induced hemoglobin reduction was performed in the IDEAL pharmacogenetic cohort.[30] Several SNPs on chromosome 20 were found to be strongly associated with protection from week-4 anemia in HCV-1 patients. The top-discovery SNP

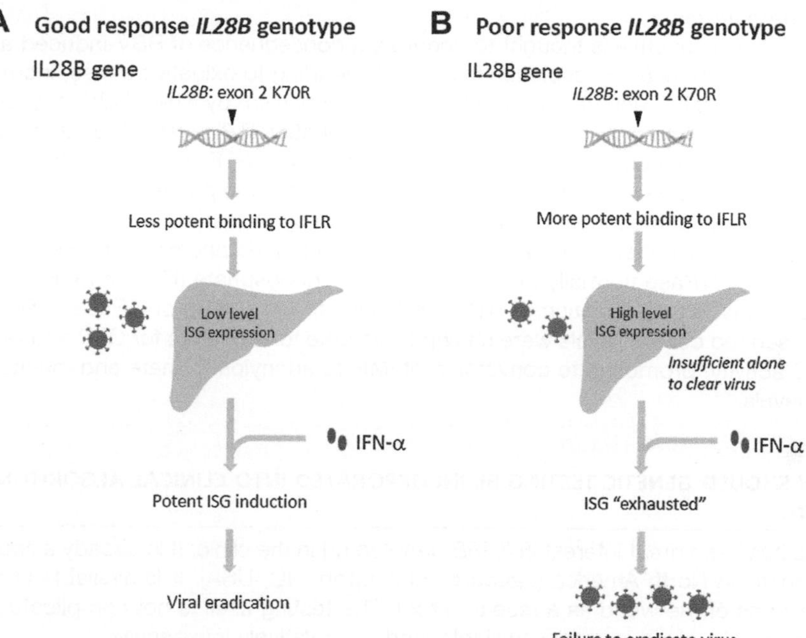

Fig. 3. Proposed hypothesis of the mechanisms of *IL28B*. Rs8103142 (K70R) is a nonsynonymous SNP located in exon 2. In (*A*), the good-responder *IL28B* genotypes, *IL28B* is less potent; this results in low levels of ISG expression. With the addition of IFN-α (more potent antiviral agent), there is potent induction of ISG leading to viral eradication. In (*B*), the poor-responder *IL28B* genotypes have more potent ISG induction with the K70R variant, leading to high levels of ISG expression, which alone is not sufficient to clear virus. With the addition of IFN-α, which has more potent antiviral activity, there is no further induction of ISG because of exhaustion, and viral eradication cannot occur.

was rs6051702 ($P = 1.1 \times 10^{-45}$, patients of European American ancestry). Genotyping of known functional variants in the region demonstrated that the association signal was entirely explained by 2 functional SNPs in the inosine triphosphatase gene (*ITPA)*, encoding inosine triphosphatase (ITPase): rs1127354 (proline to threonine substitution at position 32 in exon 8, P32T) and rs7270101 (splicing altering SNP in intron 2). The minor alleles cause ITPase deficiency and were protective against anemia. Predicted ITPase deficiency, defined according to previous functional studies of these 2 variants,[76,77] strongly protected patients against hemoglobin (Hb) reduction. In the IDEAL study cohort, 14% of patients had ITPase activity predicted to be less than or equal to 30%, and only 4% of these patients experienced a greater than 3 g/dL reduction in Hb from baseline to week 4; none had an Hb less than 10 g/dL. By contrast, in the 68% of patients predicted to have wild-type ITPase activity, the rate of Hb decline of greater than 3 g/dL was 56%. Despite the strong association with protection from anemia, the *ITPA* variants were not associated with SVR. A second study of the ViraHep-C cohort confirmed this strong association with week-4 anemia, and confirmed that the variants were associated with protection from anemia throughout the 48-week treatment course.[31] *ITPA* deficiency conferred protection from RBV dose reduction, but again no association with SVR was noted. The protection from anemia and RBV dose reduction appears to be independent of HCV genotype.[78]

ITPA mechanisms

RBV hemolytic anemia is thought to occur as a consequence of RBV-induced adenosine triphosphate (ATP) depletion in red cells, leading to oxidative stress, increased membrane fragility, and hemolysis. One major mechanism by which RBV may reduce ATP is by depletion of red cell guanosine triphosphate (GTP) levels, through inhibition of inosine monophosphate dehydrogenase (IMP DH). GTP is used as the energy source for the conversion of IMP to adenylosuccinate in the purine synthetic pathway to ATP, a reaction dependent on adenylosuccinate synthase (ADSS).[79] A mechanism for the protective effect of ITPA variants on RBV-induced anemia has recently been proposed.[79] ITPase normally hydrolyzes inosine triphosphate (ITP) and ITPase deficiency leads to accumulation of ITP in red cells. In the setting of ITPase deficiency, increased red cell ITP levels were shown to be able to substitute for GTP and restore ADSS activity, promoting to conversion of IMP to adenylosuccinate and maintaining ATP levels.

HOW SHOULD GENETIC TESTING BE INCORPORATED INTO CLINICAL ALGORITHMS?

IL28B

There has been great interest in *IL28B* genotyping in the clinic. It is already a licensed diagnostic in North America (Labcorp, Burlington, NC, USA). It is available in many other parts of the world as a research tool. The testing itself is not complicated, the technology involved is widely available, and it is relatively inexpensive.

Knowledge of a patient's *IL28B* genotype may assist in planning therapy for HCV-1. Patients with the good-response genotype can be expected to have a 70% likelihood of SVR with SOC therapy. Even when RVR was not achieved, the rate of SVR was more than 65% among Caucasians enrolled in the IDEAL study. In the absence of contraindications, it is reasonable to offer SOC therapy for 48 weeks. The incremental benefit with the addition of DAAs is expected to be small, and triple therapy will be expensive and associated with some added toxicity. In patients with a poor-response genotype, results with SOC therapy are poor (<40% SVR), and in the absence of any clinical urgency clinicians may consider deferral of treatment until the novel DAA are licensed, which is expected in the near future. The association between *IL28B* genotype and treatment outcome in HCV-2/3 appears to be attenuated, and the utility of genetic testing in this group is not yet clear. Decision models considering both viral and host predictors, including *IL28B* genotype, are being developed to further refine the accuracy of pretreatment prediction of SVR (**Fig. 4**).[80]

In patients with HIV–HCV-1 coinfection, the utility of *IL28B* genotyping appears to be similar to HCV-1 monoinfection. *IL28B* genotyping may have a place in the workup for liver transplantation in patients with hepatitis C. Recipients carrying the poor-response *IL28B* genotypes appear to have higher SVR rates if they receive a liver from a good-responder *IL28B* donor. Given the aggressive course of posttransplant HCV infection and the benefit of viral eradication,[81] consideration of whether *IL28B* genotyping can be incorporated into organ allocation protocols is warranted; this will require prospective evaluation. The role for routine *IL28B* genotyping in patients chronically infected with HCV-2/3 remains less clear at present. In acute HCV infection, *IL28B* genotyping may have a clinical role. Patients with the good-response genotype have a high likelihood of spontaneous clearance of virus, thus it is reasonable to observe for 3 months to monitor for natural clearance. However, in poor-response genotype patients, particularly anicteric patients, the chance of spontaneous viral clearance is very low. As treatment early in infection has been shown to be more effective,[82] therapy may be considered at diagnosis, rather than observing for spontaneous resolution.

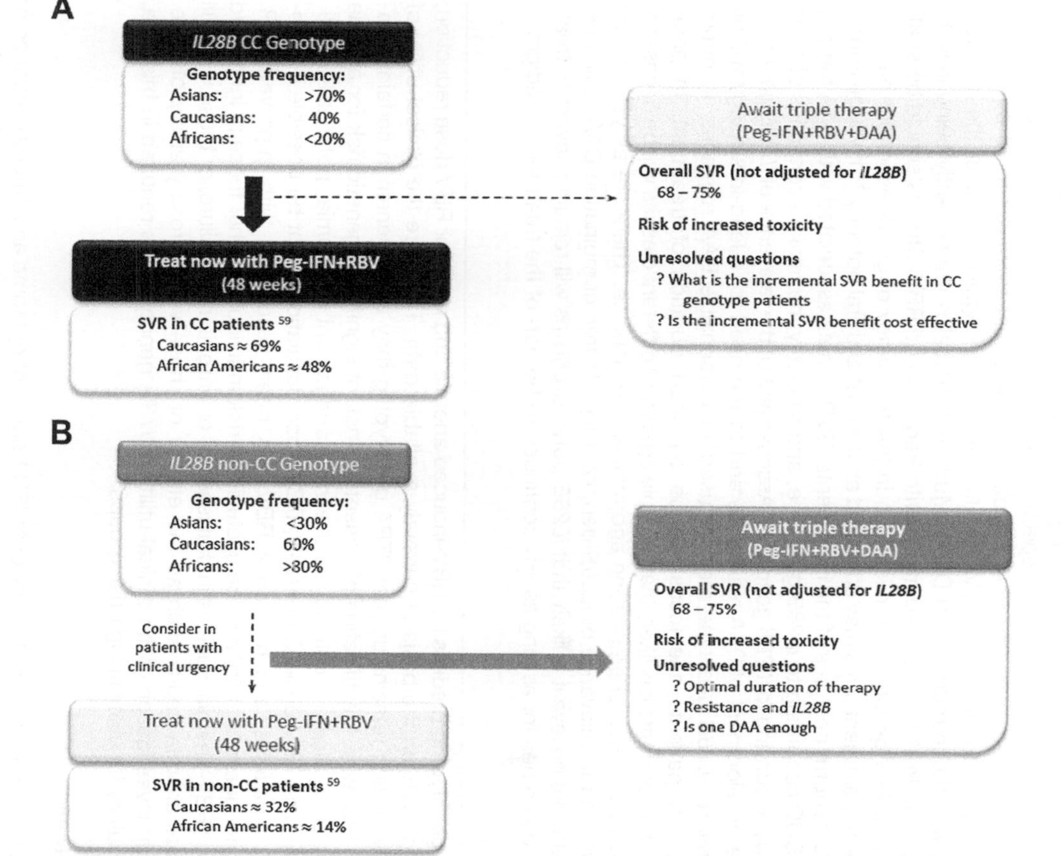
A
IL28B CC Genotype
Genotype frequency:
Asians: >70%
Caucasians: 40%
Africans: <20%
Treat now with Peg-IFN+RBV
(48 weeks)
SVR in CC patients 59
Caucasians ≈ 69%
African Americans ≈ 48%
Await triple therapy
(Peg-IFN+RBV+DAA)
Overall SVR (not adjusted for IL28B)
68 – 75%
Risk of increased toxicity
Unresolved questions
? What is the incremental SVR benefit in CC genotype patients
? Is the incremental SVR benefit cost effective
B
IL28B non-CC Genotype
Genotype frequency:
Asians: <30%
Caucasians: 60%
Africans: >80%
Consider in patients with clinical urgency
Treat now with Peg-IFN+RBV
(48 weeks)
SVR in non-CC patients 59
Caucasians ≈ 32%
African Americans ≈ 14%
Await triple therapy
(Peg-IFN+RBV+DAA)
Overall SVR (not adjusted for IL28B)
68 – 75%
Risk of increased toxicity
Unresolved questions
? Optimal duration of therapy
? Resistance and IL28B
? Is one DAA enough

Fig. 4. (*A, B*) Suggested treatment algorithms based on *IL28B* genotype. (*Data from* Refs.[33,58,59])

There are several important issues that require further study. It will be useful to assess whether *IL28B* genotype can be used to personalize treatment duration with SOC. In HCV-1, it will be important to assess whether good-responder genotype alone can be used to shorten treatment to 24 weeks, and to compare this approach to a response-guided strategy based on achievement of RVR. An *IL28B* approach would be expected to allow more HCV-1 patients to be treated for 24 weeks if RVR is achieved. An RVR strategy for shortening treatment may remain more relevant in HCV-2/3, where the rate of RVR is greater than 50% in most studies. Conversely, it will be important to explore prospectively whether HCV-2/3 non-RVR patients with poor-responder *IL28B* genotypes benefit from treatment extension to 48 weeks.

Finally, the treatment of HCV-1 is likely to change significantly over the next few years with the introduction of DAAs. Multiple candidates are currently being investigated in triple-therapy combinations with Peg-IFN and RBV. Studies should be stratified by *IL28B* genotype, as mismatch in the frequency of good-responder patients between treatment arms may confound analysis of antiviral potency.[83] It will be important to perform analyses of the incremental SVR benefit associated with DAA therapy over SOC according to *IL28B* genotype, and to justify the health economics of triple therapy according to *IL28B* genotype. Assessment of the relevance of *IL28B* genotype to the development of DAA resistance and to the need for a lead-in strategy will be necessary. *IL28B* genotype may be used to personalize DAA regimens. In good-responder patients, the focus will be on short duration of treatment. In poor-responder patients it is likely that multiple agents of different classes will be necessary to maximize rates of eradication and minimize resistance. There are as yet no data evaluating the relevance of *IL28B* genotype to IFN-free combination DAA regimens. The authors believe it is likely that *IL28B* polymorphisms will remain relevant to treatment outcomes for as long as IFN continues to be part of the treatment paradigm.

ITPA

ITPA genotyping predicts for RBV-induced anemia and need for RBV dose reduction, but not SVR on the basis of currently available data. Therefore the clinical utility of routine testing remains unclear. *ITPA* genotyping may be of benefit in certain situations, however. Identification of patients at risk of significant genetic risk for anemia might allow closer monitoring and early management of anemia, potentially maximizing total RBV dose. Conversely, RBV dose escalation might be possible in "protected" patients, and high-dose RBV has been associated with improved SVR. Second, dosing of RBV may be useful in at-risk individuals, either those at increased risk for RBV-anemia, such as in thalassemia or chronic renal failure, or those who will tolerate anemia poorly such as the elderly or those with coronary artery disease. Further investigation of the clinical utility of *ITPA* genotyping is required in this area, particularly its utility in high-risk groups.

SUMMARY

IL28B polymorphisms influence both IFN treatment outcome and natural clearance of HCV infection. *ITPA* polymorphisms have been shown to predict RBV-induced anemia, an important dose-limiting side effect of treatment. These exciting genetic discoveries are changing how we think about HCV pathogenesis, patient evaluation, and current treatment paradigms. There are, however, many questions that have been raised and several keys to the puzzle still need to be solved. Further study is required to understand the mechanism of the *IL28B* association, and to clarify how testing should be incorporated into clinical algorithms.

REFERENCES

1. Sheppard CW, Finelli L, Alter MJ. Global epidemiology of hepatitis C virus infection. Lancet Infect Dis 2005;5:558–67.
2. Thomas DL, Seeff LB. Natural history of hepatitis C. Clin Liver Dis 2005;9: 383–98, vi.
3. Yu ML, Lin SM, Chuang WL, et al. A sustained virological response to interferon or interferon/ribavirin reduces hepatocellular carcinoma and improves survival in chronic hepatitis C: a nationwide, multicentre study in Taiwan. Antivir Ther 2006;11:985–94.
4. Manns MP, McHutchison JG, Gordon SC, et al. Peginterferon alfa-2b plus ribavirin compared with IFN-2b plus ribavirin for initial treatment of chronic hepatitis C: a randomised trial. Lancet 2001;358:958–65.
5. Fried MW, Shiffman ML, Reddy KR, et al. Peginterferon alfa-2a plus ribavirin for chronic hepatitis C virus infection. N Engl J Med 2002;347:975–82.
6. Hadziyannis SJ, Sette H Jr, Morgan TR, et al. Peginterferon-alpha2a and ribavirin combination therapy in chronic hepatitis C: a randomised study of treatment duration and ribavirin dose. Ann Intern Med 2004;140:346–55.
7. Jacobson IM, Brown RS Jr, Freilich B, et al. Peginterferon alfa-2b and weight-based or flat dosed ribavirin in chronic hepatitis C patients: a randomized trial. Hepatology 2007;46:971–81.
8. Nakagawa M, Sakamoto N, Ueyama M, et al. Mutations in the interferon sensitivity determining region and virological response to combination therapy with pegylated-interferon alpha 2b plus ribavirin in patients with chronic hepatitis C-1b infection. J Gastroenterol 2010;45:656–65.
9. Shirakawa H, Mastsumoto A, Joshita S, et al. Pretreatment prediction of virological response to peginterferon plus ribavirin therapy in chronic hepatitis C patients using viral and host factors. Hepatology 2008;48:1753–60.
10. Murayama M, Katano Y, Nakano I, et al. A mutation in the interferon sensitivity-determining region is associated with responsiveness to interferon-ribavirin combination therapy in chronic hepatitis patients infected with a Japan-specific subtype of hepatitis C virus genotype 1b. J Med Virol 2007;79:35–40.
11. Akuta N, Suzuki F, Hirakawa M, et al. A matched case-controlled study of 48 and 72 weeks of peginterferon plus ribavirin combination therapy in patients infected with HCV genotype 1b in Japan: amino acid substitutions in HCV core region as predictor of sustained virological response. J Med Virol 2009; 81:452–8.
12. Kitamura S, Tsuge M, Hatakeyama T, et al. Amino acid substitutions in core and NS5A regions of the HCV genome can predict virological decrease with pegylated interferon plus ribavirin therapy. Antivir Ther 2010;15:1087–97.
13. Okanoue T, Itoh Y, Hashimoto H, et al. Predictive values of amino acid sequences of the core and NS5A regions in antiviral therapy for hepatitis C: a Japanese multi-center study. J Gastroenterol 2009;44:952–63.
14. Toyoda H, Kumada T, Tada T, et al. Association between HCV amino acid substitutions and outcome of peginterferon and ribavirin combination therapy in HCV genotype 1b and high viral load. J Gastroenterol Hepatol 2010;25:1072–8.
15. Jaeckel E, Cornberg M, Wedemeyer H, et al. Treatment of acute hepatitis C with interferon alfa-2b. N Engl J Med 2001;345:1452–7.
16. Gerlach JT, Diepolder HM, Zachoval R, et al. Acute hepatitis C: high rate of both spontaneous and treatment-induced viral clearance. Gastroenterology 2003;125: 80–8.

17. Alberti A, Boccato S, Vario A, et al. Therapy of acute hepatitis C. Hepatology 2002;36:S195–200.
18. Licata A, Di Bona D, Schepis F, et al. When and how to treat acute hepatitis C? J Hepatol 2003;39:1056–62.
19. Wiegand J, Buggisch P, Boecher W, et al. Early monotherapy with pegylated alpha-2b for acute hepatitis C infection: the HEP-NET acute-HCV-II study. Hepatology 2006;43:250–6.
20. Conjeevaram HS, Fried MW, Jeffers LJ, et al. Peginterferon and ribavirin treatment in African American and Caucasian American patients with hepatitis C genotype 1. Gastroenterology 2006;131:470–7.
21. Muir AJ, Bornstein JD, Killenberg PG. Peginterferon alfa-2b and ribavirin for the treatment of chronic hepatitis C in black and non-Hispanic whites. N Engl J Med 2004;350:2265–71.
22. Liu CH, Liu CJ, Lin CL, et al. Pegylated intergeron-alpha-2a plus ribavirin for treatment-naïve Asian patients with hepatitis C virus genotype 1 infection: a multicentre, randomized controlled trial. Clin Infect Dis 2008;47:1260–9.
23. Hepburn MJ, Hepburn LM, Cantu NS, et al. Difference in treatment outcome for hepatitis C among ethnic groups. Am J Med 2004;117:163–8.
24. Missiha S, Heathcote J, Arenovich T, et al. Impact of Asian race on response to combination therapy with pegylated interferon alfa-2a and ribavirin in chronic hepatitis C. Am J Gastroenterol 2007;102:2181–8.
25. Ge D, Fellay J, Thompson AJ, et al. Genetic variation in *IL28B* predicts hepatitis C treatment-induced viral clearance. Nature 2009;461:399–401.
26. Suppiah V, Moldovan M, Ahlenstiel G, et al. *IL28B* is associated with response to chronic hepatitis C interferon-α and ribavirin therapy. Nat Genet 2009;41:1100–4.
27. Tanaka Y, Nishida N, Sugiyama M, et al. Genome-wide association of *IL28B* with response to pegylated interferon-α and ribavirin therapy for chronic hepatitis C. Nat Genet 2009;41(10):1105–9.
28. Rauch A, Kutalik Z, Descombes P, et al. Genetic variation in *IL28B* is associated with chronic hepatitis C and treatment failure: a genome-wide association study. Gastroenterology 2010;138:1338–45.
29. Thomas DL, Thio CL, Martin MP, et al. Genetic variation in *IL28B* and spontaneous clearance of hepatitis C. Nature 2009;461:798–802.
30. Fellay J, Thompson AJ, Ge D, et al. ITPA gene variants protect against anaemia in patients treated for chronic hepatitis C. Nature 2010;464:405–8.
31. Thompson AJ, Fellay J, Patel K, et al. Variants in the ITPA gene protect against ribavirin-induced hemolytic anemia and decrease the need for ribavirin dose reduction. Gastroenterology 2010;139:1181–9.
32. McHutchison JG, Lawitz EJ, Shiffman ML, et al. Peginterferon alfa-2b or alfa-2a with ribavirin for treatment of hepatitis C infection. NEJM 2009;361(6):580–93.
33. Thompson AJ, Muir AJ, Sulkowski MS, et al. Interleukin-28B polymorphism improves viral kinetics and is the strongest pre-treatment predictor of sustained virological response in genotype 1 hepatitis C virus. Gastroenterology 2010;139:120–9.
34. Neumann A, Bibert S, Haagmans B, et al. *IL28B* polymorphism is significantly correlated with IFB anti-viral effectiveness already on first day of pegylated interferon-α and ribavirin therapy of chronic HCV infection. Vienna (Austria): EASL; 2010 [abstract: #2011].
35. Bochud PY, Bibert S, Negro F, et al. IL28B polymorphisms predict reduction of HCV RNA from the first day of therapy in chronic hepatitis C. J Hepatol 2011, in press.

36. Stättermayer AF, Stauber R, Hofer H, et al. Impact of *IL28B* genotype on the early and sustained virological response in treatment-naïve patients with chronic hepatitis C. Clin Gastroenterol Hepatol 2011;9(4):344.e2–350.e2.
37. Sarrazin C, Susser S, Doehring A, et al. Importance of *IL28B* gene polymorphisms in hepatitis C virus genotype 2 and 3 infected patients. J Hepatol 2011;54(3):415–21.
38. Kawaoka T, Hayes CN, Ohishi W, et al. Predictive value of the *IL28B* polymorphism on the effect of interferon therapy in chronic hepatitis C patients with genotypes 2a and 2b. J Hepatol 2011;54(3):408–14.
39. Scherzer TM, Hofer H, Stäettermayer AF, et al. Early virological response and *IL28B* polymorphisms in patients with chronic hepatitis C genotype 3 treated with peginterferon alfa-2a and ribavirin. J Hepatol 2011;54(5):866–71.
40. Moghaddam A, Melum E, Reinton N, et al. *IL28B* genetic variation and treatment response in patients with HCV genotype 3 infection. Hepatology 2011;53(3):746–54.
41. Yu ML, Huang CF, Huang JF, et al. Role of interleukin-28B polymorphisms in the treatment of hepatitis C virus in genotype 2 infection in Asian patients. Hepatology 2011;53(1):7–13.
42. Mangia A, Thompson AJ, Santoro R, et al. An *IL28B* polymorphism determines treatment response of hepatitis C virus genotype 2 or 3 patients who do not achieve a rapid virological response. Gastroenterology 2010;139:821–7.
43. Montes-Cano AM, García-Lozano JR, Abad-Molina C, et al. Interleukin-28B genetic variants and hepatitis virus infection by different viral genotypes. Hepatology 2010;52:33–7.
44. Rallón NI, Naggie S, Benito JM, et al. Association of a single nucleotide polymorphisms near the interleukin-28B gene with response to hepatitis C therapy in HIV/hepatitis C virus-coinfected patients. AIDS 2010;24:F23–9.
45. De Araújo ES, Dahari H, Cotler SJ, et al. Pharmacodynamics of PEG-IFN alpha-2a and HCV response as a function of *IL28B* polymorphism in HIV/HCV coinfected patients. J Acquir Immune Defic Syndr 2011;56(2):95–9.
46. Pineda JA, Caruz A, Rivero A, et al. Prediction of response to pegylated interferon plus ribavirin by *IL28B* gene variation in patients coinfected with HIV and hepatitis C virus. Clin Infect Dis 2010;51:788–95.
47. Aparicio E, Parera M, Franco S, et al. *IL28B* SNP rs8099917 is strongly associated with pegylated interferon-α and ribavirin therapy treatment failure in HCV/HIV-1 coinfected patients. PLoS One 2010;5:e13771.
48. Yilmaz N, Shiffman ML, Stravitz RT, et al. A prospective evaluation of fibrosis progression in patients with recurrent hepatitis C virus following liver transplantation. Liver Transpl 2007;13:975–83.
49. Berenguer M, Ferrell L, Watson J, et al. HCV-related fibrosis progression following liver transplantation: increase in recent years. J Hepatol 2000;32:673–84.
50. Brown RS. Hepatitis C and liver transplantation. Nature 2005;436:973–8.
51. Chalasani N, Manzarbeitia C, Ferenci P, et al. Peginterferon alfa-2a for hepatitis C after liver transplantation: two randomized, controlled trials. Hepatology 2005;41:289–98.
52. Fernández I, Meneu JC, Colina F, et al. Clinical and histological efficacy of pegylated interferon and ribavirin therapy of recurrent hepatitis C after liver transplantation. Liver Transpl 2006;12:1805–12.
53. Mukherjee S. Pegylated interferon alfa-2a and ribavirin for recurrent hepatitis C after liver transplantation. Transplant Proc 2005;37:4403–5.
54. Fukuhara T, Taketomi A, Motomura T, et al. Variants in *IL28B* in liver recipients and donors correlate with response to peg-interferon and ribavirin therapy for recurrent hepatitis C. Gastroenterology 2010;139:1577–85.

55. Charlton MR, Thompson AJ, Veldt BJ, et al. Interleukin-28B polymorphisms are associated with histological recurrence and treatment response following liver transplantation in patients with hepatitis C virus infection. Hepatology 2011;53:317–24.
56. Lange CM, Moradpour D, Doehring A, et al. Impact of donor and recipient *IL28B* rs12979860 genotypes on hepatitis C liver graft reinfection. J Hepatol 2010. [Epub ahead of press].
57. Bacon BR, Gordon SC, Lawitz E, et al. Boceprevir for treatment of chronic hepatitis C genotype 1 nonresponders. N Engl J Med 2011;54:1207–17.
58. Poordad F, McCone J Jr, Bacon BR, et al. Boceprevir with peginterferon/ribavirin for untreated chronic hepatitis C. N Engl J Med 2011;54:1195–206.
59. Jacobson IA, McHutchison JG, Dusheiko GM, et al. Telaprevir in combination with peginterferon alfa-2a and ribavirin in genotype 1 HCV treatment-naïve patients: final results of phase 3 Advance study. Boston (MA): AASLD; 2010 [abstract: 211].
60. Akuta N, Suzuki F, Hirakawa M, et al. Amino acid substitution in hepatitis C virus core region and genetic variation near the *interleukin 28B* gene predict viral response to telaprevir with peginterferon and ribavirin. Hepatology 2010;52:421–9.
61. Fried MW, Buti M, Dore GJ, et al. Efficacy and safety of TMC435 in combination with peginterferon alpha-2a plus ribavirin in treatment naive genotype 1 HCV patients: 24 week-interim results from the PILLAR study [abstract form]. Hepatology 2010;52(Suppl 1):LB5.
62. Tillmann HL, Thompson AJ, Patel K, et al. A polymorphism near *IL28B* is associated with spontaneous clearance of acute hepatitis C virus and jaundice. Gastroenterology 2010;139:1586–92.
63. Grebely J, Petoumenos K, Hellard M, et al. Potential role for interleukin-28B genotype in treatment decision-making in recent hepatitis C virus infection. Hepatology 2010;52:1216–24.
64. Kotenko SV, Gallagher G, Baurin VV, et al. IFN-lambdas mediate antiviral protection through a distinct class II cytokine receptor complex. Nat Immunol 2003;4: 66–77.
65. Sheppard P, Kindsvogel W, Xu W, et al. *IL-28, IL-29* and their class II cytokine receptor *IL-28R*. Nat Immunol 2003;4:63–8.
66. Robek MD, Boyd BS, Chisari FV. Lambda interferon inhibits hepatitis B and C virus replication. J Virol 2005;79:3851–4.
67. Muir AJ, Shiffman ML, Zaman A, et al. Phase 1b study of pegylated interferon lambda-1 with or without ribavirin in patients with chronic genotype 1 hepatitis C virus infection. Hepatology 2010;52:822–32.
68. Honda M, Sakai A, Yamashita T, et al. Hepatic ISG expression is associated with genetic variation in *IL28B* and the outcome of IFN therapy for CHC. Gastroenterology 2010;139:499–509.
69. Urban T, Thompson AJ, Bradrick SS, et al. *IL28B* genotype is associated with differential expression of intrahepatic interferon-stimulated genes in patients with chronic hepatitis C. Hepatology 2010;52:1888–96.
70. Shebl FM, Maeder D, Shao U, et al. In the absence of HCV infection, interferon stimulated gene expression in liver is not associated with *IL28B* genotype. Gastroenterology 2010;139:1422–4.
71. McHutchison JG, Gordon SC, Schiff ER, et al. Interferon alfa-2b alone or in combination with ribavirin as initial treatment for chronic hepatitis C. Hepatitis Interventional Therapy Group. N Engl J Med 1998;339:1485–92.
72. Bain VG, Lee SS, Peltekian K, et al. Clinical trial: exposure to ribavirin predicts EVR and SVR in patients with HCV genotype 1 infection treated with peginterferon alfa-2a plus ribavirin. Aliment Pharmacol Ther 2008;28:43–50.

73. Hiramatsu N, Oze T, Yakushijin T, et al. Ribavirin dose reduction raises relapse rate dose-dependently in genotype 1 patients with hepatitis C responding to pegylated interferon alpha-2b plus ribavirin. J Viral Hepat 2009;16:586–94.
74. Reddy KR, Shiffman ML, Morgan TR, et al. Impact of ribavirin dose reductions in hepatitis C virus genotype 1 patients completing peginterferon alfa-2a/ribavirin treatment. Clin Gastroenterol Hepatol 2007;5:124–9.
75. Akuta N, Suzuki F, Yawamura Y, et al. Predictive factors of early and sustained responses to peginterferon plus ribavirin combination therapy in Japanese patients infected with hepatitis C virus genotype 1b: amino acid substitutions in the core region and low-density lipoprotein cholesterol levels. J Hepatol 2007; 46:403–10.
76. Bierau J, Lindhout M, Bakker JA. Pharmacogenetic significance of inosine triphosphatase. Pharmacogenetics 2007;8:1221–8.
77. Stocco G, Choek MH, Crews KR, et al. Genetic polymorphism of inosine triphosphate pyrophosphatase is a determinant of mercaptopurine metabolism and toxicity during treatment for acute lymphocytic leukemia. Clin Pharmacol Ther 2009;85:164–72.
78. Thompson AJ, Santoro RS, Piazzolla V, et al. Inosine triphosphatase genetic variants are protective against anemia during antiviral therapy for HCV2/3 but do not decrease dose reductions of RBV or increase SVR. Hepatology 2011;53:389–95.
79. Hitomi Y, Cirulli ET, Fellay J, et al. Inosine triphosphate protects against ribavirin-induced ATP loss by restoring adenylosuccinate synthase function. Gastroenterology 2011;140(4):1314–21.
80. Kurosaki M, Matsunaga K, Hirayama I, et al. A predictive model of response to peginterferon ribavirin in chronic hepatitis C using classification and regression tree analysis. Hepatol Res 2010;40:251–60.
81. Veldta BJ, Poteruchaa JJ, Watta DS, et al. Impact of pegylated interferon and ribavirin treatment on graft survival in liver transplant patients with recurrent hepatitis C infection. Am J Transplant 2008;8:2426–33.
82. Corey KE, Mendez-Navarro J, Gorospe EC, et al. Early treatment improves outcomes in acute hepatitis C virus infection: a meta-analysis. J Viral Hepat 2010;17:201–7.
83. Thompson AJ, Muir AJ, Sulkowski MS, et al. Hepatitis C trials that combine investigational agents with pegylated interferon should be stratified by *interleukin-28B* genotype. Hepatology 2010;52:2243.

An Overview of Emerging Therapies for the Treatment of Chronic Hepatitis C

Jawad A. Ilyas, MD, MS[a,b,c], John M. Vierling, MD[a,b,c,*]

KEYWORDS

- Chronic hepatitis C • Direct-acting antivirals
- Protease inhibitors • Telaprevir • Boceprevir
- Polymerase inhibitors • Cyclophilin inhibitors
- Therapeutic vaccines

Hepatitis C virus (HCV) infection afflicts ~170 million persons worldwide and is a leading cause of chronic hepatitis, cirrhosis, liver failure, and hepatocellular carcinoma (HCC). Chronic hepatitis C (CHC) is also the leading indication for orthotopic liver transplantation in the United States and abroad.[1] The prevalence of CHC in the United States is ~1.6%, which equates to 4.1 million people with anti-HCV antibodies and 3.3 million with viremia.[2] Currently, standard of care (SOC) antiviral therapy for all HCV genotypes is pegylated interferon-α combined with weight-based ribavirin (Peg-IFN-α/R) for 24 weeks for genotypes 2 and 3 or 48 weeks for genotypes 1 and 4. Peg-IFN-α/R therapy results in variable rates of sustained virological response (SVR, defined as undetectable HCV RNA $\geq$24 weeks after cessation of antiviral therapy) depending on genotype.[3–5] SVR rates are lowest in genotype 1 infections (40%–50%) and highest in genotype 2 and 3 infections (70%–90%).[6] SOC treatment

---

Authors' disclosures: JAI is a subinvestigator and JMV is the principal investigator for clinical trials sponsored by grants from Abbott, Bristol-Meyers-Squibb, Conatus, Excalenz, Gilead, Globeimmune, Hyperion, Idenix, Ikaria, Intercept, Merck, Mochida, Novartis, Ocera, Pharmasset, Roche, Sundise, Vertex, and Zymogenetics. JMV also serves on Advisory Boards for Bristol-Meyers-Squibb, Excalenz, Gilead, Globeimmune, Hyperion, Merck, Novartis, and the Data Safety and Monitoring Board of the Drug-Induced Liver Injury Clinical Research Network, NIDDK, and NIH.

[a] Liver Center, St Luke's Episcopal Hospital, Baylor College of Medicine, 1709 Dryden, Suite 1500, Houston, TX 77030, USA

[b] Department of Medicine, Baylor College of Medicine, 1709 Dryden Street, Suite 500, Houston, TX 77030, USA

[c] Department of Surgery, Baylor College of Medicine, 1709 Dryden Street, Suite 1500, Houston, TX 77030, USA

* Corresponding author. Liver Center, 1709 Dryden, Suite 1500, Houston, TX 77030.

E-mail address: vierling@bcm.tmc.edu

Clin Liver Dis 15 (2011) 515–536

doi:10.1016/j.cld.2011.05.002

liver.theclinics.com

1089-3261/11/$ – see front matter

is also associated with multiple adverse events, such as a flulike syndrome, cytopenias (anemia, neutropenia, and thrombocytopenia), rashes, and neuropsychiatric symptoms, especially depression. The impact of CHC requires urgent development of therapies with greater efficacy, safety, and tolerability to address the unmet needs of treatment-naive patients and treatment-experienced patients who failed to achieve SVR after treatment with Peg-IFN-α/R.

Multiple novel therapies for CHC are in various stages of preclinical or clinical development. These include direct-acting antivirals (DAA), agents that specifically inhibit HCV protease or polymerase proteins, pegylated IFN-λ, inhibitors of host cyclophilins required for HCV RNA replication, inhibitors of hepatocyte apoptosis, inhibitors matrix metalloproteinases (MMPs) and therapeutic vaccines to activate HCV-specific host T-cell responses. Development of antiviral therapeutics with diverse mechanisms of action reflects recognition that the HCV lifecycle affords multiple potential therapeutic targets, the usefulness of in vitro replicon assays to screen candidate DAAs and other agents, and better appreciation of the roles of innate and adaptive T-cell immunity in both acute, self-limited infection and CHC. The purpose of this review is to summarize the status of novel therapeutics for CHC, with special emphasis on the results of phase 2 and 3 studies of the NS3 serine protease inhibitors telaprevir and boceprevir, which are expected to be approved for use in the United States and Europe this year.

HEPATITIS C LIFE CYCLE AND THERAPEUTIC TARGETS

HCV is an enveloped virus within the Flaviviridae family, genus Hepacivirus, with a 9.6-kb, single-stranded, positive-sense RNA genome.[7–9] The genome is organized into structural and nonstructural regions that encode the core and envelop structural proteins and the nonstructural proteins involved in the processing of viral proteins and RNA replication. **Fig. 1** illustrates the lifecycle of HCV, which provides multiple therapeutic targets. DAA development has primarily focused on inhibition of the HCV NS3/4A protease required to process the NS5A and NS5B, which are the key components of the replication complex. Thus, potent protease inhibition can reduce NS5A-NS5B replication complex activity and prevent RNA replication (see **Fig. 1**). Conversely, potent inhibition of NS5A-NS5B replication complex activity could completely silence RNA replication. A combination therapy with both a protease inhibitor and an NS5A-NS5B replication complex inhibitor should theoretically prevent both HCV protein processing and RNA replication and significantly reduce the probability of resistant variants.

PROTEASE (NS3/4A) INHIBITORS

Protease inhibition interrupts posttranslational processing by blocking the catalytic site of NS3 or preventing NS3/4A interaction. NS3 serine protease inhibitors can be divided into 2 chemical classes: linear tetrapeptide α-ketoamide derivatives and macrocyclic compounds. The first protease inhibitor used in humans, ciluprevir (BILN 2061),[8] provided strong evidence of proof of principle. In a randomized, double-blind, placebo-controlled proof-of-concept study, patients infected with HCV genotype 1 received ciluprevir 200 mg orally or placebo twice daily for 2 days. Ciluprevir, but not placebo, induced a rapid decline of 2 to 3 $\log_{10}$ in plasma HCV RNA in all patients within 24 to 28 hours. Development of ciluprevir was stopped because of cardiac toxicity observed in animals. Subsequently, multiple NS3 serine protease inhibitors have been synthesized and are in various stages of clinical development (**Table 1**). Phase 3 studies of the linear protease inhibitors telaprevir (VX-950)

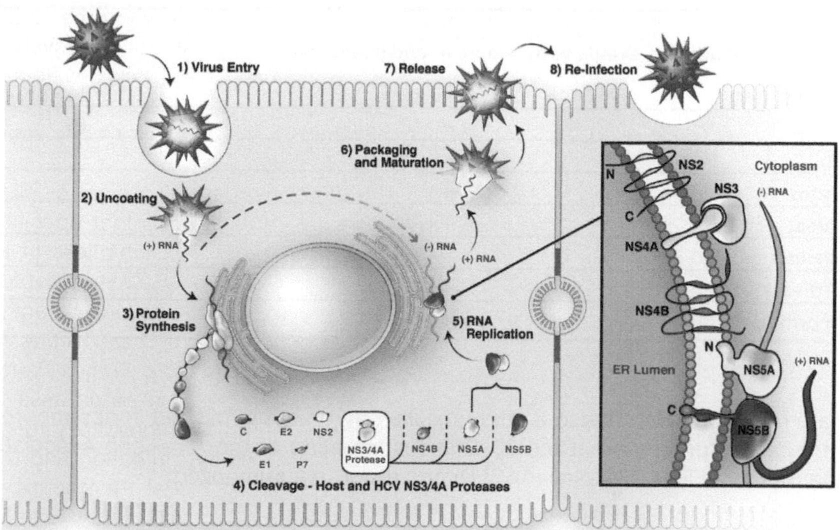

Fig. 1. HCV life cycle and multiple therapeutic targets. HCV attaches to hepatocyte-specific receptors and undergoes clathrin-mediated endocytosis and uncoating of the viral nucleocapsid. This process releases the 9.6-kb single-stranded positive-sense RNA genome into the cytoplasm, where it serves as a messenger RNA for translation of an HCV polyprotein containing ~3100 amino acids. Host proteases release the structural HCV protein core (C) and envelope 1 and 2 (E1, E2) proteins. The core protein forms the nucleocapsid-carrying E1 and E2, which are receptors for viral attachment and host cell entry. A combination of host and viral proteases process 6 nonstructural proteins (NS2, NS3, NS4A, NS4B, NS5A, and NS5B), whose enzymatic functions are obligatory for the HCV life cycle. NS2 and NS3 are viral proteases required for HCV polyprotein processing. The NS3 protein has a serine protease domain. The HCV protease enzyme is a serine proteinase with a catalytic site, 2 substrate-binding sites, an NS4A-binding site and an NS2/NS3 proteinase substrate recognition site, a helicase single-strand RNA-binding site, and a zinc-binding site. These sites offer multiple potential targets to inhibit the key NS3/NS4A protease complex required for proteolysis of the polyprotein to release NS5A and NS5B. The replication complex required for HCV RNA synthesis is shown in greater detail on the right. NS5B is the RNA-dependent RNA polymerase responsible for the synthesis of a complementary negative strand RNA from the positive-strand RNA genome. From the complementary negative-strand RNA, multiple positive-strand RNA molecules are produced and used as messenger RNAs for production of polyprotein, as new templates for negative strand synthesis, and as genomic RNA in newly formed virions. Because of the high error rates in RNA replication, numerous variants, termed HCV quasispecies, are produced. Similarly, viral proteins with amino acid substitutions are also generated. NS5A-NS5B replication complex activity requires cytosolic host cyclophilins. (*Data from* Bartenschlager R, Frese M, Pietschmann T. Novel insights into hepatitis C virus replication and persistence. Adv Virus Res 2004;63:71–180; and Moradpour D, Penin F, Rice CM. Replication of hepatitis C virus. Nat Rev Microbiol 2007;5:453–63.)

and boceprevir (SCH503034) combined with Peg-IFN-α/R have been completed in both treatment-naive and treatment-experienced patients without SVR to previous SOC treatment with P/R, and regulatory approval is anticipated in 2011.

TELAPREVIR

Telaprevir is an oral inhibitor of the NS3 protease. Phase 2 studies of safety and efficacy in treatment-naive and treatment-experienced patients have been published,

Table 1
Comparison of adverse events with telaprevir and boceprevir

Adverse Effect	Telaprevir	Boceprevir
Anemia	+	++
Rash	++	−
Pruritus	++	−
Nausea	++	+
Dysgeusia	−	++
Diarrhea	++	+
Hemorrhoids	+	−

and are reviewed later. Phase 3 study results have been published in abstract form and the results presented at the 2010 annual meeting of the American Association for the Study of Liver Diseases (AASLD) and are also summarized.

PHASE 2 STUDIES OF TELAPREVIR FOR TREATMENT-NAIVE PATIENTS

PROVE 1

This phase 2 PROVE 1[10] study randomized 250 treatment-naive, US patients with HCV genotype 1 infection to 4 treatment arms: (A) 12 weeks of telaprevir 750 mg every 8 hours plus Peg-IFN-α-2a/R followed by an additional 12 weeks of Peg-IFN-α-2a/R alone; (B) 12 weeks of telaprevir 750 mg every 8 hours plus Peg-IFN-α-2a/R followed by an additional 36 weeks of Peg-IFN-α-2a/R alone; (C) 12 weeks of telaprevir 750 mg every 8 hours plus Peg-IFN-α-2a/R; and (D) Peg-IFN-α-2a/R for 48 weeks (control arm). In telaprevir treatment arms A, B, and C, a rapid virological response (RVR, defined as undetectable HCV RNA after 4 weeks of therapy) occurred in 81%, 81%, and 59% of patients, respectively. In contrast, only 11% achieved RVR in the Peg-IFN-α-2a/R control arm D. SVR rates in telaprevir treatment arms A, B, and C were 61%, 67%, and 35%, respectively. The SVR rate of 41% in control arm D was significantly less than that in telaprevir arms A and B. Thus, addition of telaprevir to SOC Peg-IFN-α-2a/R significantly increased the SVR rates and permitted shortening the duration of therapy to 24 weeks without compromising SVR. The most common adverse events attributable to telaprevir were rash, pruritus, hemorrhoids, vomiting, and diarrhea.

PROVE 2

The PROVE 2[11] was a phase 2 trial of the safety and efficacy of telaprevir conducted in 323 treatment-naive European patients with HCV genotype 1 infection. This study had 4 treatment arms: (A) telaprevir 750 mg every 8 hours with Peg-IFN-α-2a/R for 12 weeks followed by Peg-IFN-α-2a/R alone for an additional 12 weeks; (B) telaprevir 750 mg every 8 hours with Peg-IFN-α-2a/R for 12 weeks; (C) telaprevir 750 mg every 8 hours with Peg-IFN-α-2a without ribavirin for 12 weeks; and (D) SOC Peg-IFN-α-2a/R for 48 weeks (control). The RVR rates for the 4 treatment arms were 69%, 80%, 50%, and 13%, respectively. The SVR rates were 69%, 60%, 36%, and 46%. However, only the SVR rate in arm A was statistically significantly greater than that in the control arm. The low rates of both RVR and SVR in arm C unequivocally showed that ribavirin was essential for successful therapy and prevention of emergence of viral resistance. The most common adverse event attributed to telaprevir was a maculopapular rash observed in 44% to 49% of patients.

Both PROVE 1 and PROVE 2 showed significantly increased RVR and SVR rates with triple therapy combining telaprevir and Peg-IFN-α-2a/R. However, from 12% to 21% of patients receiving telaprevir discontinued treatment because of side effects, and 30% to 40% of patients did not achieve SVR. These patients are at risk of developing viral resistance by selecting preexisting variants among the quasispecies during sustained viral replication. The primary adverse events attributed to telaprevir included rash, pruritus, hemorrhoids, vomiting, and diarrhea. Of concern, 3% to 7% of patients in PROVE 1 had severe rash, and 7% of patients in the telaprevir groups in PROVE 2 discontinued treatment because of rash. Telaprevir also increased the degree of anemia observed with ribavirin. The adverse events in studies of telaprevir and boceprevir are compared in **Table 1**.

PHASE 2 STUDIES OF TELAPREVIR FOR TREATMENT-EXPERIENCED PATIENTS

PROVE 3

PROVE 3[12] was a phase 2 study conducted in 465 treatment-experienced patients with HCV genotype 1 infection from the United States and Europe. Both nonresponders or relapsers to previous treatment with Peg-IFN-α-2a or Peg-IFN-α-2b and R were randomized into 4 treatment arms: (A) telaprevir 750 mg every 8 hours with Peg-IFN-α-2a/R for 12 weeks followed by Peg-IFN-α-2a/R alone for an additional 12 weeks; (B) telaprevir 750 mg every 8 hours with Peg-IFN-α-2a/R for 24 weeks followed by Peg-IFN-α-2a/R alone for an additional 24 weeks; (C) telaprevir 750 mg every 8 hours with Peg-IFN-α-2a without R for 24 weeks; and (D) Peg-IFN-α-2a/R for 48 weeks (control). SVR rates of 51%, 53%, 24%, and 14% were observed in groups A, B, C, and D, respectively. SVR rates were significantly greater in all 3 telaprevir groups, compared with the control group. SVR rates were substantially higher in relapsers (69%–76%) than nonresponders (38%–39%). One of the most common adverse events in the telaprevir groups was rash, which occurred in 51% of patients and was severe in 5%. Discontinuation because of adverse events was more frequent in the telaprevir groups than in the control group (15% vs 4%). As in the PROVE 2 study of treatment-naive patients, omission of R from the treatment regimen in PROVE 3 resulted in an inferior SVR. Thus, R was essential for optimal treatment responses to telaprevir for both treatment-naive and treatment-experienced patients.

ALTERNATIVE TELAPREVIR DOSING REGIMENS

An open-label, randomized phase 2 study comparing telaprevir administration every 8 hours versus every 12 hours with Peg-IFN-α-2a/R or Peg-IFN-α-2b/R was conducted in treatment-naive patients with HCV genotype 1 HCV infection.[13] This design provided data not only on the safety and efficacy of a regimen of twice-daily telaprevir but also the efficacy of telaprevir when administered with Peg-IFN-α-2b. In this trial, 161 subjects were randomized to 1 of 4 arms: (A) telaprevir 750 mg every 8 hours with Peg-IFN-α-2a (180 μg/wk) and ribavirin 1000 to 1200 mg/d (n = 40); (B) telaprevir 750 mg every 8 hours with Peg-IFN-α-2b (1.5 μg/kg/wk) and ribavirin 800 to 1200 mg/d (n = 42); (C) telaprevir 1125 mg every 12 hours with Peg-IFN-α-2a (180 μg/wk) and ribavirin 1000 to 1200 mg/d (n = 40); or (D) telaprevir 1125 mg every 12 hours with Peg-IFN-α-2b (1.5 μg/kg/wk) and ribavirin 800 to 1200 mg/d (n = 39). Patients received triple therapy for 12 weeks, followed by either 12 or 36 additional weeks of treatment with Peg-IFN-α-2a or Peg-IFN-α-2b and Peg-IFN-α/R, based on virological responses at week 4. SVR rates of 81% to 85% were observed among the 4 groups, and most patients (68%) required only 24 weeks of therapy. No statistically significant differences in SVR rates (intent-to-treat analysis) was observed among the groups, between the pooled groups that received medication every 8 hours and every 12 hours, or between the pooled groups that received Peg-IFN-α-2a or Peg-IFN-α-2b with ribavirin. The safety profile was also similar among all groups.

Although the study was underpowered to detect differences between groups receiving Peg-IFN-α-2a or Peg-IFN-α-2b with ribavirin, it did provide proof of concept that a higher dose of telaprevir administered every 12 hours could achieve an SVR rate comparable with that of a lower dose administered every 8 hours, regardless of whether telaprevir was administered with Peg-IFN-α-2a or Peg-IFN-α-2b and ribavirin.

PHASE 3 STUDIES OF TELAPREVIR

Telaprevir for Treatment-naive Patients

The results of 2 phase 3 trials of telaprevir combined with Peg-IFN-α-2a and ribavirin for the treatment of HCV genotype 1 infections in treatment-naive patients were presented at the 2010 annual meeting of the AASLD and published in abstract form.

ADVANCE

The ADVANCE[14] study was a randomized, double-blind, placebo-controlled, pivotal phase 3 trial in treatment-naive patients with CHC genotype 1, comparing the safety and efficacy of 2 response-guided regimens of telaprevir 750 mg every 8 hours with Peg-IFN-α-2a and ribavirin to that of SOC Peg-IFN-α-2a (180 μg/wk) and ribavirin (1000–1200 mg/d). A total of 1088 treatment-naive, HCV genotype 1 patients were randomized to 1 of 3 arms: (A) telaprevir in combination with Peg-IFN-α-2a and ribavirin for 8 weeks, followed by 16 additional weeks of Peg-IFN-α-2a/R (T8PR); (B) telaprevir in combination with Peg-IFN-α-2a/R for 12 weeks, followed by 12 additional weeks of Peg-IFN-α-2a/R (T12PR); or (C) Peg-IFN-α-2a/R for 48 weeks (PR48). In the telaprevir arms, patients who achieved an extended RVR (eRVR, defined as undetectable HCV RNA [<25 IU/mL] at both week 4 and 12) received a total of 24 weeks of therapy, whereas those who did not achieve eRVR received a total of 48 weeks of therapy. The rates of RVR (undetectable HCV RNA at week 4) were superior in the T8PR and T12PR arms (66% and 68%) compared with the PR48 control arm (9%). Overall, 58% of patients treated in the telaprevir arms achieved eRVR. SVR rates were statistically significantly higher in the T8PR and T12PR arms (69% and 75%) than in the PR48 control arm (44%; $P<.0001$). Conversely, the relapse rates after achieving undetectable HCV RNA at the end of treatment were less in the T8PR and T12PR arms (9% and 9%) than in the PR48 control arm (28%). Although the SVR rates were comparable for the T8PR and T12PR regimens, nevertheless the proportion of patients achieving SVR was numerically greater in the T12PR group. A subgroup analysis showed that 62% of patients with advanced fibrosis or cirrhosis achieved SVR with telaprevir regimens, compared with 33% who were treated with Peg-IFN-α-2a/R alone. Another notable finding was that 62% of African American or Black patients achieved SVR with telaprevir regimens, compared with only 25% treated with Peg-IFN-α-2a/R alone. Treatment discontinuation rates were 7% in the T12PR arm, 8% in the T8PR arm, and 4% in the control arm. Adverse events occurring in more than 25% of patients, regardless of treatment arm, included rash, fatigue, pruritus, headache, nausea, anemia, insomnia, diarrhea, influenzalike symptoms, and fever. Most adverse events were mild to moderate.

ILLUMINATE

The ILLUMINATE[15] trail was a supplemental phase 3, open-label study, in which 540 treatment-naive patients with CHC genotype 1 were treated for 12 weeks with a combination of telaprevir (750 mg every 8 hours), Peg-IFN-α-2a (180 μg/week) and ribavirin (1000–1200 mg/d) followed by either 12 or 36 weeks of Peg-IFN-α-2a/R alone. Thus, ILLUMINATE was designed to confirm the efficacy of response-guided therapy (RGT) investigated in ADVANCE and to assess whether extending therapy from 24 to 48 weeks would benefit patients achieving eRVR on T12PR. Among the 540 patients, 352 (65.2%) achieved eRVR, and 322 were randomized at week 20 to continue Peg-IFN-α-2a/R for either an additional 4 or 28 weeks (for total treatment durations of 24 or 48 weeks). Patients not achieving eRVR were assigned at 20 weeks to an additional 28 weeks of treatment, for the total treatment duration of 48 weeks. Treatment was discontinued if patients failed to achieve a $\log_{10}$ reduction of 2 or greater from baseline HCV RNA after 12 weeks of therapy or if HCV RNA was detectable at 24 weeks. Overall, SVR was achieved in 72% of patients treated with telaprevir. SVR rates for patients with eRVR who received 24 or 48 weeks of therapy (92% vs 87.5%) were comparable; thus, there was no benefit in extending therapy to 48 weeks. Subgroup analyses showed SVR rates of 60% in African American and Blacks, 67% in Latinos, and 63% in patients with advanced fibrosis or cirrhosis treated with telaprevir. However, there was no control arm of Peg-IFN-α-2a/R for comparison with SOC. The discontinuation rate was 7%, and fatigue and anemia were the most common causes of discontinuation. Adverse events occurring in more than 25% of patients were similar to those observed in the ADVANCE trial and were generally mild to moderate.

The ADVANCE and ILLUMINATE trials provide practical insights regarding telaprevir treatment in previously untreated patients with HCV genotype 1 infections. First, most patients treated with T12PR in the ILLUMINATE trial achieved eRVR. Second, patients who achieved eRVR on a regimen of T12PR had comparable SVR rates whether treated with either an additional 4 or 28 weeks of Peg-IFN-α-2a/R alone. Thus, most can achieve SVR with a T12PR regimen followed by 12 weeks of Peg-IFN-α-2a/R. Shortening the course of therapy from 48 to 24 weeks should enhance compliance and adherence, and reduce medication-related adverse events and cost. Extrapolation from the finding of comparable SVR rates in the ADVANCE trial for the T8PR and T12PR arms (69% and 75%) suggests that patients with RVRs to a combination of telaprevir and Peg-IFN-α-2a/R might achieve SVR with an even shorter course of triple therapy.

Telaprevir for Treatment-experienced Patients Who Failed to Achieve SVR with Previous Peg-IFN-α and Ribavirin Therapy

REALIZE

The REALIZE[16] study was a pivotal phase 3, randomized, double-blind, placebo-controlled study to evaluate the safety and efficacy of 2 regimens of combination therapy with telaprevir, Peg-IFN-α-2a and ribavirin in patients who did not achieve SVR after at least 1 previous treatment with IFN-based antiviral therapy. Overall, 662 patients representing all 3 types of nonresponse (null, partial, and relapse) were randomized to 3 arms: (A) 12 weeks of combination therapy with telaprevir (750 mg every 8 hours), Peg-IFN-α-2a (180 μg/wk) and ribavirin (1000–1200 mg/d) followed by 36 weeks of Peg-IFN-α-2a/R alone; (B) 4 weeks of Peg-IFN-α-2a/R alone followed by 12 weeks of combination therapy with telaprevir (750 mg every 8 hours) and Peg-IFN-α-2a/R, followed by 36 weeks of Peg-IFN-α-2a/R or (C) placebo plus Peg-IFN-α-2a/R for 12 weeks, followed by 36 weeks of Peg-IFN-α-2a/R. Overall, 65% of the 530 patients treated with telaprevir achieved SVR, compared with 17% of the 132 patients treated with Peg-IFN-α-2a/R. The overall SVR rates were 64% for the telaprevir simultaneous start arm and 66% for the delayed start arm. SVR rates varied widely, depending on the type of previous nonresponse to Peg-IFN-α and ribavirin therapy. In patients with previous null response (n = 184), the SVR rate with telaprevir therapy was 29% in the simultaneous start arm, 33% in the delayed start arm and 5% in controls. Patients with previous partial response (n = 124) had SVR rates with telaprevir treatment of 59% in the simultaneous start arm, 54% in the delayed start arm, and 15% in the control arm. Patients with relapse (n = 354) who were treated with telaprevir had the highest rates of SVR: 83% in the simultaneous start arm, 88% in the delayed start arm, and 24% in controls. The adverse events were comparable with those occurring in the phase 3 ADVANCE and ILLUMINATE studies of treatment-naive patients. Adverse events that were more common in the telaprevir treatment arms included: fatigue, pruritus, rash, flulike symptoms, nausea, and anemia. Discontinuation because of adverse events occurred in 4% of telaprevir-treated patients and 3% of controls. Rash, fatigue, and pruritus were the most notable adverse effects.

TELAPREVIR LONG-TERM STUDY

EXTEND

The EXTEND[17] study is an ongoing 3-year study of patients treated with telaprevir in the previous phase 2, PROVE 1, 2, and 3 trials. The 3 goals are to: (1) determine the durability of SVR achieved with telaprevir therapy; (2) assess the persistence of viral resistance to telaprevir; and (3) monitor for long-term complications. An interim report after a median period of 22 months showed that 99% (122/123) of patients had maintained SVR. Among patients who had not achieved SVR in the PROVE 1, 2, and 3 studies, population genetic testing of telaprevir-resistant variants was used to detect the presence of variants comprising more than 19%–24% of circulating virions. Overall, 89% of resistant variants had decreased below the 19%–24% threshhold of detection. Complications associated with advanced CHC developed in 2 patients: one developed HCC and the other hepatic encephalopathy.

BOCEPREVIR

Boceprevir is an oral inhibitor of HCV NS3 serine protease. Phase 2 and 3 studies have been completed and published as full articles or presented at the 2010 annual meeting of the AASLD and published as abstracts. Boceprevir studies have included arms with 4 weeks of lead-in therapy with Peg-IFN-α-2b (1.5 μg/kg/wk) and weight-based ribavirin 800 to 1200 mg/d. Rationales for lead-in therapy include: (1) proof of tolerability to Peg-IFN-α-2b/R before introduction of boceprevir; (2) achievement of steady-state levels of Peg-IFN-α-2b/R before introduction of boceprevir; (3) activation of host immune responses; (4) reduction of viral load and inhibition of quasispecies with pre-existing resistance mutations for boceprevir; and (5) option to withhold boceprevir in a null responder because of risk of development of boceprevir-resistant virions.

PHASE 2 STUDY OF BOCEPREVIR FOR TREATMENT-NAIVE PATIENTS

SPRINT 1

SPRINT 1[18] was a phase 2 randomized, controlled trial of the safety and efficacy of boceprevir therapy in 595 treatment-naive patients with CHC genotype 1 conducted in 2 parts. In part 1, 520 patients were randomized into 5 arms: (A) 28 weeks of therapy comprised of a 4-week lead-in with Peg-IFN-α-2b (1.5 μg/kg/wk) and weight-based ribavirin 800 to 1400 mg/d followed by addition of boceprevir to Peg-IFN-α-2b/R for 24 weeks (PR4/BPR24); (B) 48 weeks of therapy comprised of a 4-week lead-in with Peg-IFN-α-2b/R followed by addition of boceprevir to Peg-IFN-α-2b/R for 44 weeks (PR4/BPR44); (C) 28 weeks of therapy with boceprevir and Peg-IFN-α-2b/R (BPR28); (D) 48 weeks of therapy with boceprevir and Peg-IFN-α-2b/R (PR4/BPR44);

and (E) 48 weeks of therapy with Peg-IFN-α-2b/R as the SOC control (PR48). In part 2, 75 patients were randomized to receive either (A) 48 weeks of boceprevir and Peg-IFN-α-2b/R, or (B) 48 weeks of boceprevir and Peg-IFN-α-2b at full doses with lower doses of ribavirin (400–1000 mg/d).

Patients in all boceprevir groups had significantly higher SVR rates than controls: 56%, $P = 0{\cdot}005$ in the PR4/BPR24 arm; 75%, $P<0{\cdot}0001$ in the PR4/BPR44 arm; 54%, $P = 0{\cdot}013$ in the BPR28 arm; and 67%, $P<0{\cdot}0001$ in the BPR48 arm versus 38% in the PR48 control arm. SVR rates were higher in the 48-week treatment arms, and the highest rate was achieved with the PR4/BPR44 regimen. The results of part 2 showed that the lower-dose ribavirin regimen was inferior and associated with a high rate of viral breakthrough and a relapse rate similar to controls. Thus, as observed in PROVE 2, full-dose ribavirin seems essential for optimal rates of SVR. Analysis of the predictability of SVR based on the virological response to the PR4 lead-in showed that RVR was highly predictive for SVR in boceprevir and control arms. Addition of boceprevir resulted in SVR rates in the PR4/BPR24 and PR4/BPR44 arms of 29% and 44%, respectively in patients with less than 0.5 $\log_{10}$ declines in HCV RNA. Thus, absence of a significant HCV RNA decline during lead-in therapy before addition of boceprevir had a low negative predictive value for SVR. Overall discontinuation rates of 26% to 39% in the boceprevir arms were significantly higher than the 15% rate observed in controls. Adverse events observed more commonly in boceprevir treatment arms than in controls included anemia (55% vs 34%) and dysgeusia (27% vs 9%). In contrast to telaprevir studies that prohibited use of erythropoietin for anemia, SPRINT-1 allowed use of epoetin alfa at the investigator's discretion for hemoglobin less than 10 g/dL. In part 1 of the study, epoetin alfa was used in 51% of patients in the PR48 control arm and in 26% to 49% of patients in the boceprevir arms.

PHASE 3 STUDIES OF BOCEPREVIR

Boceprevir for Treatment-naive Patients

SPRINT 2

The SPRINT-2[19] trial was a phase 3, randomized, double-blind, placebo-controlled trial to assess the safety and efficacy of combination therapy with boceprevir and Peg-IFN-α-2b/R in treatment-naive patients with CHC genotype 1. A key feature of this study was the planned enrollment of a large number of African American/Black patients; however, the study was not powered to compare the rates of SVR between non-Black and Black patients. The study randomized 1097 (938 non-Black and 159 Black) patients to 3 arms: (A) 48 weeks of therapy comprised of a 4-week lead-in with Peg-IFN-α-2b (1.5 μg/kg/wk) and weight-based ribavirin 600 to 1400 mg/d followed by addition of boceprevir to Peg-IFN-α-2b/R for 44 weeks (B/PR48); (B) RGT arm with a 4-week lead-in of Peg-IFN-α-2b/R followed by addition of boceprevir to Peg-IFN-α-2b/R for 24 weeks and assignment to either cease therapy at week 28 if HCV RNA had remained undetectable (<9.3 IU/mL) between treatment weeks 8 and 24 or to continue therapy with placebo and Peg-IFN-α-2b/R for another 20 weeks (total duration 48 weeks); and (C) 48 weeks of therapy comprised of a 4-week lead-in with Peg-IFN-α-2b/R followed by addition of placebo to Peg-IFN-α-2b/R for 44 weeks (control arm). SVR rates in non-Black patients were 40% in the 48 P/R control group and 67% in the RGT arm and 68% in the B/P/R48 arm ($P<.0001$ compared with controls). In contrast, the SVR rates in Black patients were 23% in the control arm, 42% in the RGT arm, and 53% in the B/PR48 arm ($P = .004$ compared with controls). In non-Black and Black patients who had undetectable HCV RNA at weeks 8 to 24, the SVR rates were substantially higher: 97% and 96% for RGT and B/PR48 arms in non-Black patients and 87% and 95% for RGT and B/PR48 arms in Black patients. Stratification of non-Black patients into those who had less than 1 $\log_{10}$ or $\log_{10}$ decline of 1 or greater in HCV RNA after a 4-week lead-in showed substantial difference in SVR rates: 52% in controls, 82% in RGT arm, and 82% in the B/P/R48 arm with more than 1 $\log_{10}$ decline versus 5% in controls, 29% in the RGT arm and 39% in the B/P/R48 arm with less than 1 $\log_{10}$ decline. Boceprevir-resistant variants were detected in only 4% in those with $\log_{10}$ decline of 1 or greater, but in those with less than 1 $\log_{10}$ decline they were identified in 47% in the RGT arm and 35% in the B/P/R48 arm (see discussion of resistance later). Discontinuation for adverse events occurred in 16% of controls: 12% in the RGT arm and 16% in the B/P/R48 arm. The most common adverse events associated with boceprevir were anemia and dysgeusia (metallic taste). Anemia was more frequently observed in the boceprevir arms (49%) than in controls (29%). As in SPRINT-1, epoetin alfa treatment of anemia was permitted at the discretion of the investigator.

Boceprevir for Treatment-experienced Patients Who Had Partial or Relapse Responses to Treatment with Previous Peg-IFN-α and Ribavirin Therapy

RESPOND 2

The RESPOND-2[20] trial was a phase 3, randomized, double-blind, placebo-controlled trial of the safety and efficacy of boceprevir in combination with Peg-IFN-α-2b/R for the treatment of partial responders and relapsers to previous SOC therapy with Peg-IFN-α/R. Null responders to previous therapy were excluded. The study randomized 403 patients with CHC genotype 1 to 3 arms: (A) 4-week lead-in with Peg-IFN-α-2b/R followed by addition of a placebo to Peg-IFN-α-2b/R for 44 weeks (control); (B) RGT with 4-week lead-in followed by addition of boceprevir to Peg-IFN-α-2b/R with discontinuation at week 32 if HCV RNA was undetectable at week 8 or an additional 12 weeks of Peg-IFN-α-2b/R if HCV RNA was detectable at week 8; and (C) 4-week lead-in followed by 44 weeks of boceprevir and Peg-IFN-α-2b/R (B/PR48). SVR rates were significantly higher in the boceprevir arms compared with the control arm: 59% in the RGT arm, 66% in the B/PR48 arm, and 21% in controls ($P<.0001$). As observed in the telaprevir studies, SVR rates varied according to the type of previous nonresponse, being higher in relapsers (69% for RGT arm, 75% for B/PR48 arm vs 29% in controls) than in partial responders (40% for RGT arm, 52% for B/PR48 arm vs 7% for controls). SVR rates also varied between patients who had less than 1 $\log_{10}$ or $\log_{10}$ declines of 1 or greater in HCV RNA after 4 weeks of Peg-IFN-α-2b/R lead-in therapy. SVR rates for patients with 1 $\log_{10}$ declines of 1 or greater were 73% in the RGT arm, 79% in the B/PR48 arm, and 26% in controls. In contrast, SVR rates for patients with less than 1 $\log_{10}$ declines were substantially lower: 33% for the RGT arm, 34% for the B/PR48 arm, and 0% in controls. Despite exclusion of null responders to previous SOC Peg-IFN-α/R therapy, the lead-in responses indicated that many of the patients were now behaving as if they were null responders to Peg-IFN-α-2b/R by failing to achieve HCV RNA declines of $\log_{10}$ of 1 or greater; 31% of the RGT arm and 12.5% of the B/PR48 arm had less than 0.5 $\log_{10}$ declines, whereas 33% in the RGT arm and 39% of the B/PR48 arm had declines of 0.5 to less than 1 $\log_{10}$. Thus, previous partial responders or relapsers seem to have become insensitive to Peg-IFN-α/R after previous therapy. This phenomenon merits further investigation.

The most common adverse event in the boceprevir arms was anemia; others included dry skin, dysgeusia, and rash. The frequency of discontinuations caused by adverse events was 8% in the RGT arm, 12% in the B/PR48 arm, and 2.5% in controls. Investigators were allowed to treat anemia with epoetin alfa at their discretion.

Predictors of SVR in SPRINT-2 and RESPOND-2

Retrospective analyses showed that the magnitude of HCV RNA decline after 4 weeks of lead-in therapy with Peg-IFN-α-2b/R was a predictor of SVR in both the SPRINT-2 and RESPOND-2 trials.[21] Classification and regression tree analyses showed that the best predictor of SVR was approximately a 1 $\log_{10}$ decline in HCV RNA. Positive predictive values for SVR after a $\log_{10}$ decline of 1 or greater during lead-in were 80% for treatment-naive and 76% for treatment-experienced patients. However, negative predictive values were only 67% for both treatment-naive and treatment-experienced patients. Because patients with less than 0.5 $\log_{10}$ declines after lead-in had SVR rates ranging from 28% to 43%, failure to achieve a $\log_{10}$ decline of 1 or greater after lead-in should not preclude boceprevir therapy. However, such patients should be monitored closely for evidence of futility. In RESPOND-2 multivariate analysis was used to define predictors of SVR in treatment-experienced patients.[22] SVR rates in the RGT and B/PR48 arms were similar for genotypes 1a and 1b, non-Black and Black patients, mild versus severe fibrosis and whether previous therapy was with Peg-IFN-α-2a or 2b. Baseline factors significantly associated with SVR included treatment with boceprevir, classification as a relapser to previous therapy, low baseline viral load, and absence of advanced fibrosis. When decline in viral load after the 4-week lead-in was assessed, it was a stronger predictor of SVR than the type of response to previous therapy.

VIRAL RESISTANCE TO LINEAR NS3 PROTEASE INHIBITORS TELAPREVIR AND BOCEPREVIR

Mutations conferring resistance to telaprevir have been identified at 4 positions in the NS3 peptide: V36A/M/L, T54A, R155K/M/S/T, and A156S//T.[23–26] Kieffer and colleagues[27] reported viral kinetic analysis in telaprevir-resistant variants. These patients had CHC genotype 1 and received therapy for 14 days with telaprevir alone or combined with Peg-IFN-α-2a. Monotherapy with telaprevir resulted in rapid viral decline as a result of suppression of the wild-type species and viral rebound with resistant variants with R155K/T and A156/T mutations. The combination of telaprevir and Peg-IFN-α-2a prevented breakthrough of resistant mutations. The genetic barrier to resistance is greater for HCV genotype 1a than 1b. The most common mutations conferring resistance to telaprevir in phase 2 trials were V36A/M, T54A/S, R155K/M/T A156S/T/V, and the combination of V36M + R155K.[28] As noted earlier, the EXTEND[17] study indicated that most patients with telaprevir-resistant variants have the quantities decrease beneath the detection threshold of 19%–24% using population genetic testing after a median of 22 months of observation after therapy. More sensitive testing has not been performed to determine the replacement of resistant variants with wild-type virus.

Identical mutations confer viral resistance to boceprevir (**Table 2**).[28,29] During a 2-year follow-up of boceprevir-resistant mutations identified in 18 of 174 patients who did not achieve SVR, population genetic testing showed that resistant variants decreased below the detection threshold of 19% in 91% of those with V36M mutations, 71% of those with R155K mutations, and 62% of those with T54S mutations. The V36M mutation had the most rapid loss of detectability.[30]

The resistance mutations to telaprevir and boceprevir are preexisting in the HCV quasispecies and are merely selected when the antiviral regimen does not rapidly terminate HCV replication. Thus, the primary risk factor for resistance mutations is

Table 2
HCV resistance mutations associated with DAA protease inhibitors, NS5A and NS5B polymerase inhibitors, Peg-IFN-α, and ribavirin

		DAA Class								
HCV Target	**Variant**	**NS3 Linear**	**NS3 Macrocyclic**	**NS5A Inhibitor**	**NS5B Nucleoside**	**NS5B Palm**	**NS5B Thumb**	**NS5B Finger**	**IFN**	**RBV**
MS3 Protease	U36M	R	S	S	S	S	S	S	S	S
	T54A	R	S	S	S	S	S	S	S	S
	R155K	R	R	S	S	S	S	S	S	S
	A156T	R	R	S	S	S	S	S	S	S
	D168V	S	R	S	S	S	S	S	S	S
NSSA	L28V	S	S	S	S	S	S	S	S	S
	V93H	S	S	R	S	S	S	S	S	S
NS5B	S282T	S	S	S	R	S	S	S	S	S
	C316V	S	S	S	S	R	S	S	S	S
	M414T	S	S	S	S	R	S	S	S	S
	R422K	S	S	S	S	S	R	S	S	S
	M423T	S	S	S	S	S	R	S	S	S
	P495S	S	S	S	S	S	S	R	S	S

Abbreviations: R, resistance; S, sensitivity.

Data from Kieffer TL, Kwong AD, Picchio GR. Viral resistance to specifically targeted antiviral therapies for hepatitis C (STAT-Cs). J Antimicrob Chemother 2010;65:202–12.

failure to achieve an undetectable HCV RNA, and failure to eradicate replication represents a stopping rule, as does increasing viral load from a previous nadir. Because resistant variants are cross-resistant to both telaprevir and boceprevir, failure of either precludes treatment with the other. None of the resistant variants has shown greater fitness than wild-type HCV or produced a more virulent course of disease.

SECOND-GENERATION NS3 PROTEASE INHIBITORS

Multiple second-generation protease inhibitors are being developed (**Box 1**). TMC435350[31] is a novel and potent reversible NS3/4A protease inhibitor that has shown synergy with polymerase inhibitors in vitro. Monotherapy with TMC43550 200 mg once daily resulted in a rapid decline in HCV viral load in patients with genotype 1. Once-daily dosing represents a major advantage for compliance and adherence compared with the thrice-daily dosing of both telaprevir and boceprevir. The primary promise of newer NS3 protease inhibitors is their suitability to be combined with agents that disrupt RNA replication.

NS5B POLYMERASE INHIBITORS

Two classes of drugs, nucleoside polymerase inhibitors (NIs) and nonnucleoside polymerase inhibitors (NNIs), are being developed to prevent HCV RNA replication. The NI class interacts directly with the catalytic site of NS5B and by being incorporated into the elongating HCV RNA act as chain terminators of RNA synthesis (**Box 2**). In contrast, NNI agents bind to sites outside the catalytic site and inhibit NS5B function by changing the conformation of the active site (**Box 3**).[32]

NIs

Valopicitabine (NM283) and R1626 were the first NI agents studied in patients with CHC. Development of NM283 was stopped because of significant gastrointestinal adverse events and limited efficacy. In a phase 2a study of R1626, 104 treatment-naive patients with CHC genotype 1 received R1626 in combination with either Peg-IFN-α or Peg-IFN-α/R. This proof of concept study showed SVR rates of 24% to 58% among the 4 arms of the study.[33] However, development was halted because of adverse events of severe lymphopenia and visual impairment. R7128, PSI 7977,

Box 1
NS3/4A protease inhibitors

Drug Name	Company	Study Phase
Ciluprevir (BILN2061)	Boehringer Ingelheim	Stopped
Telaprevir (VX-950)	Vertex	Phase 3
Boceprevir (SCH503034)	Merck	Phase 3
TMC435350	Tibotec/Medavir/Johnson & Johnson	Phase 2
Vaniprevir (MK-7009)	Merck	Phase 2
Danoprevir (R7227/ITMN-191)	Intermune/Roche	Phase 2
Narlaprevir (SCH900518)	Schering Plough	Halted
BI201335	Boehringer Ingelheim	Phase 2
BMS-850032	Bristol Myers Squibb	Phase 1
PHX1766	Phenomix	Phase 1
ACH-1625	Achillon	Phase 1
MK-5172	Merck	Phase 1

Box 2
NS5B NIs

Drug Name	Company	Study Phase
Valopicitabine (NM283)	Idenix Novartis	Stopped
R7128	Pharmasset and Roche	Phase 2
PSI-7977	Pharmasset	Phase 2
PSI-938	Pharmasset	Phase 2
IDX-184	Idenix	Phase 2
PSI-7851	Pharmasset	Phase 1
INX-189	Inhibitex	Phase 1

PSI938, and IDX are undergoing phase 2 evaluation (see **Box 2**). Compared with NNI agents, NI agents have greater barriers to resistance, but resistance mutation S282T has been identified for the class.[34]

NNIs

Filibuvir (PF-00868554) is a potent and specific NNI for the NS5B polymerase. Filibuvir showed a good pharmacokinetic profile and oral bioavailability in preclinical animal studies and allowed twice-daily dosing in humans. In phase 1 and 2a clinical trials in treatment-naive patients with CHC genotype 1, filibuvir alone or combined with Peg-IFN-α-2b/R for up to 4 weeks significantly reduced HCV RNA levels compared with placebo or Peg-IFN-α-2b/R alone. The incidence and severity of adverse events were similar to SOC and placebo.[35] GS-9190[36] is another NNI in phase 2 testing. The safety, tolerability, and antiviral efficacy of GS-9190 given twice daily at 40 mg is being compared with placebo in combination with Peg-IFN-α/R in treatment-naive patients with CHC genotype 1. The study will randomize 200 patients (50/100/50) to 1 of 3 treatment arms: (A) Peg-IFN-α/R + placebo twice a day for 48 weeks (control); (B) Peg-IFN-α/R + GS 9190 40 mg twice a day for 48 weeks; and (C) Peg-IFN-α/R + GS 9190 40 mg twice a day for 48 weeks. However, subjects who achieve RVR (HCV RNA undetectable at week 4) in this arm and maintain that response until week 24 will stop all study drugs at week 24 and be followed for an additional 48 weeks (n = 50). The primary end point will be the rate of SVR in the 3 arms.

BILB1941, BI207127, MK-3281, VCH-759, VCH-916, VCH-922, ANA598, HCV-796, ABT-333, and IDX375 are examples of other NNI agents in clinical testing (see **Box 3**).

Box 3
NS5B NNIs

Drug Name	Company	Study Phase
BILB 1941	Boehringer Ingelheim	Stopped
BI207127	Boehringer Ingelheim	Phase 2
GS-9190	Gilead	Phase 2
Filibuvir	Pfizer	Phase 2
ANA-598	Anadys	Phase 1
VCH759	Virochem Pharma	Phase 1
VCH222	Virochem Pharma	Phase 1
ABT-333	Abbott	Phase 1
IDX-375	Idenix	Phase 1

A disadvantage of the NNI class is their lower genetic barrier to resistance. However, this disadvantage may not be an obstacle because they might be candidates for combination therapy with potent protease inhibitors. Resistance mutations vary according to the specific site of binding of the NNI (**Fig. 2**B, see **Table 2**).

NS5A INHIBITORS

BMS-790052 is a first-in-class, highly potent, once-daily inhibitor of the NS5A component of the HCV replication complex (see **Fig. 1**).[37] In a double-blind study, 48 treatment-naive patients with CHC genotype 1 were randomized 1:1:1:1 to receive placebo, 3 mg, 10 mg, or 60 mg of BMS-790052, once daily, combined with Peg-IFN-α-2a/R. The primary end point was the proportion of subjects with eRVR, defined as undetectable HCV RNA (<10 IU/mL) at both treatment weeks 4 and 12. An eRVR was achieved in 42%, 83%, and 75% of patients receiving 3 mg, 10 mg, and 60 mg BMS-790052 + Peg-IFN-α-2a/R, respectively. Only 8% achieved eRVR with Peg-IFN-α-2a/R alone. Safety was comparable for the experimental and control arms. Viral breakthrough was not observed in the 10-mg and 60-mg BMS-790052 arms to week 12. Other NS5A inhibitors in development include PPI-461, GS-5885, and BMS824393 (**Box 4**). NS5A inhibitors are prime candidates for combination therapy with potent protease inhibitors; however, resistance mutations for the class have been identified (see **Table 2**).

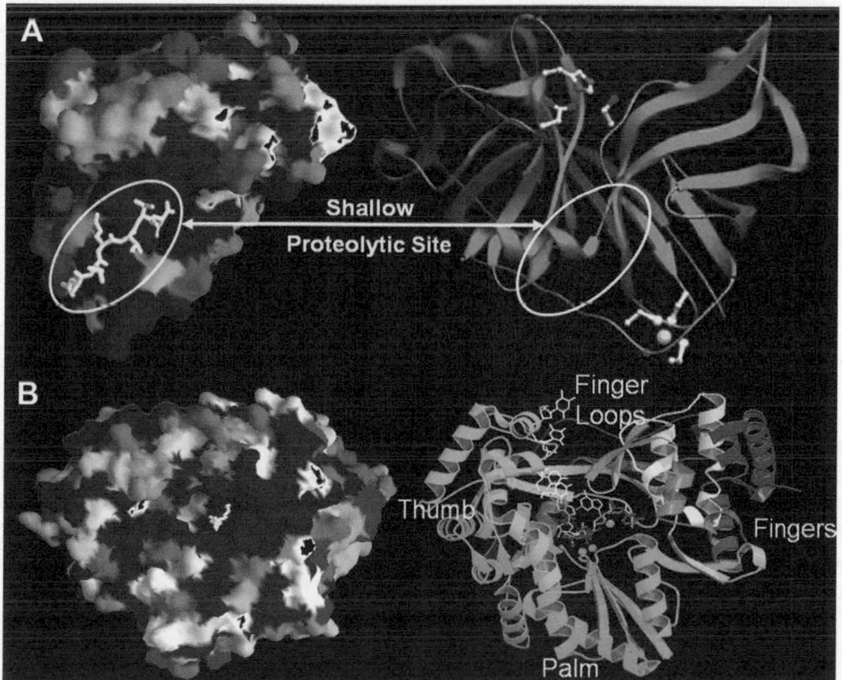

Fig. 2. (*A*) Structure of NS3 serine protease, showing shallow proteolytic site with bound linear protease inhibitor. (*B*) Structure of NS5B polymerase, showing a bound nucleoside inhibitor and regions associated with resistance mutations to nonnucleoside inhibitors, referred to as the thumb, palm, fingers, and finger loop regions.

Box 4
NS5A inhibitors

Drug Name	Company	Study Phase
BMS-790052	BMS	Phase 2
BMS 824393	BMS	Phase 1
PPI-461	Presidio	Phase 1
GS-5885	Gilead	Phase 1

STRATEGIES TO PREVENT RESISTANCE TO DAAS

The imminent introduction of combination therapy for CHC genotype 1 patients with Peg-IFN-α/R combined with either telaprevir or boceprevir will generate selection of resistant mutants from the preexisting quasispecies. Similarly, trials of NS5A or NS5B inhibitors combined with Peg-IFN-α/R may also select for resistance mutations. The primary strategy to minimize virological resistance to DAAs is to achieve rapid, sustained undetectability of HCV RNA. This strategy requires careful education and screening of patients to ensure strict compliance and frequent monitoring of viral loads. In the future, studies must strive to achieve high trough levels of the DAA 5 times or greater than the effective concentration required to prevent 90% of replication in a replicon assay. Additional studies are also required to optimize tissue distribution to prevent retention of HCV in sanctuary sites. Selection of individual DAAs with high genetic barriers to resistance is also crucial. However, the most promising approach to prevent resistance and optimize SVR rates is to combine potent DAAs acting on different targets of the HCV life cycle. Whether oral combinations of 2 to 4 DAAs can eliminate the need for either Peg-IFN or ribavirin is being addressed in clinical trials.

COMBINATION THERAPIES

Combination therapeutic strategies include addition of 2 DAA or non-DAA agents to Peg-IFN-α/R or combining 2 or more oral agents without Peg-IFN-α. The latter strategy has engendered the most excitement, especially if the regimen could omit ribavirin and its toxicity of anemia. Both strategies are now being investigated.

The first study of combination DAA therapy was the proof-of-concept INFORM-1[38] study conducted in New Zealand. This randomized, placebo-controlled trial assigned 87 patients with CHC genotype 1 to receive up to 13 days of oral combination therapy with danoprevir (RG7227), an NS3/4A protease inhibitor, and RG7128, an NI, or a combination of matched placebos. Both DAA agents had been administered previously to patients for 12 weeks in combination with Peg-IFN-α-2a/R and had resulted in profound, synergistic declines in HCV RNA. The median decline of HCV RNA from baseline was 5 $\log_{10}$, which was below the level of detection in 88% of the patients treated with the highest doses of danoprevir (900 mg twice a day) and RG7128 (1000 mg twice a day). The antiviral efficacy was similar in naive and treatment-experienced patients, including nonresponders. The rates of RVR, early virological response (EVR) at week 12, and end of treatment response (EOT) responses were markedly increased by the 2 weeks of pretreatment. In the final cohort of patients who received the highest dose of RG7227 and RG7128, 100% achieved ETR after 24 weeks of Peg-IFN-α/R treatment. No virological resistance to either DAA was observed, and no serious adverse events were reported.

In the near future, the INFORM-SVR phase 2b trial will begin enrollment of treatment-naive patients with CHC genotype 1. This is a randomized, double-blind, parallel group study that will assess the safety and efficacy of the combination of the polymerase inhibitor RO5024048 and ritonavir boosted NS3 protease inhibitor danoprevir with ribavirin or a ribavirin placebo. The primary end point is SVR. This is the first study of combination of DAAs without Peg-IFN-α and should provide valuable information about the feasibility of IFN-free regimens.[39]

OTHER ANTIVIRAL THERAPEUTICS

Pegylated IFN-λ

IFN-λ1, also known as IL-29, is a type III IFN that stimulates receptor-mediated upregulation of IFN-stimulated genes and exerting antiviral effect, similar to those of IFN-α. However, the effect of IFN-λ1 is limited to those cell types that express its unique receptor, which could significantly reduce the risk of cytopenias observed with IFN-α. IFN-λ1 was tested in a 3-part study of patients with CHC, genotype 1 infection.[40] Part 1 evaluated single-agent Peg-IFN-λ at 1.5 or 3 μg/kg administered every 2 weeks or weekly for 4 weeks in patients who had relapsed after previous IFN-α treatment. Part 2 evaluated weekly doses of Peg-IFN-λ (ranging from 0.5 to 2.25 μg/kg) combined with ribavirin for 4 weeks in relapsers. Part 3 evaluated weekly Peg-IFN-λ at 1.5 μg/kg with ribavirin for 4 weeks in treatment-naive patients. A total of 56 patients were enrolled: 24, 25, and 7 patients in parts 1, 2 and 3, respectively. Antiviral activity was observed with all Peg-IFN-λ doses. Two of 7 treatment-naive patients (29%) achieved RVR. Treatment was well tolerated with minimal flulike symptoms and no significant hematologic changes other than RBV-associated decreases in hemoglobin. The most common adverse events were fatigue (29%), nausea (12%), and myalgia (11%). Most adverse events occurred in patients with higher Peg-IFN-λ exposures. If IFN remains necessary in future regimens for the treatment of CHC, Peg-IFN-λ might prove preferable because of a more favorable side effect profile and tolerability.

Cyclophilin Inhibitors

Alisporivir (formerly known as Debio-025) is a synthetic cyclosporine analog that inhibits the binding of the host cell protein cyclophilin A to the NS5A component of the HCV replication complex. As a result, alisporivir does not induce viral resistance and is pangenotypic in its ability to suppress HCV RNA replication. A phase 2 trial included 90 patients with CHC genotypes 1 and 4 and randomized them to 1 of 5 arms: (A) Peg-IFN-α-2a and placebo; (B) Peg-IFN-α-2a and alisporivir 200 daily; (C) Peg-IFN-α-2a and alisporivir 600 mg daily; (D) Peg-IFN-α-2a and alisporivir 1000 mg daily; and (E) alisporivir 1000 mg daily. At day 29 of treatment, the Peg-IFN-α-2a plus alisporivir 200 mg daily arm showed a 4.8 $\log_{10}$ decline from baseline HCV RNA.[41]

In another phase 2 study in genotype 1 null-responders, alisporivir was generally well tolerated in combination with SOC Peg-IFN-α/R; however, increased bilirubin levels were observed in several patients. The frequency and mechanism of this reversible hyperbilirubinemia must be determined. A loading dose of alisporivir may enhance the pharmacokinetic profile; a 400-mg daily dose without loading showed delayed, albeit significant, antiviral activity.[42]

SCY-635 is a nonimmunosuppressive analog of cyclosporine A that exhibits potent suppression of HCV RNA replication in vitro by binding to human cyclophilin A. Exposure of replicon cells to SCY-635 upregulates efflux of cyclophilin A. Data from a phase 1b study were presented at EASL 2009.[43] This phase 1b clinical study was conducted to determine if treatment with SCY-635 monotherapy could suppress HCV-associated plasma RNA. SCY-635 given at 300, 600, and 900 mg daily was able to suppress HCV RNA. Maximum suppression was achieved with the 900-mg dose between days 11 and 15. Group mean and median nadir values were 2.20 and 1.82 $\log_{10}$ below baseline. A phase 2a clinical trial that involves SCY-635, Peg IFN, and ribavirin for treatment-naive CHC genotype 1 patients is under way.

CASPASE INHIBITORS

A phase 2a dose escalation study to evaluate the safety, tolerability, pharmacokinetics, and activity of GS-9450, a caspase inhibitor, in patients with CHC was recently reported.[44] In 32 patients, numerically greater reductions in alanine aminotransferase (ALT) values were observed in patients receiving GS-9450 groups compared with patients receiving placebo. The greatest percent decline (44%) occurred at the end of treatment in the 80-mg/d group. Off-treatment, ALT returned to pretreatment levels. In the 80-mg/d group, 67% of patients normalized ALT by day 14. A 26-week study of GS-9450 in HCV-infected patients assessing clinical and histologic end points is ongoing.

THERAPEUTIC VACCINE GI-5005

GI-5005 is a yeast-based therapeutic vaccine containing HCV NS3 and core antigens recognized by the CD4 and CD8 T cells of persons who spontaneously clear HCV infections.[45] The goal of the GI-5005 vaccine is to elicit HCV-antigen-specific CD4 and CD8 T-cell responses to improve the capacity of the host immune system to eliminate HCV-infected hepatocytes during concurrent therapy with other antivirals. Phase 2 data about the efficacy of GI-5005, in treatment-naive and previous nonresponder patients with CHC genotype 1, were presented at the 2010 annual meeting of the European Association for the Study of the Liver.[46] In this randomized, open-label trial 68 patients with CHC genotype 1 were randomized to arm 1 to receive 5 weekly doses of GI-5005 followed by 2 monthly doses of GI-5005 over the next 12 weeks, followed by monthly GI-5005 injections during a 48-week course of Peg-IFN-α-2a/R in treatment-naive patients or monthly GI-5005 injections during a 72-week course of Peg-IFN-α-2a/R in treatment-experienced nonresponders. In arm 2, 65 patients received Peg-IFN-α-2a/R for 48 weeks if treatment-naive or 72 weeks if treatment-experienced nonresponders. Retrospective testing of IL28B genotypes, proved to be predictive of responsiveness to IFN,[47] showed that the absence of SVR in the poorly responsive IL28 genotype TT patients treated with Peg-IFN-α-2a/R but a surprising 60% in those receiving GI-5005 vaccine and Peg-IFN-α-2a/R. The overall results of the study, presented at the 2010 annual meeting of the AASLD, showed that GI-5005 + Peg-IFN-α-2a/R was well tolerated and improved the SVR rate by 10% to 22% compared with controls.[48] GI-5005 also significantly increased HCV-antigen-specific proliferation and cytotoxic cytokine secretion of peripheral blood T cells in immunized patients, indicating that it enhanced HCV-specific immunity.[49]

MATRIX METALLOPROTEASE INHIBITORS

HCV infection increased the activities of MMPs, which may enhance HCV replication. CTS-1027 is a potent small molecule inhibitor of MMPs involved specifically in inflammation and tissue injury. The safety and efficacy of CTS-1027 is being studied in a multicenter, placebo-controlled, double-blind, randomized trial of Peg-IFN-α/R with and without CTS-1027 in patients with a null response (<2 $\log_{10}$ decline in HCV RNA at week 12) to prior treatment with Peg-IFN-α/R.[50]

SUMMARY

Advances in our understanding of the HCV lifecycle and refinement of in vitro methods to select candidate compounds with anti-HCV activity have led to development of DAA agents and other novel antiviral therapies capable of increasing the curative SVR rates in patients with CHC. The liner protease inhibitors telaprevir and boceprevir, which are expected to be approved for use with Peg-IFN-α and ribavirin in 2011, will become the new SOC for treatment of CHC genotype 1. Rapid development of new protease inhibitors, NI and NNI NS5B polymerase inhibitors, NS5A inhibitors, Peg-IFN-λ, cyclophilin inhibitors, caspase inhibitors, and therapeutic vaccines promises to provide even safer and more effective therapy. Combination therapies with 2 or more oral agents may permit elimination of Peg-IFN-α in the future. Introduction of DAA therapies will confront physicians and patients with regimens of increased complexity, a greater need for compliance, and the necessity of monitoring for virological resistance. Patients with CHC should continue to consider participation in clinical trials of new therapies to accelerate progress.

REFERENCES

1. Kim WR. The burden of hepatitis C in the United States. Hepatology 2002;36: S30–4.
2. Armstrong GL, Wasley A, Simard EP, et al. The prevalence of hepatitis C virus infection in the United States, 1999 through 2002. Ann Intern Med 2006;144:705–14.
3. Fried MW, Shiffman ML, Reddy KR, et al. Peginterferon alfa-2a plus ribavirin for chronic hepatitis C virus infection. N Engl J Med 2002;347:975–82.
4. Manns MP, McHutchison JG, Gordon SC, et al. Peginterferon alfa-2b plus ribavirin compared with interferon alfa-2b plus ribavirin for initial treatment of chronic hepatitis C: a randomised trial. Lancet 2001;358:958–65.
5. McHutchison JG, Gordon SC, Schiff ER, et al. Interferon alfa-2b alone or in combination with ribavirin as initial treatment for chronic hepatitis C. Hepatitis Interventional Therapy Group. N Engl J Med 1998;339:1485–92.
6. Zeuzem S, Hultcrantz R, Bourliere M, et al. Peginterferon alfa-2b plus ribavirin for treatment of chronic hepatitis C in previously untreated patients infected with HCV genotypes 2 or 3. J Hepatol 2004;40:993–9.
7. Bartenschlager R, Frese M, Pietschmann T. Novel insights into hepatitis C virus replication and persistence. Adv Virus Res 2004;63:71–180.
8. Lamarre D, Anderson PC, Bailey M, et al. An NS3 protease inhibitor with antiviral effects in humans infected with hepatitis C virus. Nature 2003;426:186–9.
9. Lange CM, Sarrazin C, Zeuzem S. Review article: specifically targeted anti-viral therapy for hepatitis C–a new era in therapy. Aliment Pharmacol Ther 2010;32:14–28.
10. McHutchison JG, Everson GT, Gordon SC, et al. Telaprevir with peginterferon and ribavirin for chronic HCV genotype 1 infection. N Engl J Med 2009;360:1827–38.
11. Hezode C, Forestier N, Dusheiko G, et al. Telaprevir and peginterferon with or without ribavirin for chronic HCV infection. N Engl J Med 2009;360:1839–50.
12. McHutchison JG, Manns MP, Muir AJ, et al. Telaprevir for previously treated chronic HCV infection. N Engl J Med 2010;362:1292–303.
13. Marcellin P, Forns X, Goeser T, et al. Telaprevir is effective given every 8 or 12 hours with ribavirin and peginterferon alfa-2a or -2b to patients with chronic hepatitis C. Gastroenterology 2011;140(2):459–68.

14. Jacobson IM, McHutchison JG, Dusheiko GM, et al. Telaprevir in combination with peginterferon and ribavirin in genotype 1 HCV treatment naive patients: final results of phase 3 ADVANCE study. Hepatology 2010;52:427A.
15. Sherman KE, Flamm SL, Afdhal NH, et al. Telaprevir in combination with peginterferon alfa-2a and ribavirin for 24 or 48 weeks in treatment naive genotype 1 HCV patients who achieved an extended viral response: final results of phase 3 ILLUMINATE study. Hepatology 2010;52:LB-2.
16. Vertex's and Tibotec [press release]; Cambridge (MA): Vertex Pharmaceuticals; September 7, 2010.
17. Zeuzem S, Sulkowski MS, Zoulim F, et al. Long term follow up of patients with chronic hepatitis C treated with telaprevir in combination with peginterferon alfa-2a and ribavirin: interim analysis of the EXTEND study. Hepatology 2010; 52:436A.
18. Kwo PY, Lawitz EJ, McCone J, et al. Efficacy of boceprevir, an NS3 protease inhibitor, in combination with peginterferon alfa-2b and ribavirin in treatment-naive patients with genotype 1 hepatitis C infection (SPRINT-1): an open-label, randomised, multicentre phase 2 trial. Lancet 2010;376:705–16.
19. Poordad F, McCone J, Bacon B, et al. Boceprevir with peginterferon/ribavirin for untreated chronic hepatitis C. N Engl J Med 2011;364:1195–206.
20. Bacon B, Gordon S, Lawitz E, et al. Boceprevir for treatment-resistant chronic HCV genotype 1 infection. N Engl J Med 2011;364:1207–17.
21. Vierling J, Lawitz E, Poordad F, et al. Four-week therapy with peginterferon alfa-2b/ribavirin effectively predicts sustained virologic response in treatment-naive and treatment-experienced patients with HCV-1 treated with boceprevir plus peginterferon alfa-2b/ribavirin. J Hepatol 2011;54:S197.
22. Zeuzem S, Vierling J, Estaban R, et al. Predictors of sustained virologic response among treatment-experienced patients with hepatitis C virus genotype 1 when retreated with boceprevir plus peginterferon alfa-2b/ribavirin. J Hepatol 2011;54: S199.
23. Sarrazin C, Kieffer TL, Bartels D, et al. Dynamic hepatitis C virus genotypic and phenotypic changes in patients treated with the protease inhibitor telaprevir. Gastroenterology 2007;132:1767–77.
24. Lin C, Gates CA, Rao BG, et al. In vitro studies of cross-resistance mutations against two hepatitis C virus serine protease inhibitors, VX-950 and BILN 2061. J Biol Chem 2005;280:36784–91.
25. Lin K, Kwong AD, Lin C. Combination of a hepatitis C virus NS3-NS4A protease inhibitor and α interferon synergistically inhibits viral RNA replication and facilitates viral RNA clearance in replicon cells. Antimicrob Agents Chemother 2004; 48:4784–92.
26. Lin K, Perni RB, Kwong AD, et al. VX-950, a novel hepatitis C virus (HCV) NS3-4A protease inhibitor, exhibits potent antiviral activities in HCv replicon cells. Antimicrob Agents Chemother 2006;50:1813–22.
27. Kieffer TL, Sarrazin C, Miller JS, et al. Telaprevir and pegylated interferon-α-2a inhibit wild-type and resistant genotype 1 hepatitis C virus replication in patients. Hepatology 2007;46:631–9.
28. McCown MF, Rajyaguru S, Kular S, et al. GT-1a or GT-1b subtype-specific resistance profiles for hepatitis C virus inhibitors telaprevir and HCV-796. Antimicrob Agents Chemother 2009;53:2129–32.
29. Tong X, Chase R, Skelton A, et al. Identification and analysis of fitness of resistance mutations against the HCV protease inhibitor SCH 503034. Antiviral Res 2006;70:28–38.

30. Vierling JM, Ralston R, Lawitz E, et al. Long term outcomes following combination treatment with boceprevir plus pegintron/ribavirin (P/R) in patients with chronic hepatitis C genotype 1 (CHC-G1). J Hepatol 2010;52:S470.
31. Manns MP, Reesink HW, Moreno C, et al. Safety and antiviral activity of TMC435350 in treatment naive genotype 1 HCV infected patients. Hepatology 2008;48:LB-8.
32. Beaulieu PL. Non-nucleoside inhibitors of the HCV NS5B polymerase: progress in the discovery and development of novel agents for the treatment of HCV infections. Curr Opin Investig Drugs 2007;8:614–34.
33. Pockros PJ, Nelson D, Godofsky E, et al. R1626 plus peginterferon Alfa-2a provides potent suppression of hepatitis C virus RNA and significant antiviral synergy in combination with ribavirin. Hepatology 2008;48:385–97.
34. Kieffer TL, Kwong AD, Picchio GR. Viral resistance to specifically targeted antiviral therapies for hepatitis C (STAT-Cs). J Antimicrob Chemother 2010;65:202–12.
35. Shi ST, Herlihy KJ, Graham JP, et al. Preclinical characterization of PF-00868554, a potent nonnucleoside inhibitor of the hepatitis C virus RNA-dependent RNA polymerase. Antimicrob Agents Chemother 2009;53:2544–52.
36. Safety, Tolerability, and Antiviral Activity of 24 or 48 Weeks of GS-9190 in Combination With Peginterferon Alfa 2a and Ribavirin for the Treatment of Genotype-1 Chronic HCV Infection. 2011. Available at: http://Clinicaltrials.gov. Accessed February 25, 2011.
37. Pol S, Everson G, Ghalib S, et al. Once daily NS5A Inhibitor(BMS-790052) plus peginterferon-α 2a and ribavirin produces high rates of extended rapid virologic response in treatment naive HCV genotype 1 subjects: phase 2a trial. Hepatology 2010;52:S462.
38. Gane EJ, Roberts SK, Stedman CA, et al. Oral combination therapy with a nucleoside polymerase inhibitor (RG7128) and danoprevir for chronic hepatitis C genotype 1 infection (INFORM-1): a randomised, double-blind, placebo-controlled, dose-escalation trial. Lancet 2010;376:1467–75.
39. A study on the combination of RO5024048 and ritonavir-boosted danoprevir with and without Copegus (Ribavirin) in interferon-naïve patients with chronic hepatitis C genotype 1 (INFORM-SVR). 2011. Available at: http://clinicaltrials.gov/ct2/show/NCT01278134. Accessed February 25, 2011.
40. Muir AJ, Shiffman ML, Zaman A, et al. Phase 1b study of pegylated interferon λ 1 with or without ribavirin in patients with chronic genotype 1 hepatitis C virus infection. Hepatology 2010;52:822–32.
41. Flisiak R, Feinman SV, Jablkowski M, et al. The cyclophilin inhibitor Debio 025 combined with PEG IFNα2a significantly reduces viral load in treatment-naive hepatitis C patients. Hepatology 2009;49:1460–8.
42. Nelson D, Ghalib R, Sulkowski M, et al. Efficacy and safety of the cyclophilin inhibitor DEBIO 025 in combination with pegylated interferon α 2a and ribavirin in previously null-responder genotype 1 HCV patients. J Hepatol 2010;50(Suppl 1):S40.
43. Hopkins S, Heuman D, Gavis E, et al. Safety, plasma pharmacokinetics and antiviral activity of SCY-635 in adult patients with chronic hepatitis C virus infection. J Hepatol 2009;50(Suppl 1):S36.
44. Manns M, Lawitz E, Hoepelman A. Short term safety, tolerability, pharmacokinetics and preliminary activity of GS-9450, a selective caspase inhibitor in patients with chronic HCV infection. J Hepatol 2010;52(Suppl 1):S114–5.
45. Available at: http://www.globeimmune.com/products/gi-5005/. Accessed February 25, 2011.

46. Jacobson S, McHutchison J, Boyer T. GI-5005 therapeutic vaccine plus PEG-IFN/Ribavirin significantly improves virologic response and ALT normalization at end of treatment and improves SVR24 compared to PEG-IFN/Ribavirin in genotype 1 chronic HCV patients. J Hepatol 2010;52(Suppl 1):S465–6.
47. Ge D, Fellay J, Thompson A, et al. Genetic variation in IL28B predicts hepatitis C treatment-induced viral clearance. Nature 2009;461:399–401.
48. Pockros P, Jacobson I, Boyer T, et al. GI-5005 therapeutic vaccine plus Peg-IFN/ribavirin improves sustained virological response versus Peg-IFN/Ribavirin in prior non-responders with genotype 1 chronic HCV infection. Hepatology 2011; 52:404A.
49. Vierling J, McHutchison J, Jacobson I, et al. GI-5005 therapeutic vaccine improves deficit in cellular immunity in IL28B Genotype T/T, treatment naive patients with Chronic hepatitis C genotype 1 when added to standard of care(SOC) PEG-IFN-α-2a/Ribavirin. Hepatology 2011;52:1258A.
50. Available at: http://www.conatuspharma.com/products/cts-1027-for-liver-disease.htm. Accessed February 25, 2011.

Boceprevir: A User's Guide

Paul Y. Kwo, MD*, Rong Zhao, MD, PhD

KEYWORDS

- Hepatitis C virus • Protease inhibitor • Boceprevir
- Direct-acting antiviral • Resistance

Chronic hepatitis C virus (HCV) affects about 170 million people worldwide.[1] HCV, the most common blood-borne infection in the United States, is a major cause of chronic liver disease leading to death from liver failure or hepatocellular carcinoma. Hepatitis C is the most common indication for liver transplantation worldwide, and is a major cause of the increased incidence of hepatocellular cancer in the United States.[2,3] Approximately 500,000 patients die annually from complications of HCV-related end-stage liver disease.[4]

HCV VIRION AND ITS LIFE CYCLE

HCV is a small enveloped virus with a 9.6 kb positive-sense single-stranded RNA genome that encodes a unique large polyprotein, which is processed by cellular and virally encoded proteases to produce at least 10 mature structural and nonstructural (NS) proteins (**Fig. 1**).[3,5] Among the structural proteins the two envelope glycoproteins, E1 and E2, are essential components of the HCV virion envelope, and are necessary for viral entry and fusion with cellular membrane.[6] The latter is an important step for the release of HCV nucleocapsid in the cell cytoplasm and initiation of HCV polyprotein translation in a membranous web made of the NS proteins and host cell proteins called the "replication complex," located in close contact with perinuclear membranes.[5] HCV 5′-nontranslated region contains a highly structured element, called the internal ribosome entry site (IRES), which is essential for the initiation of HCV polyprotein translation.[7] Among the NS proteins, the NS3 serine-like protease and the RNA-dependent RNA polymerase (RdRp), which is encoded by the NS5 region, are essential for viral maturation and replication, and therefore represent ideal targets for the development of direct-acting antiviral (DAA) compounds.[8,9] Genome encapsidation occurs in the endoplasmic reticulum, and nucleocapsids are enveloped and matured in the Golgi apparatus before they are released in the pericellular space by exocytosis.[10]

Liver Transplantation, Gastroenterology/Hepatology Division, Indiana University School of Medicine, 975 West Walnut, IB 327, Indianapolis, IN 46202-5121, USA
* Corresponding author.
E-mail address: pkwo@iupui.edu

Clin Liver Dis 15 (2011) 537–553
doi:10.1016/j.cld.2011.05.005
liver.theclinics.com

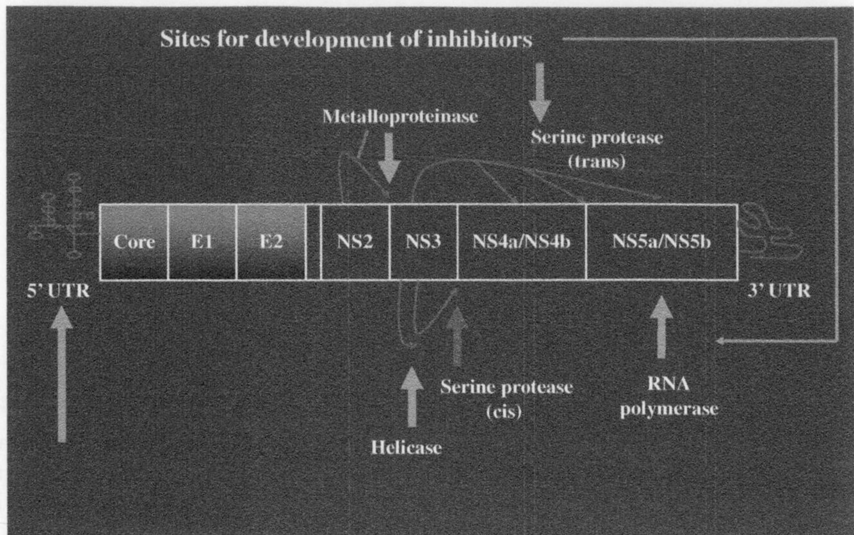

Fig. 1. The HCV genome and potential sites for inhibition. UTR, untranslated region.

CURRENT TREATMENT OF HEPATITIS C

Up until now, treatment for this disease has consisted of therapies to stimulate the immune system and interfere in a nonspecific manner with viral replication. Standard of care (SOC) treatment of genotype-1 HCV is pegylated interferon (PEG-IFN)-α and ribavirin for 48 weeks, which results in sustained virological response (SVR) in about 40% to 50% of individuals.[11–14] SVR rates for black patients treated with SOC are substantially lower; in two studies undertaken almost exclusively in genotype-1 individuals, 19% to 28% of black persons achieved SVR versus 52% of non-Hispanic white persons.[15,16] Those who achieve SVR can have long-term benefits with improvement in degrees of liver fibrosis, reduction in complications of chronic liver disease, and improved quality of life. Studies have shown that response-guided therapy can allow tailoring of duration of treatment, with week-4 viral clearance (rapid virological response) allowing shorter duration of therapy than for those who clear virus at week 12 (complete early virological response).[17]

PROTEASE INHIBITORS

With better understanding of HCV infection and the viral life cycle, new agents targeting HCV entry, HCV RNA translation, and virus assembly and release are showing promising antiviral efficacy in preclinical and early clinical trials. This review focuses on the NS3/4A protease inhibitor, boceprevir, and discusses the mechanism of action, anti-HCV effect, and viral resistance of this novel agent.

Hepatitis C viral protein synthesis is mediated by an internal ribosome-entry site that binds directly to ribosomes, and RNA is translated into a polyprotein of 3000 amino acids that is proteolytically cleaved into 4 structural and 6 NS proteins (see **Fig. 1**).[18] The structural proteins are used to assemble new viral particles, and the NS proteins support viral RNA replication.

The NS3/4A is a serine protease (NS3) and cofactor (NS4A) that catalyzes the post-translational processing of NS proteins from the polyprotein, which is important for viral replication. The NS3 protease cleaves NS4A-NS4B, NS4B-NS5A, and NS5A-NS5B junctions. The products released go on to form a replicative complex responsible for forming viral RNA. Given its essential role in the process of HCV replication, NS3/4A provides an ideal target for antiviral therapy.

Characterization of peptide substrates led to the observation that the N-terminal peptide product was able to inhibit the enzyme.[19,20] This proved to be a useful starting point for inhibitor design, first by optimizing the sequence of a peptide inhibitor[21] and subsequently using nonpeptidic substituents.

A major limitation in the development of anti-HCV compounds was the lack of a virus replication system. This hurdle was finally overcome with the development of a novel replicon system that directed persistent replication in a cell culture system.[22] In 1999, Lohmann and colleagues[22] described a reliable method of HCV replication with subgenomic HCV RNA in a hepatoma cell line. Based on the finding that in other viral replication models structural proteins are not required for RNA replication, the HCV RNA genome was modified. Structural proteins were replaced with a selectable marker, in this case, a gene encoding neomycin phosphotransferase (NPT), which inactivates the cytotoxic drug G418. The hepatoma cells were then transfected with the subgenomic RNA replicon and placed in a medium containing G418. Only cells in which the replicon amplified sufficiently were able to produce NPT and confer G418 resistance. The surviving cells were isolated to form colonies of cell clones that carry stable replicating HCV replicons. This technique has allowed evaluation of therapeutic agents that inhibit viral replication and characterization of resistant mutants.[18] Using such a system, it was possible to demonstrate antiviral activity of an NS3/4A inhibitor in a cell culture assay, and demonstrate potency on par with interferon-α treatment.[23] In the first clinical application of an NS3 protease inhibitor, the protease inhibitor BILN 2061 provided "proof of concept" data with marked direct antiviral activity in a genotype-1 population; however, further investigation in humans was stopped because of cardiac toxicity in animals.[24,25]

EARLY CLINICAL RESULTS: BOCEPREVIR (SCH 503034)

Boceprevir is a structurally novel peptidomimetic ketoamide HCV NS3 protease inhibitor that forms a covalent and reversible bond to the NS3 active site.[26] Malcolm and colleagues[26] demonstrated a robust antiviral activity of boceprevir on HCV replicons. Treatment of HCV replicons resulted in a 1.5- to 2-log decline in RNA levels at 72 hours and a 3.5- to 4-log drop by day 15. No toxic hepatocyte effects were seen. Cells treated with boceprevir and interferon-α had greater HCV replicon suppression than either agent alone, and this effect appeared to be additive rather than synergistic. These promising in vitro data allowed boceprevir to enter clinical trials.

Phase 1 Studies

Boceprevir/peginterferon-α2b combination study

A subsequent phase 1b study compared boceprevir monotherapy with PEG-IFN–α2b monotherapy and PEG-IFN–α2b plus boceprevir therapy in a nonresponder population.[27]

In this randomized, double-blind crossover study, 26 patients with HCV genotype 1a or 1b, who previously did not achieve an early virologic response (EVR) with PEG-IFN–α2b with or without ribavirin, were enrolled and randomized to a 3-way crossover study with 2 doses of boceprevir. Treatment consisted of boceprevir monotherapy (200 or 400 mg 3 times a day) for 1 week, PEG-IFN–α2b (1.5 mcg/kg) weekly for 2 weeks, and combination PEG-IFN–α2b plus boceprevir for 2 weeks. At least 2 weeks between treatments was allowed for washout of the therapies. Combination therapy yielded greater reductions in viral load than either drug given as monotherapy. In the nonresponder patients treated with PEG-IFN–α2b and boceprevir 200 mg 3 times a day, a maximum mean change in HCV RNA of -2.28 ± 1.03 $\log_{10}$ was observed. In those treated with PEG-IFN–α2b and boceprevir 400 mg 3 times a day, a maximum mean change in HCV RNA of -2.68 ± 1.12 $\log_{10}$ was observed. In the monotherapy arms, single-week therapy with boceprevir 200 or 400 mg only, 3 times daily resulted in viral load reductions of -1.08 ± 0.22 $\log_{10}$ and -1.61 ± 0.21 $\log_{10}$, respectively. Two-week monotherapy with PEG-IFN–α2b yielded RNA reductions of -1.08 to -1.26 $\log_{10}$. Four patients did not complete the study, and no new adverse events were seen. In addition, there was no difference in safety parameters in patients treated with 200 or 400 mg boceprevir TID as compared with PEG-IFN–α2b. Pharmacokinetic phase 1 data did not reveal significant interaction between PEG-IFN–α2b and boceprevir, with area-under-the-curve values for each drug yielding similar results for monotherapy (boceprevir or PEG-IFN–α2b) and combination therapy, suggesting little interaction. Boceprevir was well tolerated alone and in combination with PEG-IFN–α2b. Viral breakthrough resulting from selection of preexisting resistant mutants was observed in some patients, in particular during boceprevir monotherapy.[28]

Phase 2 Studies

Boceprevir and peginterferon-α2b with and without ribavirin

With these preliminary data, a phase 2 dose-finding boceprevir study was initiated with multiple aims: to determine the optimal boceprevir dose, whether ribavirin is required in combination with PEG-IFN–α2b and boceprevir, and what the optimal duration would be in a null responder population.[29] In this study, 357 null responders who either failed to achieve EVR or failed to clear virus with more than 12 weeks of PEG-IFN–α2b/ribavirin therapy were enrolled and treated with PEG-IFN–α2b/ribavirin plus placebo, PEG-IFN–α2b plus boceprevir in ascending doses (100/200/400/800 mg) 3 times daily, or PEG-IFN–α2b/boceprevir 400 mg 3 times a day plus ribavirin. After an interim analysis by the Data Safety Monitoring Board, the protocol was amended, and all responding patients (defined as <10,000 IU/mL on original therapy) were assigned to receive PEG-IFN–α2b, ribavirin, and boceprevir 800 mg 3 times a day for 24 weeks. Although the overall sustained response rate was low, this trial established several important concepts in the treatment of HCV nonresponders with boceprevir. First, for treatment of null responders, ribavirin is required for optimal response in combination with NS3 protease inhibitors such as boceprevir. Second, the optimal boceprevir dose was determined in this study at 800 mg 3 times a day, a dose that no patient initially received. In addition, more rapid time to undetectable HCV RNA and longer duration of therapy with undetectable HCV RNA predicted sustained response. Finally, null responders randomized to the PEG-IFN–α2b/ribavirin without boceprevir arm (control) who demonstrated interferon responsiveness (1–2 log reduction at week 13) were more likely to go on to sustained response with the addition of boceprevir.

SPRINT-1

These preliminary results led to the design of a phase 2 clinical trial, HCV Serine Protease Inhibitor Therapy 1 (SPRINT-1), evaluating boceprevir in combination with PEG-IFN and ribavirin in HCV genotype 1 treatment-naïve patients. In this international, multi-arm trial, genotype-1 subjects were randomized to receive PEG-IFN–α2b, weight-based ribavirin, and boceprevir therapy, 800 mg 3 times a day for 28 (PRB28) or 48 weeks (PRB48), or a lead-in strategy with 4 weeks of PEG-IFN–α2b and ribavirin followed by boceprevir 800 mg 3 times a day with PEG-IFN–α2b and ribavirin for 24 (PR4PRB24) or 44 weeks (PR4PRB44), and these treatment arms were compared with standard therapy for PEG-IFN–α2b and ribavirin for 48 weeks (PR48) (**Fig. 2**). Finally, a low-dose ribavirin arm (400–1000 mg) was included with PEG-IFN–α2b and boceprevir, and compared with PRB48.

The rationale for the potential benefit of a lead-in strategy is based on the fact that both PEG-IFN–α2b and ribavirin reach steady-state concentrations by week 4, and with the lead-in strategy, patients have the protease inhibitor added when the backbone drug levels have been optimized and the patient's immune system has been activated. This approach may minimize the period of time when there is a "functional monotherapy" with a DAA, potentially reducing the likelihood for the development of resistance. This strategy may also have the potential to reduce the likelihood of the development of resistance by identifying patients who are responders to interferon and ribavirin before giving them a protease inhibitor or other DAA drug. The low-dose ribavirin arm was added to determine whether SVR rates could be preserved while reducing potential anemia.

In this multicenter, international trial, approximately 100 subjects were enrolled in each arm and were stratified for the presence of cirrhosis and black race.[30] The demographic data are shown in **Table 1**. In this trial, 14% to 17% of individuals in part 1 of the study were black, and 6% to 9% had cirrhosis. The SVR rates for the SPRINT-1 trial are shown in **Table 2**. Regardless of treatment arm, in part 1 of the study SVR rates were higher with the addition of boceprevir to PEG-IFN–α2b/ribavirin compared with PEG-IFN–α2b/ribavirin alone. The SVR rates after 28 weeks of triple-treatment arms were 56% for PR4/PRB24 and 54% with PRB28 (**Fig. 3**). In the 48-week treatment arms, SVR rates were 75% for PR4/PRB44 and 67% with PRB48. In a subgroup analysis, up to 53% of African American patients treated with boceprevir achieved SVR. Although the number of patients was small, this represents a considerable improvement over the 21% to 23% SVR previously reported after 48 weeks of standard therapy with PEG-IFN and ribavirin in large United States trials.[11,16] The results from the low-dose ribavirin arm established that full-dose ribavirin is required for optimal response with PEG-IFN–α2b and boceprevir.

Achieving rapid virologic response (RVR) was highly predictive of SVR with the addition of boceprevir. Compared with standard therapy with PEG-IFN–α2b/ribavirin, significantly more patients in the triple-therapy groups achieved an RVR. RVR, defined as undetectable virus at week 4 of treatment, predicts high SVR rates with shorter duration of therapy with PEG-IFN and ribavirin. In this study, RVR and complete EVR (cEVR) were defined by the week of boceprevir therapy, thus in the lead-in arm, the week-4 and week-12 RVR and cEVR results were at weeks 8 and 16 of total therapy. In the 28-week treatment groups, the RVR was 60%, and 39%, for PR4/PRB24, and PRB28, respectively. In the 48-week treatment groups, the RVR rates were 64% PR4/PRB44 and 37% for PRB48 with PR48 group RVR of 8%. Regardless of treatment arm, achieving RVR was highly predictive of SVR, with 82% and 74% of patients in the PR4/PRB24 and PRB28 and 94% and 84% of patients achieving SVR in the PR4/PRB44 and PRB48 arms, respectively. cEVR, defined as undetectable virus at week 12 of boceprevir therapy, was also predictive of SVR. Participants who cleared virus between weeks 4 and 12 of boceprevir therapy were more likely to go on to SVR if they received 48 weeks of treatment rather than 28 weeks in the lead-in arms (see **Table 2**). In the lead-in arms, nearly two-thirds of patients achieved undetectable HCV RNA levels at week 4 of boceprevir therapy after PR4, and these individuals were treated for 28 weeks with high SVR. An additional 19 patients in both lead arms went on to achieve undetectable HCV RNA between weeks 4 and 12 of boceprevir therapy, and 15 of 19 went on to achieve SVR with PEG-IFN–α2b, ribavirin, and boceprevir in the 48-week treatment arm.

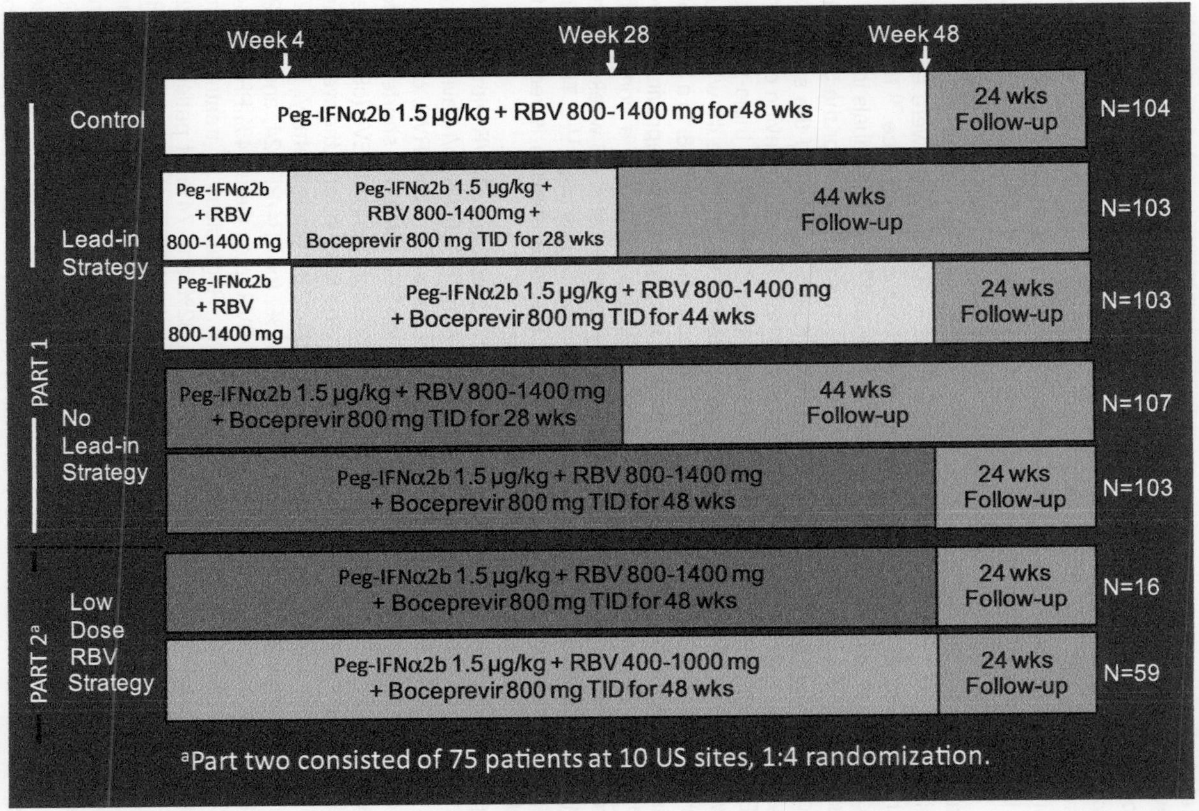

Fig. 2. SPRINT-1 trial design. P, peginterferon-α2b; R, ribavirin; B, boceprevir.

Table 1
Baseline characteristics for SPRINT-1 trial

	PART 1					PART 2	
	P/R Control 48 wk, N = 104	P/R/B 28 wk, N = 107	P/R 4 wk→ P/R/B 24 wk, N = 103	P/R/B 48 wk, N = 103	P/R 4 wk→ P/R/B 44 wk, N = 103	P/R/B 48 wk, N = 16	P/Low-Dose R/B 48 wk, N = 59
Gender							
Male (%)	67	59	50	61	56	56	69
Race							
Caucasian (%)	80	80	83	84	83	75	73
Black (%)	15	17	15	14	15	25	27
Mean age (y)	48.3	46.4	47.7	46.7	47.6	50.3	48.7
Mean weight (kg)	83.4	83.4	79.9	80.0	78.4	81.4	88.5
HCV subtype (%)							
1a	51	63	51	53	58	44	66
1b	40	28	36	35	34	44	31
1 (no subtype)	9	9	13	12	8	13	3
Viral load mean (log_{10} IU/mL)	6.53	6.64	6.53	6.54	6.53	6.43	6.47
HCV RNA >600,000 IU/mL (%)	90	92	87	91	90	81	83
Cirrhosis (%)	8	7	7	9	6	0	7

Abbreviations: P, peginterferon-α2b; R, ribavirin; B, boceprevir.

Table 2
Effect of treatment duration on SVR

Time to First PCR-negative HCV RNA	P/R Control 48 wk, % (n/N)	P/R 4 wk→P/R/B 24 wk, % (n/N)	P/R 4 wk→P/R/B 44 wk, % (n/N)
≤4 wk	100 (8/8)	82 (54/66)	94 (62/66)
>4 wk– ≤12 wk	83 (24/29)	21 (4/19)	79 (15/19)
>12 wk	30 (7/23)	0 (0/1)	0 (0/1)

Abbreviation: PCR, polymerase chain reaction.

The addition of boceprevir after the 4-week lead-in period demonstrated that SVR could be predicted by the degree of PEG-IFN/ribavirin responsiveness achieved during the initial 4 weeks of therapy. If a greater than 1.5 $\log_{10}$ was achieved during the lead-in, high rates of SVR were achieved with boceprevir addition regardless of treatment duration. However, even those who were poorly PEG-IFN–α2b/ribavirin responsive with less than 1 $\log_{10}$ reduction at week 4 of lead-in could achieve SVR with boceprevir addition with a total treatment duration of 48 weeks, leading to better SVR rates (55%) than the 28-week treatment duration (28%) in these poorly interferon-responsive patients. Thus the lead-in may also be used to assess during therapy the degree of PEG-IFN/ribavirin responsiveness, and can help predict SVR with boceprevir addition.

Relapse rates were comparable in the 28-week treatment arms at 24% (PR4/PRB24) and 30% (PRB28), the presence of RVR in either arm markedly reducing relapse rates (**Fig. 4**). In the 48-week treatment arms, relapse rates were lower at 3% (PR4/PRB44) and 7% (PRB48), though not significantly different between the lead-in and non–lead-in arms. A modest reduction in breakthrough in the lead-in arms was noted, though again this did not reach statistical significance. Treatment discontinuation rates were higher in the triple-therapy groups as compared with the standard therapy (26%–40% vs 15%). Response guided therapy was not tested in this phase 2 study.

The most common side effects related to boceprevir were anemia, nausea, vomiting, and dysgeusia. Adverse events were more common in the boceprevir groups than in PEG-IFN–α2b/ribavirin treatment groups (11%–15% vs 8%) and were largely due to anemia and dysgeusia, with no new adverse events noted. Most hemoglobin reductions were grade 1 and 2 (World Health Organization criteria), and no increase in skin or subcutaneous disorders was noted. Higher rates of both anemia and dysgeusia were noted in the boceprevir-containing regimens than in the controls, although stopping treatment for anemia was rare. A recent publication suggested that anemia may be a surrogate marker of ribavirin exposure, with higher rates of anemia.[31] Indeed, in this study anemia and use of erythropoietin were associated with higher SVR rates (**Fig. 5**), and the role of erythropoietin as an adjuvant in patients receiving PEG-IFN and ribavirin in addition to therapy with DAA agents is being explored in a large randomized trial.

Phase 3 Studies

In the SPRINT-2 (Serine Protease Inhibitor Therapy 2) trial, 1097 treatment-naïve patients achieved overall SVR rates of 63% (68% in nonblack patients and 53% in blacks compared with controls [40% and 23%, respectively]; $P = .004$ and $P = .044$) with a regimen that used a 4-week lead-in of PEG-IFN/ribavirin followed by

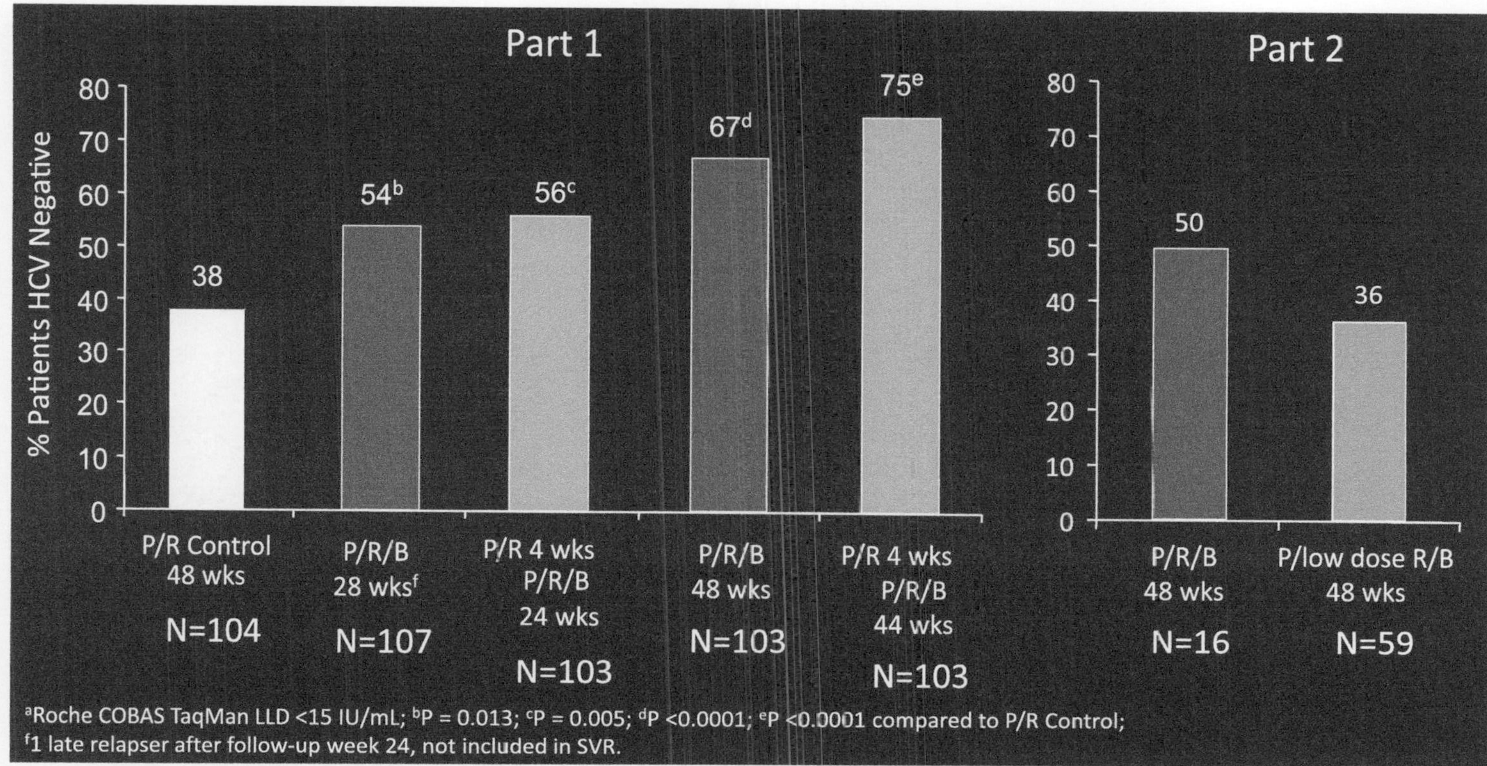

Fig. 3. SVR rates of SPRINT-1. Combination therapy of boceprevir and peginterferon-α2b + ribavirin (RBV) in treatment-naïve genotype-1 patients.

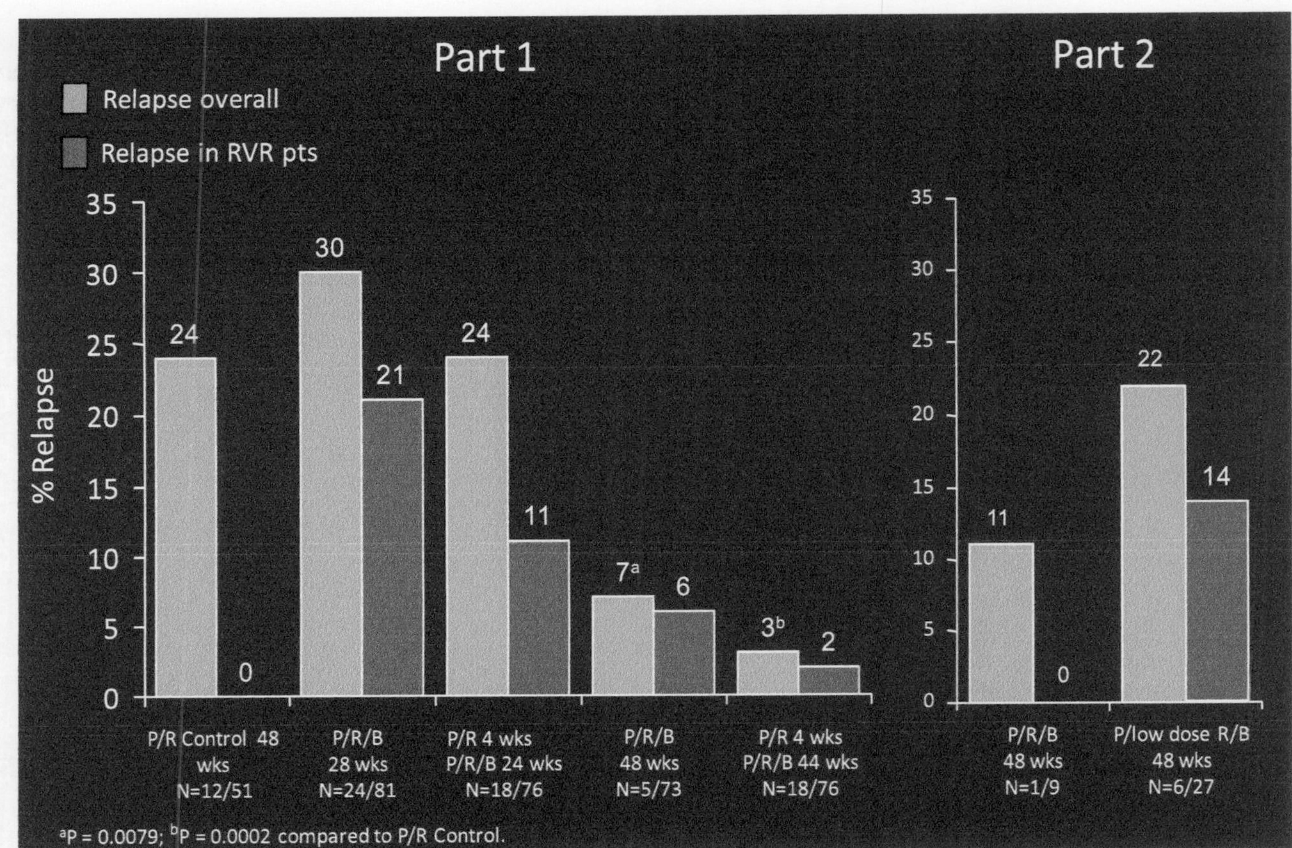

Fig. 4. Relapse rates in Parts 1 and 2 of SPRINT-1 are demonstrated.

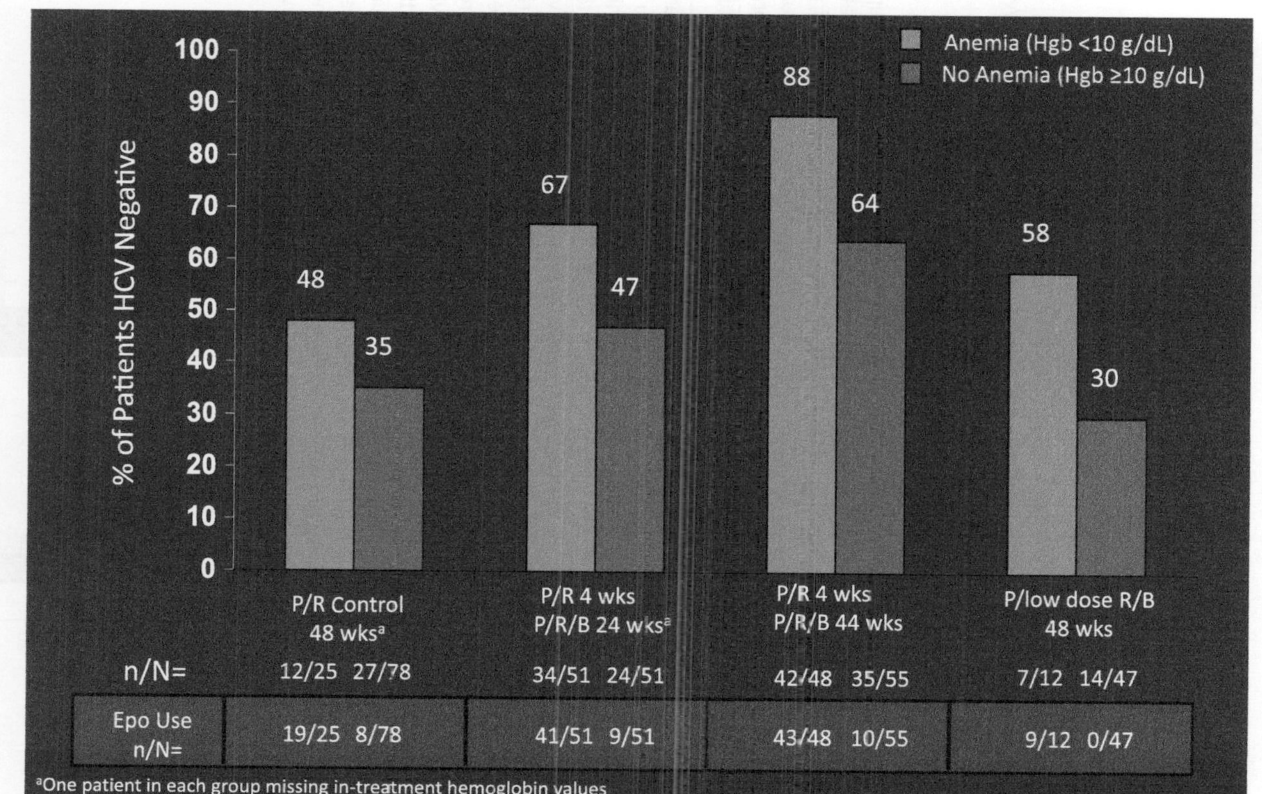

Fig. 5. The association of anemia and EPO use to SVR in SPRINT-1 is demonstrated.

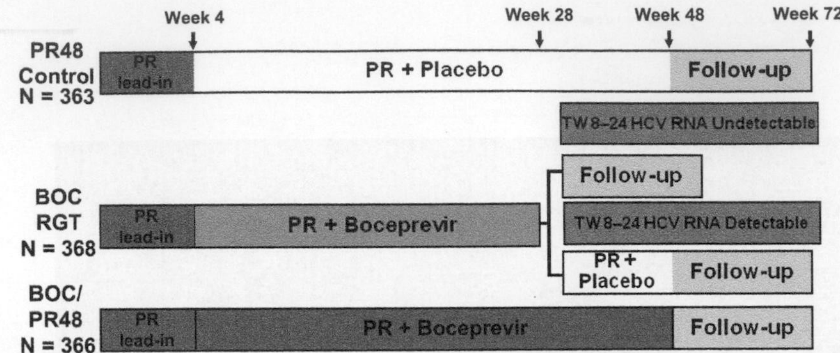

Fig. 6. Trial design of SPRINT-2. BOC, boceprevir; PR48, pegylated interferon α-2b 1.5 μg/kg/wk plus ribavirin 600 to 1400 mg daily; RGT, response-guided therapy.

the addition of boceprevir for 24 weeks (**Figs. 6** and **7**).[32] A response-guided therapy paradigm was then used to determine ultimate length of PEG-IFN/ribavirin of 28 weeks or 48 weeks based on viral negativity at and beyond week 8. Just under half of all patients qualified for the shortened duration (28 weeks of therapy); after discontinuations for adverse events, for predefined stopping rules, and other discontinuations, approximately 25% received 24 weeks of boceprevir and 48 weeks of PEG-IFN/ribavirin.

In the RESPOND (Retreatment with HCV Serine Protease Inhibitor Boceprevir and Peginteron/Rebetol)-2 trial, SVR rates in 403 previous treatment failures was 66% in the 48-week arm and 59% in the response-guided arm, both of which were significantly better than control (21%) (*P*<.0001) (**Figs. 8** and **9**).[33] The study was limited to previous relapsers and those who had demonstrated some interferon responsiveness, having achieved at least a 2-log decline of virus with PEG-IFN/ribavirin. Surprisingly, one-quarter of patients during the 4-week lead-in had less than a 1-log decline in virus before beginning boceprevir. These patients who had poor current interferon response had SVR rates of only 34% compared with 73% to 79% in patients with some interferon response at the end of lead-in. The 4-week lead-in did predict the risk of resistance-associated variants (RAVs), with fewer than 10% of patients developing variants if they had PEG-IFN/ribavirin responsiveness compared with at least one-third developing RAVs if they did not. As with the phase 2 trials, anemia, defined as hemoglobin below 10 g/dL, occurred in half of the patients exposed to boceprevir.

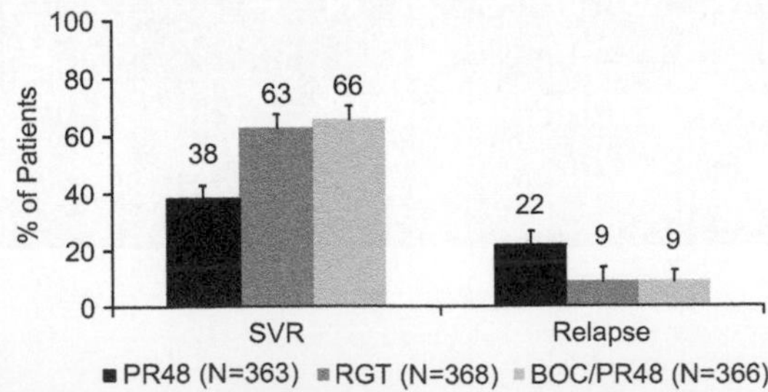

Fig. 7. Sustained virologic response (SVR) and relapse rates in SPRINT-2.

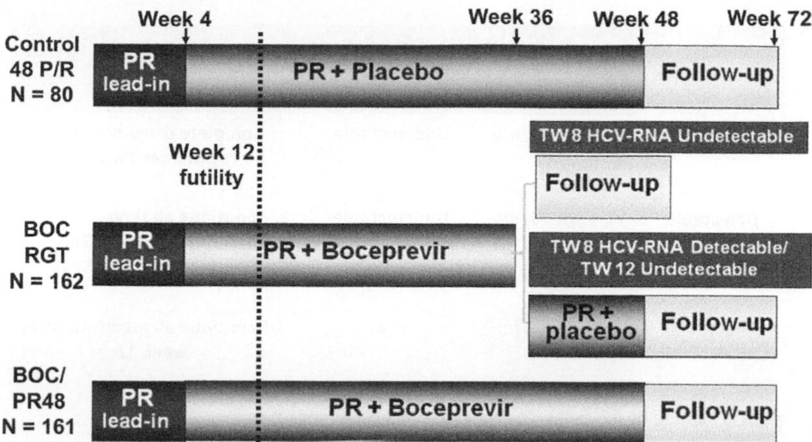

Fig. 8. Trial design of RESPOND 2.

Possibly due to erythropoietin use, fewer than 2% of patients discontinued as a consequence of anemia.

In clinical practice, the use of the lead-in may have utility in predicting likelihood of response and resistance. This approach may be particularly useful in helping risk stratify patients not likely to respond, and treating only on an as-needed case-by-case basis. It may also be used in health care systems concerned with cost containment, as patients with rapid response may have a high chance of achieving SVR even without boceprevir. It is expected that response-guided therapy (RGT) will be the treatment paradigm for patients, receiving shorter durations of therapy if they show early viral responsiveness. The futility rules will be further defined, but will likely incorporate both week-12 and week-24 time points, which have become accepted and familiar to clinicians from the recently published SPRINT-2 and RESPOND-2 studies (**Figs. 6–9**; **Fig. 10**). Some subsets of patients may benefit from particular treatment durations and strategies, but this may need further elucidation. It is expected that postmarketing studies will answer many of these questions.

VIRAL RESISTANCE TO BOCEPREVIR

A major concern with the addition of DAA molecules such as boceprevir to PEG-IFN and ribavirin is the development of drug-resistant mutations. In the early phase 2 study

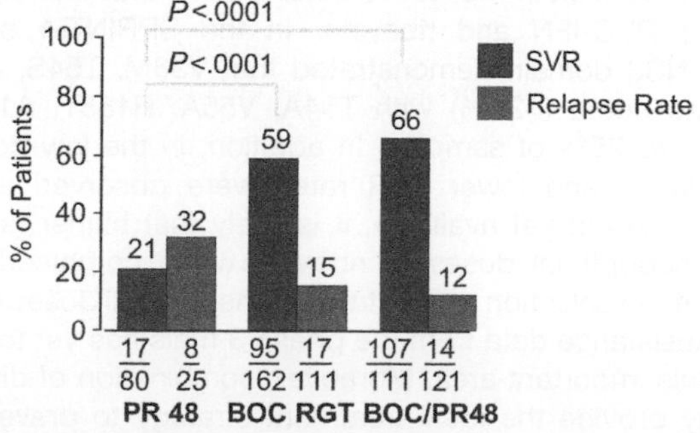

Fig. 9. SVR and relapse rates in the RESPOND 2 trial.

A

Week 8 HCV RNA*	Week 12 HCV RNA	Week 24 HCV RNA*	ACTION
Undetectable¶	VL < 100 IU/mL	Undetectable	Complete three-medicine regimen at TW36
Detectable	VL < 100 IU/mL	Undetectable	1. Continue all three medicines until TW36; 2. Continue PR until TW48
Detectable/ undetectable	VL > 100 IU/mL	n/a	Discontinue all medications at week 12

¶ 46% of patients eligible for shorter duration therapy in RESPOND-2.

* PCR Assay LLQ should be < 25 IU/mL

B

Week 8 HCV RNA*	Week 12 HCV RNA	Week 24 HCV RNA*	ACTION
Undetectable	VL < 100 IU/mL	Undetectable	Complete three-medicine regimen at TW28
Detectable	VL < 100 IU/mL	Undetectable	1. Continue all three medicines and finish through TW36; 2. Administer peginterferon alfa and ribavirin and finish through TW48
Detectable/ undetectable	VL > 100 IU/mL	n/a	Discontinue all 3 drugs

* PCR Assay LLQ should be < 25 IU/mL

Fig. 10. (*A*) Stopping rules for boceprevir in previous partial responders and relapsers. (*B*) Stopping rules for boceprevir in non-cirrhotic naïve patients.

using lower (suboptimal dose) doses of boceprevir with combinations of PEG-IFN–α2b without ribavirin, boceprevir-resistant mutants were noted in most patients not achieving SVR.[29] Ideally, optimally dosed therapy with boceprevir, PEG-IFN, and ribavirin will allow viral suppression before the emergence or dominance of resistant strains or will allow reduction in replicative fitness, such that the resistant strains will retain sensitivity to PEG-IFN and ribavirin. In the SPRINT-1 study, population sequencing of the NS3 domain demonstrated that V36M, T54S, and R155K were the major mutations noted (>25%) with T54A, V55A, R155T, A156S, V158I, and V170A noted in 5% to 25% of samples. In addition, in the low-dose ribavirin arm, higher rates of relapse and lower SVR rates were observed and, though final sequencing studies are not yet available, it is likely that higher rates of resistance will be seen with suboptimal doses of ribavirin when combined with DAAs and PEG-IFN. To prevent the selection of resistant strains optimal doses of ribavirin should be administered. Resistance data from the phase 3 trials has yet to be reported, but will further define this important area. Moreover, combination of different classes of DAA therapies may provide the ideal treatment strategy to prevent emergence of viral-resistant strains.

SUMMARY

Standard therapy for HCV genotype 1 leads to sustained response rates of approximately 40%. The addition of DAA molecules to PEG-IFN and ribavirin has been shown to improve the SVR rate in addition to shortening the duration of treatment in genotype-1 individuals. Thus far, the protease inhibitors boceprevir and telaprevir have shown substantial promise. In vitro and in vivo data have demonstrated viral suppression with boceprevir and superior suppression with boceprevir in combination with PEG-IFN–α2b. An early phase 2 study established that optimal response to boceprevir depends on ribavirin therapy and PEG-IFN–α2b responsiveness in nonresponders. The SPRINT-1 trial results are notable for several findings. The study suggests that a lead-in strategy with PEG-IFN/ribavirin therapy may reduce relapse and prevent breakthrough while optimizing antiviral response by allowing the PEG-IFN/ribavirin backbone to achieve a steady state before boceprevir is added. In SPRINT-2, both the 28-week and 48-week treatment arms, SVR rates were improved over PEG-IFN/ribavirin control and indeed, the SVR rate of 63% to 66% represents a dramatic increase in SVR over 38% control in genotype-1 patients. Boceprevir is generally well tolerated with a safety profile tested over 48 weeks. Finally, response rates in African Americans and cirrhotic patients, who typically have poor response to standard therapy, were also substantially higher than has been previously reported with PEG-IFN and ribavirin therapy. As with the resistance seen in the development of human immunodeficiency virus therapy, the emergence of resistance to protease inhibitors will be an important consideration. As newer therapies emerge, the true significance of resistant variants will become clearer. In the immediate future, the addition of boceprevir to PEG-IFN and ribavirin will be an important advance in the treatment of genotype-1 patients.

REFERENCES

1. Thomas DL. Hepatitis C. Epidemiologic quandaries. Clin Liver Dis 2001;5(4): 955–68.
2. Verna EC, Brown RS Jr. Hepatitis C virus and liver transplantation. Clin Liver Dis 2006;10(4):919–40.
3. Lauer G, Walker B. Hepatitis C virus infection. N Engl J Med 2001;345(1):41–52.
4. Wasley A, Alter MJ. Epidemiology of hepatitis C: geographic differences and temporal trends. Semin Liver Dis 2000;20(1):1–16.
5. Penin F, Dubuisson J, Rey FA, et al. Structural biology of hepatitis C virus. Hepatology 2004;39(1):5–19.
6. Nielsen SU, Bassendine MF, Burt AD, et al. Characterization of the genome and structural proteins of hepatitis C virus resolved from infected human liver. J Gen Virol 2004;85(Pt 6):1497–507.
7. Pisarev AV, Shirokikh NE, Hellen CU. Translation initiation by factor-independent binding of eukaryotic ribosomes to internal ribosomal entry sites. C R Biol 2005;328(7):589–605.
8. Lee G, Piper DE, Wang Z, et al. Novel inhibitors of hepatitis C virus RNA-dependent RNA polymerases. J Mol Biol 2006;357(4):1051–7.
9. Biswal BK, Wang M, Cherney MM, et al. Non-nucleoside inhibitors binding to hepatitis C virus NS5B polymerase reveal a novel mechanism of inhibition. J Mol Biol 2006;361(1):33–45.
10. Kunkel M, Lorinczi M, Rijnbrand R, et al. Self-assembly of nucleocapsid-like particles from recombinant hepatitis C virus core protein. J Virol 2001;75(5):2119–29.

11. McHutchison JG, Lawitz EJ, Shiffman ML, et al. Peginterferon alfa-2b or alfa-2a with ribavirin for treatment of hepatitis C infection. N Engl J Med 2009;361(6): 580–93.
12. Manns MP, McHutchison JG, Gordon SC, et al. Peginterferon alfa-2b plus ribavirin compared with interferon alfa-2b plus ribavirin for initial treatment of chronic hepatitis C: a randomised trial. Lancet 2001;358(9286):958–65.
13. Fried MW, Shiffman ML, Reddy KR, et al. Peginterferon alfa-2a plus ribavirin for chronic hepatitis C virus infection. N Engl J Med 2002;347(13):975–82.
14. Sulkowski M. Treatment of hepatitis C in HIV-infected persons: a work in progress. J Hepatol 2008;48(1):5–7.
15. Conjeevaram HS, Fried MW, Jeffers LJ, et al. Peginterferon and ribavirin treatment in African American and Caucasian American patients with hepatitis C genotype 1. Gastroenterology 2006;131(2):470–7.
16. Muir AJ, Bornstein JD, Killenberg PG, et al. Peginterferon alfa-2b and ribavirin for the treatment of chronic hepatitis C in blacks and non-Hispanic whites [see comment] [Erratum appears in N Engl J Med 2004;351(12):1268]. N Engl J Med 2004;350(22):2265–71.
17. Mangia A, Minerva N, Bacca D, et al. Individualized treatment duration for hepatitis C genotype 1 patients: a randomized controlled trial. Hepatology 2008;47(1): 43–50.
18. Bartenschlager R. Hepatitis C virus replicons: potential role for drug development. Nat Rev Drug Discov 2002;1(11):911–6.
19. Llinas-Brunet M, Bailey MD, Bolger G, et al. Structure-activity study on a novel series of macrocyclic inhibitors of the hepatitis C virus NS3 protease leading to the discovery of BILN 2061. J Med Chem 2004;47(7):1605–8.
20. Steinkuhler C, Biasiol G, Brunetti M, et al. Product inhibition of the hepatitis C virus NS3 protease. Biochemistry 1998;37(25):8899–905.
21. Ingallinella P, Altamura S, Bianchi E, et al. Potent peptide inhibitors of human hepatitis C virus NS3 protease are obtained by optimizing the cleavage products. Biochemistry 1998;37(25):8906–14.
22. Lohmann V, Körner F, Koch J, et al. Replication of subgenomic hepatitis C virus RNAs in a hepatoma cell line. Science 1999;285(5424):110–3.
23. Pause A, Kukolj G, Bailey M, et al. An NS3 serine protease inhibitor abrogates replication of subgenomic hepatitis C virus RNA. J Biol Chem 2003;278(22): 20374–80.
24. Hinrichsen H, Benhamou Y, Wedemeyer H, et al. Short-term antiviral efficacy of BILN 2061, a hepatitis C virus serine protease inhibitor, in hepatitis C genotype 1 patients. Gastroenterology 2004;127(5):1347–55.
25. Lamarre D, Anderson PC, Bailey M, et al. An NS3 protease inhibitor with antiviral effects in humans infected with hepatitis C virus. Nature 2003;426(6963):186–9.
26. Malcolm BA, Liu R, Lahser F, et al. SCH 503034, a mechanism-based inhibitor of hepatitis C virus NS3 protease, suppresses polyprotein maturation and enhances the antiviral activity of alpha interferon in replicon cells. Antimicrob Agents Chemother 2006;50(3):1013–20.
27. Sarrazin C, Rouzier R, Wagner F, et al. SCH 503034, a novel hepatitis C virus protease inhibitor, plus pegylated interferon alpha-2b for genotype 1 nonresponders [see comment]. Gastroenterology 2007;132(4):1270–8.
28. Sarrazin C, Kieffer TL, Bartels D, et al. Dynamic hepatitis C virus genotypic and phenotypic changes in patients treated with the protease inhibitor telaprevir. Gastroenterology 2007;132(5):1767–77.

29. Schiff E, Poordad E, Jacobson I, et al. Boceprevir (B) combination therapy in null responders (NR): response dependent on interferon responsiveness. J Hepatol 2008;48:S46.
30. Kwo PY, Lawitz EJ, McCone J, et al. Efficacy of boceprevir, an NS3 protease inhibitor, in combination with peginterferon alfa-2b and ribavirin in treatment-naïve patients with genotype 1 hepatitis C infection (SPRINT-1): an open-label, randomised, multicentre phase 2 trial. Lancet 2010;376(9742):705–16.
31. Sulkowski M, Shiffman ML, Afdhal NH, et al. Decline in hemoglobin is associated with sustained virologic response (SVR) among HCV genotype 1-infected persons treated with peginterferon (PEG)/ribavirin (RBV): analysis from the ideal study. Gastroenterology 2010;139:1602–11.
32. Poordad F, McCone J, Bacon B, et al. Boceprevir with peginterferon/ribavirin for untreated chronic hepatitis C. N Engl J Med 2011;364:1195–206.
33. Bacon B, Gordon S, Lawitz E, et al. Boceprevir for treatment-resistant chronic HCV genotype 1 infection. N Engl J Med 2011;364:1207–17.

Telaprevir User's Guide

AnnMarie Liapakis, MD, Ira Jacobson, MD*

KEYWORDS

• Telaprevir • Hepatitis C virus • User's guide • Interferon
• Ribavirin • Protease inhibitor

Approximately 3 to 4 million persons in the United States and 170 million worldwide are infected with the hepatitis C virus (HCV),[1] and up to 75% of new infections progress to chronic infection, which is a major cause of chronic liver disease.[2,3] HCV is the leading cause of death from liver disease and the most frequent indication for liver transplant in the United States.[4]

For a decade, standard therapy for patients with genotype 1 chronic HCV (HCV G1) consisted of pegylated interferon (Peg-IFN) alfa-2a or Peg-IFN alfa-2b, combined with ribavirin, for 48 weeks in patients with HCV G1 or 24 weeks for those with genotypes 2 or 3.[5] Despite the improvement in efficacy over previous regimens when this therapy was introduced, the overall sustained virologic response (SVR) rate in patients with HCV G1 was still only 40% to 50%.[6]

TELAPREVIR: MECHANISM OF ACTION

Determination of the structure of HCV proteins, the development of a subgenomic replicon system, and a cell culture model that enables productive HCV infection have facilitated the development of direct-acting antiviral agents (DAAs).[7,8] These agents have the potential to substantially increase rates of SVR and to truncate the duration of therapy.

Each step of the HCV life cycle offers a potential target for DAA therapy.[9] Polyprotein processing is one step. Two viral peptidases are involved in the posttranslational processing of HCV proteins NS2 and NS3/4A. NS3 is a multifunctional viral protein containing a serine protease domain in its *N*-terminal third (approximately 180 amino acids) and a helicase/NTPase domain in its *C*-terminal two-thirds. NS3 has a typical chymotrypsin-like fold, and NS4A is a cofactor of its proteinase activity. The NS3/4A serine protease catalyzes HCV polyprotein cleavage. NS3 must assemble with its cofactor NS4A to catalyze *cis*-cleavage at the NS3–NS4A junction and *trans*-cleavage at all downstream junctions, including NS4A–NS4B, NS4B–NS5A, and

Division of Gastroenterology and Hepatology, Weill Cornell Medical College, 1305 York Avenue, 4th Floor, New York, NY 10021, USA
* Corresponding author.

Clin Liver Dis 15 (2011) 555–571
doi:10.1016/j.cld.2011.05.013
liver.theclinics.com
1089-3261/11/$ – see front matter

Key Points

- The NS3/4A serine protease of HCV plays a critical role in the HCV life cycle through cleaving most of the nonstructural proteins from the polypeptide formed during translation of the viral mRNA.
- Telaprevir is an orally bioavailable inhibitor of NS3/4A.

NS5A–NS5B. VX-950, or telaprevir, is a NS3/4A serine protease inhibitor produced by Vertex Pharmaceuticals (Cambridge, MA, USA). Telaprevir is a potent covalent orally bioavailable peptidomimetic inhibitor of NS3/4A with an alpha ketoamide moiety that anchors at the enzyme active site (**Fig. 1**).[9]

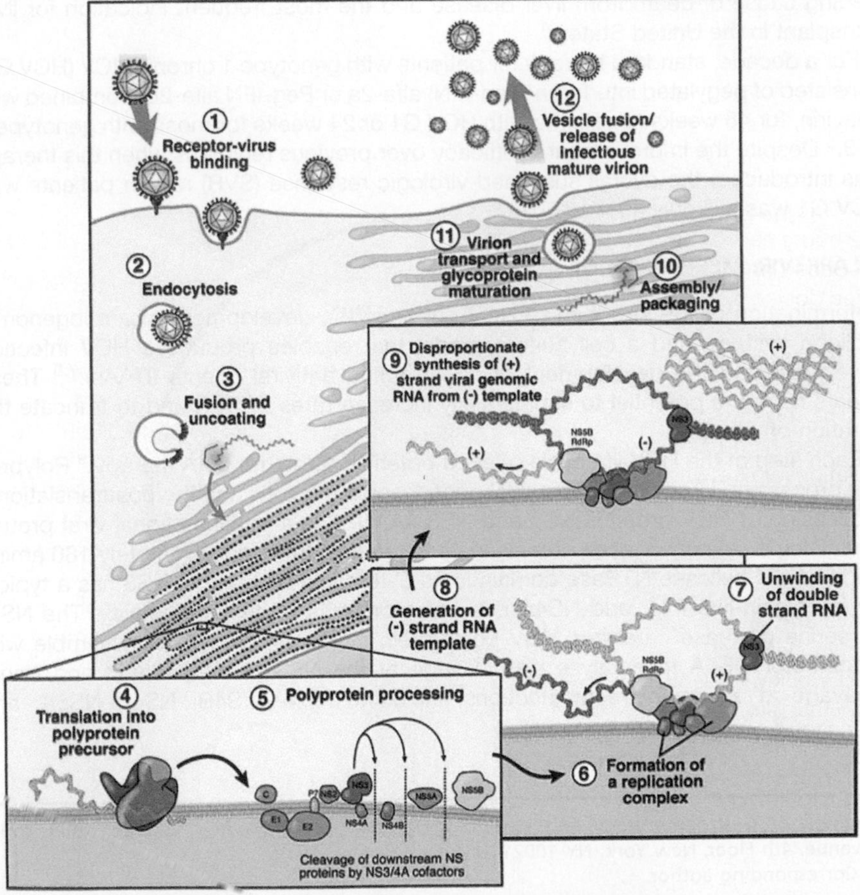

Fig. 1. Life cycle of HCV with potential drug targets. The polyprotein processing stage is the point at which telaprevir acts. (*From* Pawlotsky JM. The hepatitis C viral life cycle as a target for new antiviral therapies. Gastroenterology 2007;132:1979–98; with permission.)

PHASE I STUDIES

The phase I clinical trials for telaprevir were initially conducted in two parts at two collaborative sites in The Netherlands and one in Germany in 2004 to 2005.[10–12] In the first part of the initial trial, 24 healthy subjects received doses of 450 mg or 750 mg, every 8 hours, or 1250 mg every 12 hours for 5 days. Telaprevir was well tolerated and no serious adverse events were reported. The second part of the trial was conducted to evaluate the safety and tolerability of ascending multiple doses of telaprevir in patients with chronic hepatitis C and to investigate its pharmacokinetics and antiviral activity. Median HCV RNA levels in the telaprevir dose groups substantially and rapidly decreased. The median maximum change was $-3.46\ \log_{10}$ IU/mL in the 450-mg group, $-4.77\ \log_{10}$ IU/mL in the 750-mg group, and $-3.49\ \log_{10}$ IU/mL in the group that received 1250 mg of telaprevir every 12 hours. All subjects in the telaprevir groups had at least a 2-$\log_{10}$ decrease from baseline in HCV RNA. All subjects in the 750-mg group had at least a 3-$\log_{10}$ decrease. All three telaprevir dose groups showed similar declines in median HCV RNA up to day 3 of dosing. A further decrease was not evident in the groups who received telaprevir at 450 mg every 8 hours and 1250 mg every 12 hours, and median HCV RNA levels in those two dose groups increased at the end of the dosing period.[10]

The initial rapid decline in HCV RNA was related to maximal exposure to telaprevir, and the second phase of the viral decline was sustained by trough concentrations (C_{trough}) of telaprevir. Subjects who received telaprevir, 750 mg, every 8 hours had an average C_{trough} of 1054 ng/mL and $\geq$4-$\log_{10}$ decrease in HCV RNA, whereas subjects who received telaprevir, 450 mg, every 8 hours had an average C_{trough} of 781 ng/mL with a $\geq$3-$\log_{10}$ decrease in HCV RNA, and subjects who received telaprevir, 1250 mg, every 12 hours had an average C_{trough} of 676 ng/mL with a $\geq$3-$\log_{10}$ decrease in HCV RNA.[10]

Based on these data, telaprevir at a dose of 750 mg every 8 hours emerged as the lead dosing regimen for further trials. The virologic breakthroughs that occurred during the dosing period were related to selection of viral variants with decreased sensitivity to telaprevir, and confirmed that telaprevir would need to be used in combination therapy.[10]

The resistant variants were well characterized in subsequent studies, which differentiated high-level from low-level resistant variants and defined a generally inverse relationship between degree of resistance conferred by a mutation and the replicative fitness of the resulting viral variant.[11]

Further study was undertaken to compare telaprevir monotherapy and combination therapy with telaprevir and Peg-IFN. Twenty HCV G1 treatment–naïve patients were randomized to one of three treatment regimens: placebo every 8 hours orally for 14 days and Peg-IFN weekly for 2 weeks (four patients); telaprevir every 8 hours orally for 14 days (eight patients); or telaprevir every 8 hours orally for 14 days and Peg-IFN weekly for 2 weeks (eight patients).[12] Telaprevir was dosed at 1250 mg once, and then subsequent doses were 750 mg every 8 hours. Telaprevir/Peg-IFN combination therapy resulted in a more significant viral decline during the study period, with a median change in HCV RNA from baseline to day 15 of $-5.49\ \log_{10}$ versus $-3.99\ \log_{10}$ for telaprevir monotherapy, and $-1.09\ \log_{10}$ for Peg-IFN monotherapy.[11,12] Analysis of viral kinetics during the study period showed a biphasic viral decline. The rapid first phase was similar in the Peg-IFN/telaprevir and the telaprevir group. The second phase of decline was more sustained in the Peg-IFN/telaprevir combination group. In the telaprevir monotherapy group, four patients experienced continued decline, and four had viral decline followed by rebound.[12] In the four patients who had viral rebound on telaprevir alone, R155K/T- and A156V/T-resistant variants were detected with sequence analysis during the initial steep decline but were replaced by V36(M/A)/R155(K/T) double mutant variants during the rebound phase. This V36(M/A)/R155(K/T) double mutant variant was shown in in vitro analysis to confer both higher levels of resistance and higher relative fitness.[11] All patients enrolled in the trial were offered continued therapy off-study with Peg-IFN and ribavirin after the study period, of which 19 accepted. All 8 patients initially treated in the combination Peg-IFN/telaprevir group had undetectable HCV RNA at week 12 while receiving standard therapy with Peg-IFN/ribavirin, versus 5 of 8 patients initially treated with telaprevir monotherapy. At week 24 on standard therapy, all patients who initially received Peg-IFN/telaprevir or telaprevir alone had undetectable HCV RNA, thereby showing that telaprevir-resistant variants are sensitive to Peg-IFN and ribavirin.[11,12]

In logical progression, further phase I study was conducted using telaprevir in combination with the current Peg-IFN/ribavirin standard therapy.[13] Twelve treatment-naïve subjects with chronic G1 HCV were treated with telaprevir, 750 mg, every 8 hours, Peg-IFN 180 μg/wk, and ribavirin, 1000 or 1200 mg/d for 28 days, and then could continue treatment with Peg-IFN and ribavirin for up to 44 weeks. All subjects experienced a decrease from baseline of at least 4 log_{10}, and 10 subjects had a decrease greater than 5 log_{10}. No viral breakthrough was seen. Viral sequencing analysis showed no evidence of previously identified telaprevir-resistant mutations in 10 subjects during study drug dosing. Although resistant mutations were noted in 2 subjects, their viral load continued to decline, again indicating sensitivity to Peg-IFN/ribavirin. HCV RNA was undetectable in 2 subjects within 8 days, and was undetectable in all at 28 days. All 12 subjects continued therapy, 8 of whom experienced an SVR, 2 of whom had viral breakthrough, and 2 of whom were lost to follow-up. All subjects experienced at least one adverse event, with influenza-like illness, fatigue, headache, nausea, anemia, depression, and pruritus the most frequent.[13]

Based on this background, the PROVE (PROtease inhibition for Viral Evaluation) phase II trials were initiated.

Key Points

- Telaprevir, 750 mg, every 8 hours results in maximal trough concentrations, and therefore optimized sustained HCV decline and the least viral breakthrough relative to the two other monotherapy doses studied.
- Early studies established that viral breakthrough secondary to resistance precludes consideration of use of telaprevir as monotherapy.
- Telaprevir-resistant variants are sensitive to Peg-IFN and ribavirin.

PHASE II STUDIES

PROVE 1

PROVE 1 studied the safety and efficacy of telaprevir in combination with Peg-IFN and ribavirin (PR) in treatment-naïve patients with HCV G1 without cirrhosis aged 18 to 65 years old in the United States.[14] It was designed as a phase IIb, randomized, double-blind, placebo-controlled, multicenter (37 centers) study. Exclusion criteria included infection with hepatitis B virus or HIV, cirrhosis on biopsy within 2 years, decompensated liver disease, hepatocellular carcinoma, another cause of clinically significant liver disease, absolute neutrophil count less than 1500/μL, and platelets less than

90,000/μL. Most study subjects were middle-aged (mean age, 48 years), white (77%), and male (63%), and 87% had a viral load greater than 800,000 IU/mL. Subjects were stratified by weight (>75 kg or ≤75 kg) and race (black or other). The study design included four treatment groups: (1) T12PR12 (telaprevir, 1250 mg on day 1 and then 750 mg every 8 hours thereafter for 12 weeks, and Peg-IFN, 180 μg/wk, and ribavirin, 1000–1200 mg/d, for the same 12 weeks; n = 17); (2) T12PR24 (telaprevir, 1250 mg, on day 1 and then 750 mg every 8 hours thereafter for 12 weeks, with Peg-IFN and ribavirin and then an additional 12 weeks of Peg-IFN and ribavirin; n = 79); (3) T12PR48 (telaprevir, 1250 mg on day 1 and then 750 mg every 8 hours thereafter for 12 weeks, with Peg-IFN and ribavirin, and then an additional 36 weeks of Peg-IFN and ribavirin; n = 79); (4) PR48 (control group receiving standard of care; n = 75). Standard stopping rules applied in the PR48 control group (2-log decline in HCV RNA by week 12 of treatment and undetectable viral load at week 24). Subjects in the T12PR24 and T12PR12 groups were required to have a rapid virologic response (RVR) (ie, HCV RNA undetectable) to stop therapy at 24 or 12 weeks, respectively. If they did not have an RVR at 4 weeks, they were treated to 48 weeks. If breakthrough occurred (>100 IU/mL after being undetectable or increase in RNA of 1-$\log_{10}$ unit) during the first 12 weeks, then telaprevir or placebo was discontinued and standard therapy was continued. If breakthrough did occur and the viral load was greater than 1000 IU/mL, then sequencing of the NS3/4A region was performed.[14]

SVR rates were 41% for the standard of care regimen (PR48), 35% for T12PR12, 61% for T12PR24, and 67% for T12PR48. Rates of RVR were also better in patients treated with telaprevir: 8% for PR48 versus 59% for T12PR12, 81% for T12PR24, and 81% for T12PR48. Relapse was less common in subjects treated with telaprevir for at least 24 weeks: 2% for T12PR24, 6% for T12PR48 versus 33% for T12PR12, and 23% for PR48. The rate of virologic breakthrough in patients treated with telaprevir was 7%, with most of the breakthroughs occurring in patients who had never cleared HCV RNA completely. In patients experiencing breakthrough, resistant variants were detected, with mutations including V36M, R155K (genotype 1a), or A156T (genotype 1b).[14] V36M and R155K/T variants are observed in patients with genotype 1a because of a lower genetic barrier; these mutations require only one nucleotide change in the triplet codon at the 36 and 155 positions compared with two changes required in genotype 1b.[11] The V36M and R155K/T variants are more fit than the A156T variant noted in patients with genotype 1b.[11]

The telaprevir-based groups had a higher rate of discontinuation of the overall treatment regimen because of adverse events compared with controls (21% vs 11%), with an increased frequency of rash, pruritus, nausea, diarrhea, and anemia. Twelve patients (7%) who received telaprevir developed severe rash and discontinued therapy versus one (1%) control. Erythropoiesis-stimulating agents were prohibited during the trial. The mean decline in hemoglobin was 3 g/dL in the control group, with an incremental rate of hemoglobin decline of 0.5 to 1 g/dL more in telaprevir-treated patients. After telaprevir was discontinued the hemoglobin increased.[14]

PROVE 1 showed superiority of combination therapy over standard of care and illustrated that a shorter treatment course could be considered with combination therapy. It suggested RVR as a required criterion for stopping therapy at earlier time points than the standard 48 weeks. Rash and anemia emerged as the most common side effects of therapy.[14]

PROVE 2

PROVE 2 was the European counterpart to PROVE 1. It evaluated the safety and efficacy of telaprevir in combination with Peg-IFN with or without ribavirin in treatment-naïve patients with HCV G1 without cirrhosis.[15] It was designed as a multicenter, randomized, partially double-blind, placebo-controlled phase IIb trial.

This trial had four treatment groups (total n = 334), including T12PR12, T12PR24, T12P12 (telaprevir and Peg-IFN only), and PR48. The ribavirin-free arm (T12P12) was distinct from PROVE 1, as was the equivalent number of patients in all four treatment arms. An RVR was not required for patients to stop therapy at the predefined stopping point in each treatment arm. Instead, patients in the T12PR24, T12PR12, and T12P12 groups were required to have undetectable HCV RNA levels at the last study visit before the planned end of treatment, which was week 10 for T12PR12 and T12P12 and week 20 for the T12PR24 group, or they went on to continue Peg-IFN/ribavirin for 48 weeks. SVR rates were 46% in the control group (PR), 36% in T12P12, 60% in T12PR12, and 69% in T12PR24. RVR rates were 13% in PR48, 50% in T12P12, 69% in T12PR24, and 80% in T12PR12. Relapse occurred in 22% of controls, 48% of patients treated without ribavirin (T12P12), 14% of patients in the T12PR24 group, and 30% of those in the T12PR12 group. A multivariate analysis showed that treatment group and baseline HCV RNA were the only two variables significantly associated with an SVR.[15]

HCV with low-level resistance was found at baseline in 1% of subjects. Among subjects with viral breakthrough who had sequencing performed, wild-type virus was noted in 5%, low-level resistance in 41%, and high-level resistance in 55%. Among subjects with relapse who had sequencing performed, wild-type virus was noted in 5%, low-level resistance in 79%, and high-level resistance in 17%.[15]

The median time to appearance of rash of any severity in the telaprevir-based groups was 9 to 12 days. Severe (grade 3) rash was found in 7% of patients (6 of 81) in the T12PR24 group, 6% (5 of 82) in the T12PR12 group, and 3% (2 of 78) in the T12P12 group, but was not seen in the PR48 group. Of the 163 patients in the combined T12PR24 and T12PR12 groups, 12 (7%) discontinued treatment because of rash.[15]

Key Points

- Telaprevir/Peg-IFN/ribavirin combination therapy is superior to the current standard treatment (Peg-IFN/ribavirin) of HCV in treatment-naïve patients without cirrhosis.
- Ribavirin is an essential component of combination therapy for HCV, even when telaprevir is used.
- The addition of telaprevir to standard therapy seems to permit a shorter treatment course of 24 weeks in treatment-naïve patients with chronic HCV G1 without cirrhosis (SVR = 61% for T12PR24 in PROVE 1, SVR = 69% for T12PR24 in PROVE 2)
- An SVR can be attained in substantial numbers of patients given triple therapy for 12 weeks, but higher rates of relapse and lower overall SVR rates led to exclusive focus on 24-week regimens in the phase III development program (see later discussion).
- Viral breakthrough is associated with resistance conferred by mutations, including V36M, R155K (genotype 1a), or A156T (genotype 1b)
- RVR was identified by PROVE 1 as a requirement for shortening the duration of therapy to 24 weeks.
- Baseline HCV viral load is predictive of response to telaprevir combination therapy.
- An increased frequency of rash and anemia is associated with telaprevir-based combination therapy

PROVE 2 confirmed that telaprevir is effective and has an acceptable tolerability profile when used in combination therapy for treatment-naïve patients with HCV G1, and that the clinical viral breakthrough that occurred during the dosing period was related to selection of viral variants with decreased sensitivity to telaprevir. It highlighted the importance of ribavirin in the treatment regimen. It showed that baseline viral load was predictive of response even with telaprevir therapy.[15]

PROVE 3

PROVE 3 was undertaken to evaluate the efficacy of telaprevir in patients with HCV infection who had not experienced a sustained response to an initial full course of treatment with Peg-IFN and ribavirin (ie, prior treatment failures).[16] PROVE 3 was an international, randomized, partially placebo-controlled, partially double-blind, phase II study. The study population included subjects with HCV G1 aged 18 to 70 years who were previously treated with Peg-IFN/ribavirin for at least 12 weeks and did not experience an SVR. They were stratified by type of treatment failure: nonresponse, relapse, or breakthrough. Of the subjects, 57% were considered to previously have experienced nonresponse, 36% relapse, and 7% breakthrough. Exclusion criteria included chronic hepatitis B virus, HIV, decompensated liver disease, hepatocellular carcinoma, another cause of clinically significant liver disease, absolute neutrophil count less than 1500/μL, and platelet count less than 100,000/μL. Subjects were required to have had a liver biopsy within 3 years. Unlike PROVE 1 and 2, PROVE 3 included patients with cirrhosis, which constituted 16% of the study population. Four treatment groups were included: (1) T12PR24, (2) T24PR48, (3) T24PR24, and (4) PR48. Those in the control group (PR48) were allowed to roll over and receive telaprevir after study conclusion. Telaprevir was dosed at 1125 mg on day 1 and then 750 mg orally every 8 hours. Stopping rules included breakthrough between weeks 4 and 24; less than 1-log drop by week 4 in the control group; HCV greater than 30 IU/mL at week 4 in the telaprevir-treated subjects; less than 2-log decline at week 12; and detectable virus at week 24.[16]

The T12PR24 and T24PR48 regimens were most efficacious and not statistically different from one another, with SVR rates of 51% and 53%, respectively, versus 24% with T24P24 and 14% with PR48. However, discontinuation of therapy because of adverse events was less common in the T12PR24 group than in the T24PR48 group. Rates of SVR were higher among subjects who had previously experienced a relapse (T12PR24, 69%; T24PR48, 76%; T24P24, 42%; and PR48, 20%) than among those who had not experienced a response to previous treatment (T12PR24, 39%; T24PR48, 38%; T24P24, 11%; and PR48, 9%). Fewer relapses occurred among the subjects in the T12PR24 and T24PR48 arms, with rates of 30% and 13% respectively, versus 53% in both the T24P24 and PR48 groups. For subjects in the T24PR48 group who actually completed treatment, relapse rates were 4% overall, 4% for patients with no previous response, 20% for those with previous breakthrough, and 0% for those with a previous relapse. More breakthroughs were seen among patients with genotype 1a then 1b, with rates of 24% versus 11%. In a subanalysis of this study, patients with cirrhosis had equivalent rates of SVR as those without cirrhosis.[16]

Logistic regression analysis showed that a sustained virologic response was significantly associated with assignment to the T12PR24 or T24PR48 group, an undetectable HCV RNA level during a previous period of treatment with Peg-IFN alpha and ribavirin, and low baseline viral load (<800,000 IU/mL). Most subjects who discontinued therapy because of a stopping rule had the V36M/R155K double variant; all but one of the subjects were infected with HCV genotype 1a.[16]

The overall efficacy and safety results indicate that the T12PR24 regimen seems to provide a better risk/benefit profile than the T24PR48 group.[16] This observation raised the question of whether selected patients who are tolerating treatment and have a significant risk of relapse (eg, genotype 1a patients) might optimize their treatment with a total of 48 weeks of therapy, perhaps with a total of 48 weeks of total therapy with an initial 12 weeks of telaprevir. This question is, in fact, what was studied in phase III (**Figs. 2–4**).

Key Points

- Telaprevir/Peg-IFN/ribavirin combination therapy is superior to a course of retreatment with Peg-IFN/ribavirin alone in patients infected with HCV for whom a course of standard therapy has failed.
- Patients with history of relapse after Peg-IFN/ribavirin have a higher SVR rate with telaprevir combination therapy than those with a prior nonresponse (69% vs 39% for T12PR24).
- Telaprevir/Peg-IFN/ribavirin combination therapy is safe and effective in patients with compensated cirrhosis.
- In prior treatment-experienced patients receiving telaprevir, viral breakthrough is more common among patients with genotype 1a infection than 1b infection (24% vs 11%), consistent with a lower genetic barrier to resistance for genotype 1a.

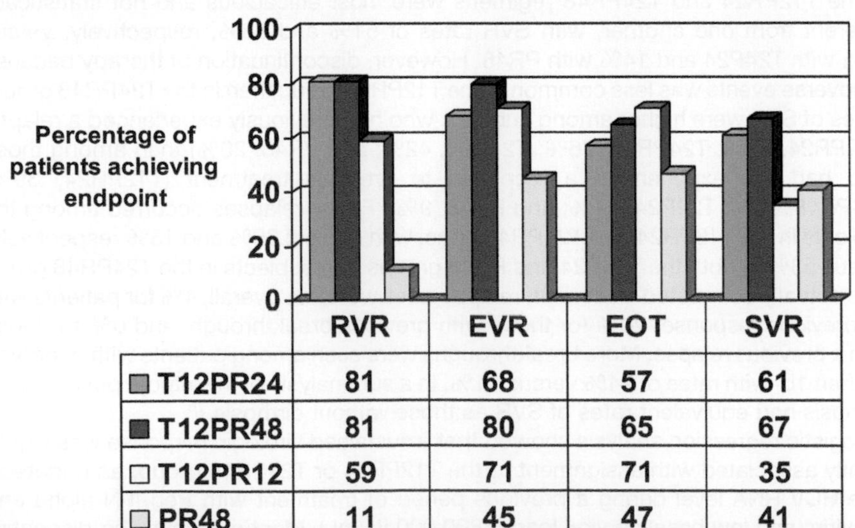

	RVR	EVR	EOT	SVR
T12PR24	81	68	57	61
T12PR48	81	80	65	67
T12PR12	59	71	71	35
PR48	11	45	47	41

Fig. 2. PROVE 1 efficacy data. EVR, early virologic response; EOT, end of treatment; RVR, rapid virologic response; SVR, sustained virologic response. Data reported are percentages.

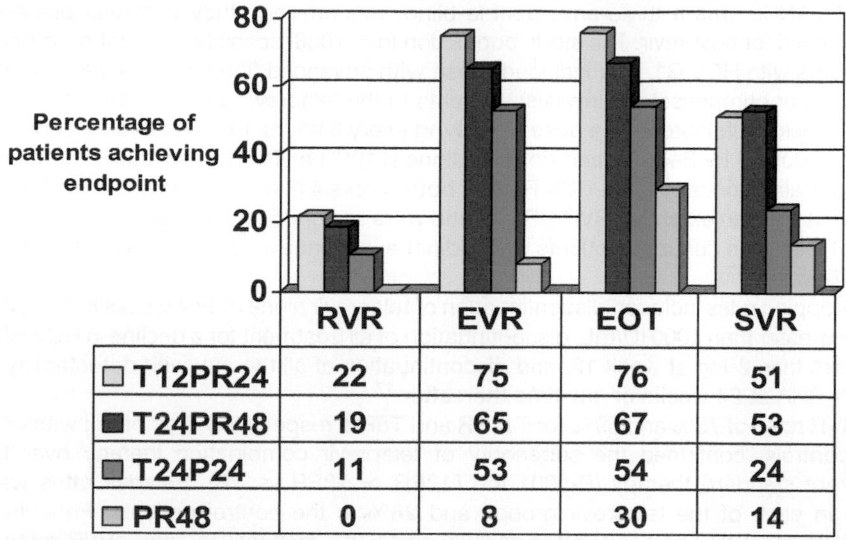

Fig. 3. PROVE 3 efficacy data. EVR, early virologic response; EOT, end of treatment; RVR, rapid virologic response; SVR, sustained virologic response.

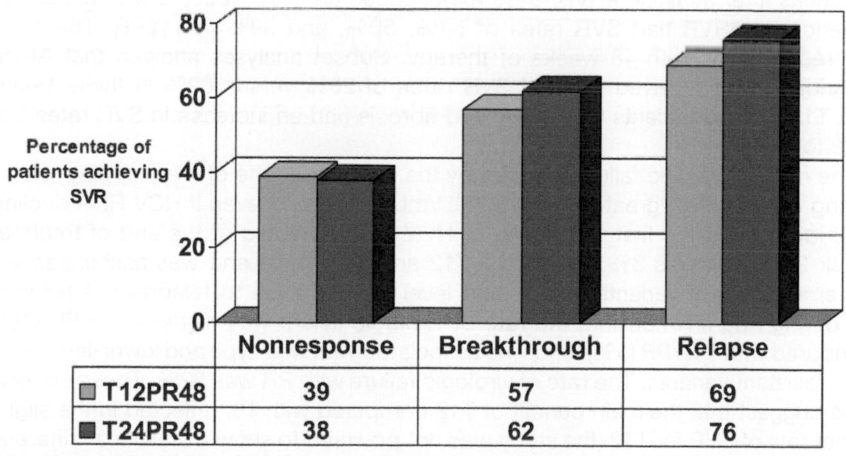

Fig. 4. PROVE 3 SVR according to prior treatment response.

PHASE III STUDIES

ADVANCE

ADVANCE was the pivotal phase III trial of telaprevir in treatment-naïve patients infected with HCV G1.[17,18] In addition to establishing the safety and efficacy of telaprevir for purposes of registration, it had two important goals: first, to explore an 8-week rather than 12-week course of telaprevir to assess whether the incidence or severity of side effects, particularly rash, could be reduced while preserving efficacy; and second, to assess the capacity to truncate therapy to 24 weeks in patients with robust viral responses and still attain high rates of SVR with minimal relapse.

ADVANCE was a three-arm, double-blind, randomized study that was placebo-controlled for telaprevir. The study population (n = 1088) consisted of treatment-naïve patients with HCV G1, and included those with advanced fibrosis (21%) (ie, bridging fibrosis or compensated cirrhosis). Patients in the telaprevir arms received either 12 or 8 weeks of telaprevir at a dose of 750 mg every 8 hours, Peg-IFN alfa-2a and ribavirin, followed by Peg-IFN and ribavirin alone (T12PR or T8PR, respectively). Patients who attained undetectable HCV RNA at both weeks 4 and 12 were defined as having experienced an extended RVR (eRVR), and were assigned to stop after total treatment of 24 weeks. In contrast, patients who did not experience an eRVR were treated for up to 48 weeks.[17]

Stopping rules included discontinuation of telaprevir alone after 4 weeks if HCV RNA was greater than 1000 IU/mL, discontinuation of all treatment for a decline in HCV RNA of less than 2-log at week 12, and discontinuation of all therapy with detectability of HCV RNA at 24 weeks or any time thereafter.[17]

SVR rates of 75% and 69% for T12PR and T8PR, respectively, compared with 44% in controls, confirmed the superiority of telaprevir combination therapy over the current standard therapy ($P<.001$ for T12PR or T8PR vs PR). Relapse rates were 9% in each of the telaprevir groups and 28% in the control patients. Patients in T12PR and T8PR had RVR rates of 68% and 67%, respectively, and eRVR rates of 58% and 57%, versus only 9% and 8% of controls. The patients with an eRVR were those assigned to 24 weeks of treatment; these patients had SVR rates of 89% (T12PR) and 83% (T8PR). Of the small number of patients who received PR for 48 weeks after attaining eRVR, 97% experienced an SVR. Patients who did not experience an eRVR had SVR rates of 54%, 50%, and 39% in T12PR, T8PR, and PR, respectively, with 48 weeks of therapy. Subset analyses showed that African Americans who received PR had SVR rates of 25% versus 62% in those treated with T12PR, and patients with advanced fibrosis had an increase in SVR rates from 33% to 62%.[17,18]

The rate of virologic failure, defined by the meeting of one of the stopping rules or having an HCV RNA greater than 1000 IU/mL at week 12 even if HCV RNA declined by 2 logs during the first 12 weeks, or HCV RNA detected at the end of treatment (week 24 or 48), was 3% in both the T12 and T8 groups and was associated with the emergence of variants with a high level of resistance to telaprevir. After week 12, during Peg-IFN/ribavirin, the rate of virologic failure was higher in T8/PR (10%) compared with T12/PR (5%), and was associated with wild-type and lower-level telaprevir-resistant variants. The rate of virologic failure with PR was 32%. These observations suggest that the main benefit of T12 compared with T8, reflected in the slightly higher rate of SVR for T12 (the study was not powered to show a statistical difference between T12 and T8), was more efficient clearance of wild-type and low-level telaprevir-resistant variants with the additional 4 weeks of telaprevir.[18]

Overall rates of treatment discontinuation for adverse events occurred in 10%, 10%, and 7% of patients in T12PR, T8PR, and PR, respectively. During the first 12 weeks of therapy, telaprevir/placebo alone was stopped in 11%, 7%, and 1%, respectively, because of adverse events overall. Telaprevir was associated with an increase in rash, anemia, diarrhea, pruritus, and nausea. Grade 3 rash occurred in 6%, 4%, and 1% of patients, respectively. The rash was primarily eczematous clinically and histologically. Severe rash was managed by sequentially discontinuing telaprevir, followed by ribavirin 7 days later if considered necessary, and then Peg-IFN for continued progression. Severe rash events led to discontinuation of telaprevir/placebo alone in 7%, 5%, and 1%, respectively. In contrast, discontinuation of all study drugs for rash events seldom occurred (1.4%, 0.5%, and 0%, respectively). The rash resolved on discontinuation.[17] The rash management plan was credited with a lower rate of overall treatment discontinuation for rash than occurred in the phase II programs.

A nadir hemoglobin of less than 10 g/dL occurred in 38% of patients treated with telaprevir and 14% of controls, whereas nadir hemoglobin less than 8.5 g occurred in 9% of patients treated with telaprevir and 2% of controls. As per the protocol, anemia was managed with ribavirin dose modifications, and erythropoiesis-stimulating agents were not allowed. Discontinuation of all drugs because of anemia events occurred in 1%, 3%, and 1% of patients in T12PR, T8PR, and PR, respectively; 4%, 2%, and 0% of patients, respectively, discontinued telaprevir/placebo only. By 24 weeks of therapy, hemoglobin levels were comparable among patients who had initially received telaprevir and controls. Treatment with 8 weeks of telaprevir, compared with 12 weeks, was associated with a similar rate of treatment discontinuation of the entire treatment regimen for adverse events during the first 12 weeks (8% vs 7%) (**Fig. 5**).[17]

ILLUMINATE

The ADVANCE study strongly suggested that 24 weeks of total therapy was sufficient in patients with eRVR, an inference derived from the high rates of SVR and low rates of relapse in patients with eRVR treated for 24 weeks. To support this concept, the supportive phase III, open-label, multicenter (N = 540) ILLUMINATE trial was undertaken.[19] Treatment-naïve patients with HCV G1 treated with 12 weeks of triple therapy (telaprevir, Peg-IFN, and ribavirin) and those who experienced an eRVR were randomized at week 20 to receive either 24 or 48 weeks of total Peg-IFN/ribavirin therapy to show noninferiority of the 24-week treatment course. Patients who did not experience an eRVR continued 48 weeks of therapy. The study population included patients with cirrhosis (11%).[19]

Noninferiority of the 24-week treatment regimen among subjects who experienced an eRVR was established by SVR rates of 92% for 24 weeks versus 88% for 48 weeks of therapy. Overall SVR rate in the intention-to-treat analysis was 72%. Permanent discontinuation of therapy because of adverse events occurred in 17.4% of subjects and was more common in the 48-week treatment group. ILLUMINATE affirmed the

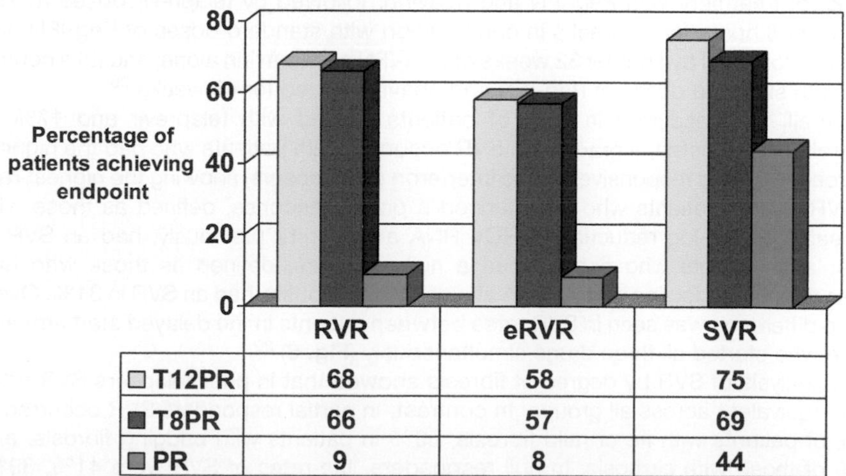

	RVR	eRVR	SVR
T12PR	68	58	75
T8PR	66	57	69
PR	9	8	44

Fig. 5. ADVANCE efficacy data. eRVR, extended rapid virologic response; RVR, rapid virologic response; SVR, sustained virologic response.

Key Points

- The phase III trials confirmed the significantly superior efficacy of telaprevir plus Peg-IFN and ribavirin versus Peg-IFN and ribavirin alone for HCV G1 infection.
- Response-guided therapy is valid for telaprevir/Peg-IFN/ribavirin combination therapy of treatment-naïve patients with G1 HCV. Patients who experience an eRVR may be successfully treated with 24 weeks of total therapy (telaprevir 750 mg orally every 8 hours in combination with Peg-IFN and ribavirin for 12 weeks, followed by Peg-IFN and ribavirin alone for an additional 12 weeks).
- Shortening telaprevir treatment from 12 to 8 weeks is associated with a reduced frequency of severe rash and slightly decreases the frequency of telaprevir discontinuation but does not affect the rate of overall discontinuation of therapy.
- Shortening telaprevir treatment from 12 to 8 weeks increases the rate of virologic failure during the peginterferon/ribavirin phase.
- The rash associated with telaprevir is generally eczematous. Severe rash should be managed by sequentially discontinuing telaprevir, ribavirin 7 days later as necessary, and then Peg-IFN if further progression.
- Telaprevir therapy results in an incremental rate of hemoglobin decline of approximately 1 g/dL more than Peg-IFN/ribavirin. Anemia was managed by ribavirin dose reduction alone, with erythropoiesis-stimulating agents being prohibited in the phase III trials.

foundation for response-guided therapy in telaprevir-containing combination treatment of HCV.[19]

REALIZE

The REALIZE trial (Re-treatment of Patients with Telaprevir-based Regimen to Optimize Outcomes) was conducted to further define telaprevir-based therapy in subjects for whom a previous course of Peg-IFN and ribavirin failed.[20] This trial included three treatment arms: (1) telaprevir dosed at 750 mg every 8 hours for 12 weeks in combination with standard doses of Peg-IFN and ribavirin, followed by 36 weeks of treatment with Peg-IFN and ribavirin alone; (2) a delayed-start arm, consisting of 4 weeks of treatment with Peg-IFN and ribavirin, followed by telaprevir dosed at 750 mg every 8 hours for 12 weeks in combination with standard doses of Peg-IFN and ribavirin, followed by another 32 weeks of Peg-IFN and ribavirin alone; and (3) a control arm with standard doses of Peg-IFN and ribavirin dosed for 48 weeks.[20]

Overall, SVR occurred in 65% of patients treated with telaprevir and 17% of controls. As expected, a gradient of SVR occurred, with patients who had the highest degree of intrinsic responsiveness to interferon (ie, relapsers) showing the highest rate of SVR (86%). Patients who experienced a partial response, defined as those with a greater than 2-log reduction in HCV RNA at week 12 previously, had an SVR in 57%; and patients who experienced a null response, defined as those who had a less than 2-log decline in HCV RNA at week 12 previously, had an SVR in 31%. Overall, no difference was seen in SVR rates between patients in the delayed start arm and those who started all three drugs simultaneously (**Fig. 6**).[20]

An analysis of SVR by degree of fibrosis showed that in prior relapsers SVR rates were equivalent across all groups. In contrast, in partial responders SVR occurred in 72% of patients with no or mild fibrosis, 56% in patients with bridging fibrosis, and 34% of those with cirrhosis. In null responders, the rates of SVR were 41%, 39%, and 14%, with 10% of the control patients who were null responder cirrhotics having SVR. Patients with genotype 1b had somewhat higher rates of SVR among partial

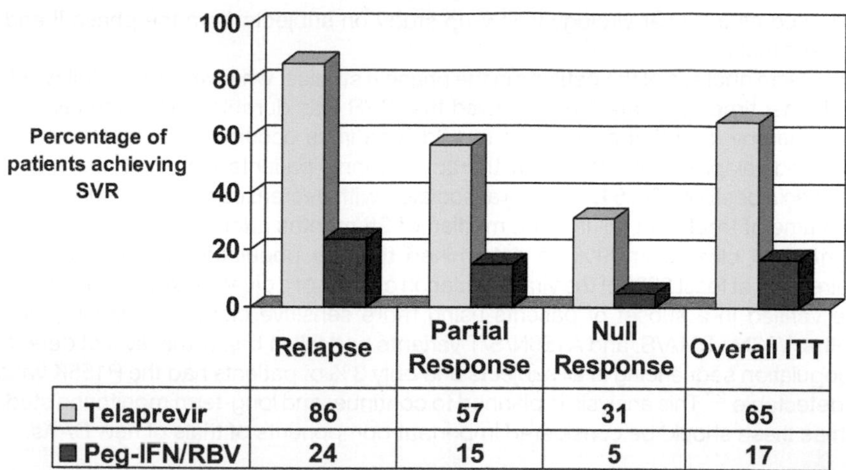

Fig. 6. REALIZE SVR according to prior treatment response. ITT, intention-to-treat; RBV, ribavirin.

and null responders than patients with genotype 1a. In the delayed start or lead-in arm, relapsers with HCV RNA reduction of less than 1 log after 4 weeks of Peg-IFN and ribavirin treatment had SVR of 62% versus 94% in those with greater degrees of viral decline; in partial responders SVR occurred in 56% and 59%; while in null responders those less than 1 log decline at week 4 of lead-in treatment had SVR in 15% versus 54% of those with better response at week 4.[21]

EXTEND

The capacity of HCV to become resistant to DAAs in general, including protease inhibitors, manifests itself in the resistant variants that are frequently detectable in patients with virologic failure or virologic breakthrough on therapy with telaprevir. Considerable concern has been expressed about the long-term fate and clinical impact of these resistant variants. If these variants are persistent, they could theoretically have an adverse impact on treatment outcomes if patients for whom a prior course of therapy with a protease inhibitor failed are being considered for retreatment with the same or similar drugs in future regimens of which they are a component. The EXTEND trial was

Key Points

- Telaprevir-based therapy offers a substantial chance of SVR in patients for whom prior treatment failed.
- A gradient of SVR is seen in retreated patients, with prior relapsers, partial responders, and null responders experiencing decreasing rates of SVR with 48 weeks of therapy. Prior null responders had the lowest SVR rates at 31%, but only 14% in null responders with cirrhosis.
- Currently no evidence shows that lead-in dosing with Peg-IFN and ribavirin, followed by triple therapy with telaprevir, affects treatment outcomes in treatment-experienced patients.
- SVR from telaprevir/Peg-IFN/ribavirin is durable.
- Resistant virus tends to revert to wild-type virus over time after discontinuation of therapy.

conducted as a 3-year virology follow-up study on subjects from the phase II and III telaprevir trials.[22]

An interim analysis of the patients in the phase II studies, who were hence followed up for a longer time as of late 2010, showed that SVR was durable (99%) with telaprevir-based therapy, and that a reversion to wild-type virus occurred in subjects who had developed telaprevir resistance on therapy. Among patients who had viral variants (amino acid positions 36, 54, 155, 156) associated with decreased telaprevir susceptibility at the time of treatment failure, at a median of 25 months after treatment the resistant variants had cleared in 89% as determined through population sequencing, which requires that at least 20% of the viral population consist of a given variant.[22] These results were verified in a subset of patients using more sensitive clonal sequencing. By 36 months, V36M, T54A/S, and A156N/S/T variants had fallen below the level of detection by population sequencing in all subjects and only 3% of patients had the R155K variant still detectable.[22] This analysis is planned to continue, and long-term monitoring studies such as these should be considered important components of trials of new DAAs.

TREATING WITH TELAPREVIR

The use of a protease inhibitor in conjunction with Peg-IFN and ribavirin can be considered the new standard of care in patients infected with HCV G1. Treatment-naïve patients with HCV G1 can undergo treatment in a response-guided fashion. However, as stated in the telaprevir package insert "treatment-naive patients with cirrhosis who have undetectable HCV-RNA at weeks 4 and 12 of telaprevir combination treatment may benefit from an additional 36 weeks of peginterferon alfa and ribavirin (48 weeks total)".[23] This is based on the small number of cirrhotics in the treatment-naive pivotal trials, making it difficult to formulate definitive conclusions about response-guided therapy in this population, and on the ILLUMINATE data which showed that in cirrhotics SVR rates were 67% (12/18) for the T12PR24 group and 92% (11/12) for the T12PR48 group.[19] Patients who have relapsed after a previous course of Peg-IFN/ribavirin are also eligible for response-guided therapy.

If telaprevir is chosen as the protease inhibitor with which a patient should be treated, triple therapy should be initiated simultaneously with telaprevir, followed by 750 mg (two 375 mg tabs) orally every 7–9 hours dosed with food containing approximately 20 gms of fat, Peg-IFN and, ribavirin 1000 to 1200 mg orally daily. Telaprevir monotherapy should never be used, because it will result in the emergence of resistant variants and lead to treatment failure.[10–12] As illustrated by PROVE2, ribavirin-free treatment is much less effective and more likely to lead to viral resistance.[15]

HCV RNA should be determined at week 4 of therapy. If HCV RNA remains greater than 1000 IU/mL, the entire treatment regimen should be discontinued.[23] At week 12, telaprevir should be discontinued, an HCV RNA assay should be performed, and Peg-IFN/ribavirin should be continued alone. However, if the HCV RNA is greater than 1000 IU/ml at week 12, the entire regimen should be discontinued. Note the difference between these stopping rules, as reflected in the telaprevir package insert, from those applied in the pivotal trials.

Moreover, the stopping rules are identical for treatment-naive and treatment experienced patients.

If an eRVR has been achieved with undetectable HCV RNA for treatment-naive patients and relapsers at both weeks 4 and 12, then the planned treatment duration can be reduced to a total of 24 weeks and 12 further weeks of Peg-IFN/ribavirin given. If an eRVR has not been achieved, then the planned treatment duration should remain at a total of 48 weeks and 36 further weeks of Peg-IFN/ribavirin given, provided that

HCV RNA is undetectable by week 24 and remains so throughout the treatment course. If HCV RNA is detectable at week 24, treatment should be discontinued.[17,19] Note that in clinical trials HCV-RNA in plasma was measured using a COBAS Taqman assay with a lower limit of quantification of 25 IU/mL and a limit of detection of 10 IU/mL; "detectable but below limit of quantification" should not be considered equivalent to an "undetectable".

Patients should be monitored during therapy with follow-up visits and laboratory testing, including complete blood cell count at 2 and 4 weeks and at least every 4 weeks during telaprevir treatment with periodic chemistries, liver function tests, and thyroid-stimulating hormone assessment. A greater mean level of hemoglobin decline than traditionally seen with Peg-IFN and ribavirin should be anticipated.[14,17] Anemia should be managed with ribavirin dose reductions. Although erythropoiesis-stimulating agents were not allowed in the phase III telaprevir development program and are not approved by the US Food and Drug Administration, they can be considered in patients on an individualized basis.

An eczematous rash can be expected to occur commonly. Severe rash (eg, rash involving over 50% of body surface area) should be managed with sequential discontinuation of telaprevir, followed by ribavirin 7 days later as necessary, and Peg-IFN as needed. Therapy need not be stopped all at once unless necessary in the clinician's judgement.[17] As indicated in the package insert, treatment of rash with oral antihistamines and/or topical corticosteroids may provide symptomatic relief but effectiveness of these measures has not been established and treatment of rash with systemic corticosteroids is not recommended. Although 12 weeks of telaprevir therapy is preferred, it may be discontinued at week 8 or thereafter with at most a slight impact on the subsequent chance of SVR.[17,18]

Telaprevir treatment should be discontinued for confirmed viral breakthrough during the first 12 weeks. Although the emergence of resistant viral variants is associated with treatment failure, evidence shows a tendency to reversion to wild-type after treatment discontinuation, which may allow for the possibility of later DAA therapy incorporating protease inhibitors.[22]

Currently data are insufficient to support telaprevir/Peg-IFN/ribavirin response-guided therapy in the treatment of patients with HCV G1 for in whom HCV RNA never became undetectable (ie, nonresponders). The phase III REALIZE trial was conducted without a response-guided component; all patients were assigned to 48 weeks of treatment. The approval for response guided therapy for relapsers is based upon phase 2 data showing, across two trials, SVR in 49/52 relapsers who were treated for 24 weeks after attaining RVR, in addition to the documented high level of responsiveness of relapsers.[20,23]

The treatment of prior null responders with telaprevir deserves particular mention. The success rates of just over 30% reported in these patients represent a more efficacious option than any prior treatment regimen. Unfortunately, for those who are in the greatest need of treatment, the cirrhotic null responders, SVR rates are lower at 14% per REALIZE).[20] Moreover, the price of treatment failure with telaprevir (or any protease inhibitor) is a substantial likelihood that the patient will be left with resistant variants. As with all patients in the new treatment era, the concept of resistance, and the basic aspects of what is understood about its potential implications, must be conveyed to patients in an understandable manner. Ultimately, we will need retreatment studies in patients who have failed protease inhibitor therapy to assess the long term impact of resistant variants. In the interim, the encouraging data on the decline in resistant variants over time indicate that no group of patients should be categorically denied therapy on the basis of resistance concerns.

It should be noted that the geriatric population was excluded from clinical study and therefore there was an insufficient number of patients aged 65 and over to determine whether they respond differently from younger patients.

Drug-drug interactions are an important theme with protease inhibitors, including telaprevir. The clinician must be familiar with the information in the package insert regarding these documented or potential interactions. Telaprevir is an inhibitor of CYP3A4. Therefore, co-administration of drugs that are dependent on CYP3A4 for clearance and have a narrow therapeutic margin may result in toxicity. Examples include certain statins (lovastatin, simvastatin, and atorvastatin) alfuzosin, ergot derivatives, and others. Drugs that induce CYP3A4 may result in reduced exposure to telaprevir. Finally, exposure to certain other drugs may be reduced by co-administration with telaprevir. An example of the latter is ethinyl estradiol, accounting for the guideline that hormonal contraceptives are not adequate as one of the two required methods of contraception for women of child bearing age during hepatitis C therapy while telaprevir is being given and for 2 weeks after telaprevir has been discontinued. The reader is reminded that for both female and male patients at least 2 forms of birth control must be used during treatment with Peg-IFN and ribavirin and for 6 months thereafter.

REFERENCES

1. Dienstag JL, McHutchinson JG. American Gastroenterological Association technical review on the management of hepatitis C. Gastroenterology 2006;130: 231–64.
2. World Health Organization. Hepatitis C. World Health Organization. 2000. Available at: http://www.who.int/mediacentre/factsheets/fs165/en. Accessed April 1, 2011.
3. El-Serag HB, Mason AC. Rising incidence of hepatocellular carcinoma in the United States. N Engl J Med 1999;340:745–50.
4. Kim WR. The burden of hepatitis C in the United States. Hepatology 2002; 36(Suppl):S30–4.
5. Ghany MG, Strader DB, Thomas DL, et al. AASLD practice guidelines: diagnosis, management, and treatment of hepatitis C: an update. Hepatology 2009;49: 1335–74.
6. Jacobson IM. Treatment options for patients with chronic hepatitis C not responding to antiviral therapy. Clin Gastroenterol Hepatol 2009;7:921–30.
7. Lohmann V, Körner F, Koch J, et al. Replication of subgenomic hepatitis C virus RNAs in a hepatoma cell line. Science 1999;285:110–3.
8. Lindenbach BD, Evans MJ, Syder AJ, et al. Complete replication of hepatitis C virus in cell culture. Science 2005;309:623–6.
9. Pawlotsky JM, Chevaliez S, McHutchison JG. The hepatitis C viral life cycle as a target for new antiviral therapies. Gastroenterology 2007;132:1979–98.
10. Reesink HW, Zeuzem S, Weegink CJ, et al. Rapid decline of viral RNA in hepatitis C patients treated with VX-950: a phase 1b, placebo-controlled, randomized study. Gastroenterology 2006;131:997–1002.
11. Kieffer TL, Sarrazin C, Miller JS, et al. Telaprevir and pegylated interferon-alpha-2a inhibit wild-type and resistant genotype 1 hepatitis c virus replication in patients. Hepatology 2007;46:631–9.
12. Forestier N, Reesink HW, Weegink CJ, et al. Antiviral activity of telaprevir (VX-950) and peginterferon alfa-2a in patients with hepatitis C. Hepatology 2007;46:640–8.
13. Lawitz E, Rodriguez-Torres M, Muir AJ, et al. Antiviral effects and safety of telaprevir, peginterferon alfa-2a, and ribavirin for 28 days in hepatitis C patients. J Hepatol 2008;49:163–9.

14. McHutchison JG, Everson GT, Gordon SC, et al. Telaprevir with peginterferon and ribavirin for chronic HCV genotype 1 infection. N Engl J Med 2009;360(18): 1827–38.
15. Hezode C, Forestier N, Dushieko G, et al. Telaprevir and peginterferon with or without ribavirin for chronic HCV infection. N Engl J Med 2009;360(18):1839–50.
16. McHutchison JG, Manns MP, Muir AJ, et al; PROVE3 Study Team. Telaprevir for previously treated chronic HCV infection. N Engl J Med 2010;362(14):1292–303.
17. Jacobson IM, McHutchison JG, Dusheiko G, et al. Telaprevir for previously untreated chronic hepatitis C virus infection. N Eng J Med 2011;364:2405–16.
18. Kieffer TL, Bartels D, Sullivan J, et al. Clinical virology results from telaprevir phase 3 study ADVANCE. 61st Annual Meeting of the American Association for the Study of Liver Disease (AASLD 2010). Boston (MA), October 29 to November 2, 2010 [abstract: ID#LB-11].
19. Sherman KE, Flamm SL, Afdhal NH, et al. Telaprevir in combination with peginterferon alfa2a and ribavirin for 24 or 48 weeks in treatment-naïve genotype 1 HCV patients who achieved an extended rapid viral response: final results of phase 3 ILLUMINATE study. 61st Annual Meeting for the American Association for the Study of Liver Disease (AASLD 2010). Boston (MA), October 29 to November 2, 2010 [abstract: ID#LB2].
20. Zeuzem S, Andreone P, Pol S, et al. Telaprevir for retreatment of HCV infection. N Eng J Med 2011;364:2417–28.
21. Foster GR, Zeuzem S, Andreone P, et al. Subanalyses of the telaprevir lead-in arm in the REALIZE Study: response at week 4 is not a substitute for prior null response categorization. J Hepatology 2011;54(Suppl 1):S3.
22. Zeuzem S, Sulkowski MS, Zoulim F, et al. Long term follow-up of patients with chronic hepatitis C treated with telaprevir in combination with peginterferon alfa-2a and ribavirin: interim analysis of the EXTEND study. Presented at: 61st Annual Meeting of the American Association for the Study of Liver Diseases (AASLD 2010). Boston (MA), October 29 to November 2, 2010 [abstract: 227].
23. Telaprevir (INCIVEK™) Package Insert, Vertex Pharmaceuticals.

Management of the Treatment-Experienced Patient Infected with Hepatitis C Virus Genotype 1: Options and Considerations

Omer Khalid, MD, Bruce R. Bacon, MD*

KEYWORDS

- Hepatitis C • Consensus interferon • Genotype 1
- NS3 protease inhibitor • Boceprevir • Telaprevir
- IL-28B polymorphism • Difficult-to-treat patients

An estimated number of 170 million people in the world are infected with hepatitis C virus (HCV). These individuals are at risk for cirrhosis and/or hepatocellular carcinoma (HCC). Prevalence of HCV infection has been recorded to be high in certain parts of the world like Africa and South East Asia and is considerably lower in the United States, with an estimated rate of around 1.8% of the population with positive HCV antibodies and an estimated number of 3.1 million individuals having active HCV infection.[1–3] Treatment of HCV infection has undergone several revisions over the past 15 years and continues to evolve. The current major advance is with the protease inhibitors in addition to pegylated interferon and ribavirin.

With the approval of peginterferon and ribavirin in 2001 by the Food and Drug Administration, this combination has become the standard of care for patients infected with HCV. Historically, sustained virologic response (SVR) rates for patients infected with genotype 1 receiving treatment with pegylated interferon and ribavirin

---

Omer Khalid, MD, has nothing to disclose. Bruce R. Bacon, MD, is a speaker, consultant, and a member of the Advisory Boards and the Data and Safety Monitoring Board with Merck, Roche Laboratories, Gilead Sciences, Bristol-Myers Squibb, Three Rivers Pharmaceuticals, Vertex, ISIS, Wyeth, and Romark Laboratories.

Division of Gastroenterology and Hepatology, St Louis University School of Medicine, 3635 Vista Avenue at Grand Boulevard, St Louis, MO 63110-0250, USA
* Corresponding author.
E-mail address: baconbr@slu.edu

Clin Liver Dis 15 (2011) 573–583
doi:10.1016/j.cld.2011.05.001
1089-3261/11/$ – see front matter

were 40% to 50%. SVR rates are even lower in difficult-to-treat patients, such as African Americans, with high baseline viral load or those with human immunodeficiency virus coinfection. The fact that more than one-third of the patients are classified as peginterferon/ribavirin nonresponders is becoming a major public health concern. These patients are at a higher risk for chronic liver disease, including decompensated cirrhosis and HCC. With the advancement of liver disease and development of HCC, the need for liver transplantation is growing along with a substantial economic burden.[4–9] The likelihood of achieving an SVR can be predicted by viral and host factors. Viral factors include genotype and viral level. Genotype does not predict the natural history of infection but, however, does predict the likelihood of treatment response and, in many cases, determines the duration of treatment. In most prospective studies, genotype is the strongest predictor of response; however, recently it has been shown that rapid virologic response (RVR) is a stronger predictor of SVR than genotype.[10] SVR rates are higher in patients infected with HCV genotypes 2 or 3 and lower pretreatment HCV RNA levels. Host factors of poor response include male sex, age at infection, duration of infection, race or ethnicity, presence of hepatic steatosis, genetic factors, and poor immune response.[11–16]

TREATMENT OVERVIEW

There are several potential approaches to the management of peginterferon/ribavirin nonresponders. Some clinicians are using the watchful waiting approach, whereas others are waiting for new antiviral therapies to emerge. Although the wait and watch approach seems reasonable for some patients, there are few a concerns that have to be kept in mind. There has to be ongoing monitoring of liver function, which should be done at appropriate regular intervals. If the patient has advanced fibrosis/cirrhosis, surveillance for HCC with routine imaging studies should be performed. The optimal approach to peginterferon/ribavirin nonresponders has not been established. In patients who have failed peginterferon/ribavirin–based therapy, limited data exist on retreatment with peginterferon and ribavirin. Retreatment with peginterferon and ribavirin has shown to be of benefit in patients who have previously failed therapy with conventional interferon and ribavirin therapy. However, current guidelines advise against the use of peginterferon and ribavirin for retreatment of patients who have once failed therapy with the same drugs.[17] Poynard and colleagues[18] conducted an open-label study evaluating the efficacy of pegylated interferon alfa-2b and weight-based ribavirin in patients with chronic HCV infection with significant fibrosis/cirrhosis who had previously failed treatment with interferon alfa/ribavirin. In total, 2312 patients were enrolled in the study, with 1425 patients who had received prior therapy with nonpegylated interferon/ribavirin and 865 patients who had previously been treated with peginterferon/ribavirin. Almost two-thirds of patients were nonresponders to previous therapy, 28% were relapsers, and 11% were treatment failures. Patients received 1.5 μg/kg/wk of peginterferon alfa-2b and daily weight-based ribavirin for 48 weeks. Patients with detectable HCV RNA at week 12 were offered randomization into maintenance studies. Overall, 22% of patients achieved SVR. Further analysis showed that patients, specifically nonresponders and relapsers, who were previously treated with nonpegylated interferon and ribavirin responded better to treatment than those who were previously treated with peginterferon and ribavirin. Similarly, relapsers responded better to retreatment than nonresponders, irrespective of previous treatments. Fifty-six percent of patients who had undetectable virus at week 12 achieved SVR. In contrast, only 12% of patients achieved SVR whose viral load dropped by 2 logs but was still detectable at week 12. Jensen and colleagues[19] studied the effects of extended treatment with pegylated interferon and ribavirin in patients who previously failed to respond to peginterferon-based therapy. Nine hundred fifty patients were randomized to 4 treatment groups: group A—received peginterferon alfa-2a (360 μg/wk) and ribavirin for 12 weeks, followed by peginterferon alfa-2a (180 μg/wk) plus ribavirin to complete 72 weeks of treatment; group B—received peginterferon alfa-2a (360 μg/wk) plus ribavirin for 12 weeks, followed by peginterferon alfa-2a (180 μg/wk) for 48 weeks in total; group C—received peginterferon alfa-2a (180 μg/wk) plus ribavirin for 72 weeks; and group D—received peginterferon alfa-2a (180 μg/wk) and ribavirin for 48 weeks. About 90% of patients enrolled in the study were white, and a similar percentage had HCV genotype 1 infection. Data analysis showed that treatment for 72 weeks increased the chances of SVR compared with that for 48 weeks. SVR rate in group A was 16% compared with 9% in group D. It also showed that the proposed fixed-dose induction therapy with peginterferon and ribavirin did not improve outcomes compared with the standard-dose regimen. Fifty-seven percent of patients had complete viral suppression at week 12 and achieved SVR after 72 weeks of treatment, compared with 35% of patients who were treated for 48 weeks, supporting the concept that viral negativity at week 12 was a strong predictor of SVR which was supported by less than 5% of patients achieving SVR who were noted to have a positive result for HCV at week 12 of therapy.

Consensus interferon (CIFN) is a genetically engineered molecule developed to have higher biologic activity than naturally occurring type 1 interferon alfa. As noted in previous studies, retreatment with peginterferon has yielded dismal SVR rates. Studies have been conducted to assess CIFN as a mode of treatment in patients who have not responded to peginterferon and ribavirin. A study by Kaiser and colleagues[20] evaluated response to extended treatment duration of 72 weeks in patients with genotype 1 with CIFN who had experienced a relapse after 48 weeks of treatment with peginterferon and ribavirin. Patients were randomized to receive either 9 μg/d of CIFN or 180 μg/wk of peginterferon alfa-2a for 72 weeks, both in combination with weight-based ribavirin. SVR rates were observed in 69% of patients who received CIFN versus 42% of those who received peginterferon, indicating a significantly higher SVR rate among those who were retreated with CIFN.

Leevy[4] evaluated the use of CIFN for retreatment of patients not responding to peginterferon. All patients who failed to exhibit a 2-log drop by week 12 were eligible and were switched to 15 μg of CIFN daily along with weight-based ribavirin. If patients had positive HCV RNA levels after 12 weeks of treatment, they were switched to daily CIFN for 3 months, than thrice-weekly injections of CIFN, whereas those who had greater than a 2-log drop by week 12 but still positive viral levels were continued on standard of care. Thirty-seven percent of CIFN-treated patients achieved an SVR with a relapse rate of only 14%. A phase 3 study, the DIRECT (daily dose CIFN and ribavirin) trial was conducted investigating the effect of 15 μg CIFN daily for retreatment of patients who did not respond to prior standard of care therapy with peginterferon and ribavirin. Patients were enrolled to receive either CIFN 9 μg/d (group 1) or 15 μg/d (group 2) plus weight-based ribavirin or a control group who did not receive any treatment (group 3). Five hundred forty-one patients were randomized for this study from multiple sites within the United States and Puerto Rico. The overall SVR rates for groups 1, 2, and 3 were 7%, 11%, and 0%, respectively. There was no statistical difference for SVR rates between groups 1 and 2. Further analysis showed that patients who demonstrated early virologic response had a higher likelihood of achieving SVR. In group 1, 81.3% of patients and 63.6% of patients in group 2 who achieved a complete early virologic response (CEVR) achieved an SVR. Patients who still had positive viral levels at week 12 but had a greater than 2-log drop in HCV RNA levels achieved 12% and

35% SVR rates in groups 1 and 2, respectively. Those patients who exhibited the greatest viral reduction on previous treatment with peginterferon and ribavirin had the best chance of achieving an SVR rate when receiving treatment with CIFN. SVR rates also varied with respect to the stage of fibrosis and, as expected, were lower in patients with higher levels of fibrosis as documented on pretrial biopsies. This trial demonstrated that patients with a high pretreatment viral load and advanced fibrosis had a lower chance of achieving SVR, whereas those who exhibited an early virologic response by week 12 have an excellent chance of achieving SVR.[9]

With the ongoing efforts to better understand treatment responses and variations, especially among African Americans, the recent discovery of polymorphism in the interleukin (IL)-28B gene have given new insight into the matter. Variations in the gene have been linked to variable response rates in people with chronic HCV infection. The IL-28 gene encodes IL-28, also known as interferon lambda, a cytokine with antiviral activity. Thompson and colleagues[21] evaluated 1671 patients who were genotyped as CC, CT, and TT for the IL-28B polymorphism and evaluated the on-treatment virologic response and SVR rates in patients infected with genotype 1. HCV RNA levels were checked at weeks 2 and 4 to detect ultrarapid virologic response and RVR and at week 12 to detect complete early virologic response (CEVR). The CC genotype was more frequently observed in Caucasians (37%) than Hispanics (29%) or African Americans (14%). The TT genotype was more commonly observed among African Americans (37%) than Hispanics (22%) and Caucasians (12%). The CC genotype was associated with improved early viral kinetics and viral suppression among all races such that the median reduction in viral load by week 2 of treatment was more than 2 logs.

Preliminary results presented at the 2011 European Association for the Study of Liver Diseases Congress correlated IL-28B polymorphisms and SVR rates in patients being treated with triple therapy using pegylated interferon, ribavirin, and boceprevir. A proportion of patients from 2 phase 3 trials (SPRINT-2 and RESPOND-2) who received boceprevir were tested for polymorphism in the IL-28B gene. In treatment-naive patients, SVR rates were higher by 50% in the CC patients compared with CT or TT, whereas in the boceprevir arms, they were 27% higher in the CC genotype compared with the CT and TT genotypes. For patients with prior treatment failure, there was a clear advantage for boceprevir in all categories. Multivariate analysis showed that IL-28B genotype was a stronger predictor than other baseline variables; however, it was not a stronger predictor when the week 4 response to pegylated interferon and ribavirin was included in the analysis. At present, IL-28B is being considered as one of the strongest pretreatment predictors of SVR, and further exploratory studies are ongoing at this time.[22]

NS3 PROTEASE INHIBITORS

With better understanding of the HCV life cycle and structural features of the HCV proteins, there has been a shift in investigational focus toward direct-acting antivirals (DAAs) that inhibit HCV proteins, which are essential for intracellular viral replication. The first 2 DAAs to emerge are the protease inhibitors boceprevir and telaprevir.[23,24]

Telaprevir is an orally bioavailable NS3 protease inhibitor that belongs to the alfa-ketoamides and binds to the enzyme covalently but reversibly. Two landmark phase 2 studies, PROVE-1 (conducted in the United States) and PROVE-2 (conducted in Europe), showed an excellent response to therapy in treatment-naive patients infected with genotype 1. Results showed SVR rates of up to 70% when telaprevir was added to the regimen consisting of peginterferon and ribavirin.[25,26] Subsequent (ADVANCE and ILLUMINATE) studies have been conducted evaluating SVR rates with telaprevir-based triple therapy in treatment-naive patients infected with genotype 1. Both the ADVANCE and

ILLUMINATE trials evaluated the possibility of tailoring treatment based on achieving early viral response, whereby those patients succeeding to exhibit such a response would be entitled to have a shorter duration of treatment, thus helping to minimize unnecessary drug exposure and stopping rules to minimize chances of resistance-associated variants. Thus, all such patients who achieve RVR and remain undetectable until week 12 (extended RVR) are eligible for 12 weeks of telaprevir with 24 weeks of pegylated interferon and ribavirin, whereas those who have a small amount of virus at week 4 but have negative viral load by week 12 will receive 12 weeks of telaprevir and 48 weeks of pegylated interferon and ribavirin.[27,28]

The PROVE-3 study was conducted with 453 patients enrolled in 53 international sites. Patients enrolled had not achieved SVR (including nonresponders, relapsers, and those with breakthrough) after having received a full course of therapy with peginterferon/ribavirin.[29] Patients were assigned to 4 treatment groups as follows: arm 1—patients received telaprevir/peginterferon/ribavirin for 12 weeks followed by placebo/peginterferon/ribavirin for another 12 weeks; arm 2—patients received telaprevir/peginterferon/ribavirin for 24 weeks followed by just peginterferon/ribavirin for an additional 24 weeks; arm 3—tested the effects of treatment without ribavirin and patients received telaprevir and peginterferon for 24 weeks; and arm 4—this was the control group in which patients received placebo/peginterferon/ribavirin for 24 weeks followed by only peginterferon/ribavirin for another 24 weeks. Peginterferon was provided as a subcutaneous injection of 180 μg/wk peginterferon alfa-2a, and ribavirin was dosed according to a weight-based regimen. Telaprevir was dosed at 750 mg every 8 hours, following an initial loading dose of 1125 mg. Several stopping rules were implemented in this study; all patients who had a viral breakthrough from week 4 through week 24 (increase in HCV RNA level of more than 100 IU/mL after being undetected) or a nonresponse by week 4 (a drop less than 1 log from baseline) or a nonresponse at week 12 (a drop less than 2 logs in HCV RNA from baseline) or for the control arm, detectable HCV RNA level at week 24 were taken off treatment. SVR rates were similar in arms 1 and 2: 51% and 53%, respectively. They were considerably lower in arm 3 with no ribavirin on board: 24% in arm 3 and 14% in the control group. When the data were evaluated by prior response to treatment, patients who were considered nonresponders exhibited SVR rates of 39%, 38%, 11%, and 9% in the arms 1 to 4 respectively. Patients with prior relapse to treatment had a much more successful response to telaprevir-based therapy, with 69% and 76% SVR rates in arms 1 and 2, and 42% and 20% in arms 3 and 4, respectively. Patients with cirrhosis also did well with the treatment, with similar results compared with those without advanced fibrosis. SVR rates of 53% in arm 1 and 45% in arm 2 were documented. Results show benefit for all patients who completed telaprevir-based therapy because SVR rates were maintained at 48 weeks after the end of treatment. The phase 3 REALIZE study showed overall SVR rates of 66% and specifically 86% in relapsers (24% control), 57% in partial interferon responders (15% control), and 31% in null responders (5% control). A lead-in arm was evaluated in this study, showing a 2% higher SVR rate. Patients not achieving at least a 1-log decline in virus achieved an SVR of 33%.[30]

Boceprevir is a structurally novel peptidomimetic ketoamide HCV NS3 protease inhibitor that binds reversibly to the NS3 active site. It is the other protease inhibitor that will be making its way to the main stream along with telaprevir. Initial phase 2 studies that were conducted in the Unites States and Europe (SPRINT-1) showed promising data for treatment-naive patients infected with genotype 1. They used a lead-in strategy with a hypothesis that both peginterferon and ribavirin reach a steady-state concentration in 4 weeks, allowing the patient's immune system to be optimally activated before the addition of a protease inhibitor. This approach was hypothesized to minimize the likelihood for the development of resistance. This strategy may also have the potential to define a patient's interferon responsiveness before adding the DAA.[23,24]

The phase II study (SPRINT-1) was conducted in treatment-naive patients infected with HCV genotype 1. Patients who received boceprevir had higher SVR rates compared with the control, and after 48 weeks of treatment, SVR rates of 75% were noted.[23,24] A phase III study (SPRINT-2) evaluated the effects of boceprevir in treatment-naive patients infected with HCV genotype 1 with 2 different cohorts: black and nonblack.[30] A response-guided arm was explored in this study and allowed roughly half of the patients to be treated with a 4-week lead-in followed by 24 weeks of triple therapy with boceprevir.[31] Response rates were again noted to be higher in patients who received boceprevir compared with the control group. SVR rates in non-blacks were close to 70%, whereas they were as high as 53% in the black cohort. These data confirmed that addition of boceprevir increased SVR rates among all patients, irrespective of race. In addition, this trial showed that the treatment duration could be tailored to individual patients who exhibit RVR in an attempt to minimize exposure to medication beyond necessity.

A nonresponder phase 3 study (RESPOND-2) (**Fig. 1**) was conducted to observe the effects of boceprevir on retreatment of patients infected with HCV genotype 1 who

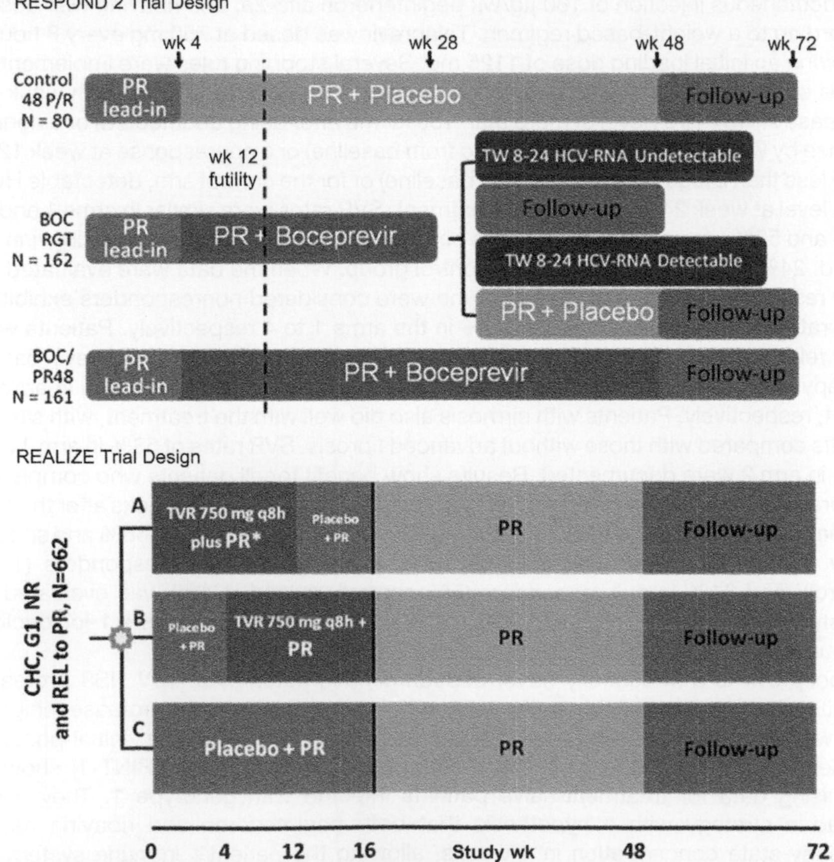

Fig. 1. Trial designs for RESPOND-2 and REALIZE trials.

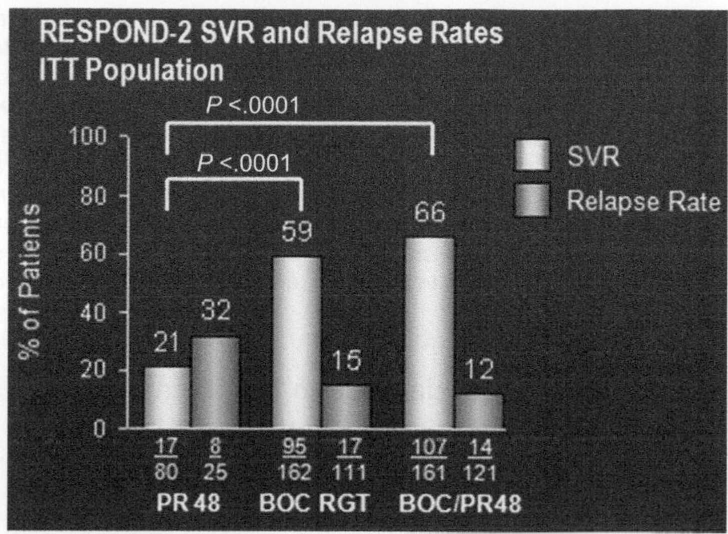

Fig. 2. SVR for RESPOND 2 trial.

had shown a partial response or had experienced relapse to previous treatment with standard therapy with interferon and ribavirin. In total, 403 patients were enrolled in this study and were assigned to 1 of the 3 arms. All patients received a 4-week lead-in with peginterferon and ribavirin. Patients in arm 1 received placebo plus

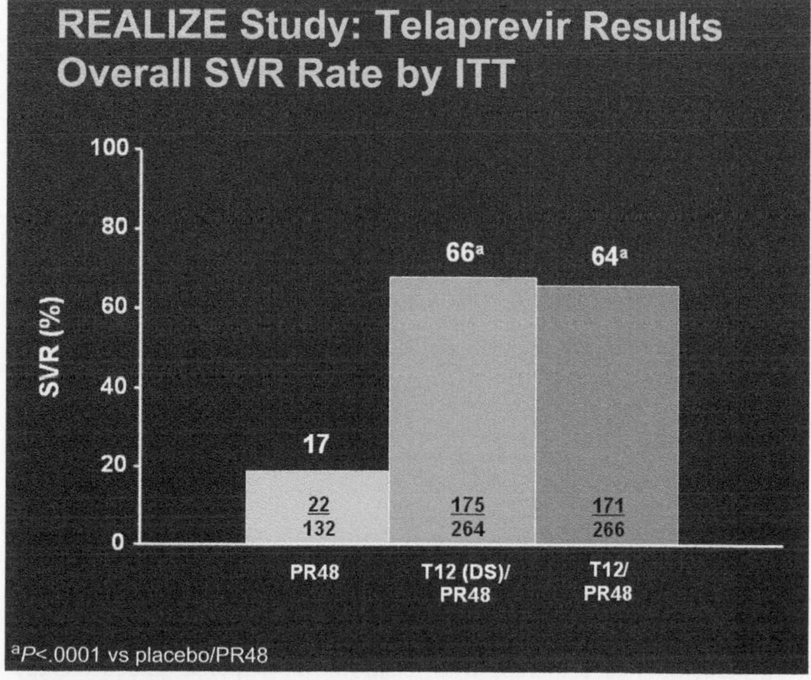

Fig. 3. REALIZE SVR results.

peginterferon and ribavirin for 44 weeks; arm 2 was the response-guided therapy arm in which patients who had undetectable HCV RNA at week 8 received a total of 36 weeks of therapy (lead-in with peginterferon/ribavirin followed by the addition of boceprevir for 32 weeks) and those who had detectable HCV RNA levels at week 8 but undetectable at treatment week 12 stopped boceprevir at week 36 but received an additional 12 weeks of peginterferon and ribavirin for a total treatment duration of 48 weeks. Patients in arm 3 received boceprevir with interferon and ribavirin for 44 weeks. SVR rates were significantly higher in patients receiving boceprevir compared with those being treated with interferon and ribavirin alone, with overall rates of 21%, 59%, and 66% (**Fig. 2**), respectively, in arms 1, 2, and 3. There was a higher incidence

A RGT With Telaprevir in Treatment-experienced Patients

Prior Relapsers (Same RGT as Naives):

HCV RNA	Triple Therapy: TVR + PegIFN/RBV	Dual Therapy: PegIFN/RBV	Total Treatment Duration
Undetectable at wk 4 and 12	First 12 wk	Additional 12 wk	24 wk
Detectable (1000 IU/mL or less) at wk 4 and/or 12	First 12 wk	Additional 36 wk	48 wk

Prior Partial or Null Responders:

HCV RNA	Triple Therapy: TVR + PegIFN/RBV	Dual Therapy: PegIFN/RBV	Total Treatment Duration
All Prior Partial and Null responders	First 12 wk	Additional 36 wk	48 wk

B Stopping Rules for Boceprevir in Previous Partial Responders and Relapsers

wk 8 HCV RNA*	wk 12 HCV RNA	wk 24 HCV RNA*	ACTION
Undetectable¶	**VL < 100 IU/mL**	**Undetectable**	**Complete three-medicine regimen at TW36**
Detectable	**VL < 100 IU/mL**	**Undetectable**	**1. Continue all three medicines until TW36; 2. Continue PR until TW48**
Detectable/ undetectable	**VL > 100 IU/mL**	**n/a**	**Discontinue all medications at wk 12**

¶ 46% of patients eligible for shorter duration therapy in RESPOND-2.

* PCR Assay LLQ should be < 25 IU/mL

Fig. 4. (*A*) Response guided therapy with telaprevir. (*B*) Response guided therapy with boceprevir.

of anemia noted in the boceprevir-containing regimens (43%–47%) compared with controls (20%); however, discontinuation rates because of anemia were infrequent, with 0%, 0%, and 3.1% in the respective arms (see **Fig. 1**).[31]

The REALIZE trial is the phase 3 trial of nonresponders using telaprevir and studied 2 telaprevir-based regimens compared with a peginterferon alfa-2a/ribavirin control. The main study arm was 12 weeks of telaprevir with 48 weeks of peginterferon and ribavirin. The other study arm used an exploratory lead-in of 4 weeks of peginterferon and ribavirin followed by 12 weeks of telaprevir and continuation of peginterferon and ribavirin up to 48 weeks. The control arm had an SVR rate of 17%, whereas the 2 study arms had SVR rates of 64% and 66% (**Fig. 3**). In a pooled analysis of both the study arms, relapsers had an SVR of 86%, partial responders 57%, and null responders 31%, all superior to controls.[32]

These data demonstrate that the addition of boceprevir or telaprevir to peginterferon and ribavirin leads to higher rates of SVR in patients who had previous therapy failures. Furthermore, patients who had experienced relapse to prior standard therapy experienced an SVR rate of 75% to 86%. Similarly, patients who did not respond to previous standard therapy were noted to have reasonable SVR rates up to 57%. The response-guided therapy concept was only used with boceprevir in treatment-experienced patients, allowing just less than half of the patients to have shortened therapy with 36 weeks of therapy rather than a 48-week backbone of peginterferon and ribavirin (**Fig. 4**).[33]

SUMMARY

These are exciting times for patients who have previously failed therapy with standard of care of peginterferon and ribavirin. Treatment with both boceprevir and telaprevir has proven to increase SVR rates by at least 20% more than the standard therapy of 48 weeks of peginterferon and ribavirin. The previous relapsers and those with some interferon responsiveness will clearly benefit from protease inhibitor–based therapy. Patients with little interferon response may not be ideally suitable for these regimens but can be treated based on careful selection on a case-by-case basis. The emergence of resistance needs to be monitored carefully as these newer and more potent drugs are added to the interferon and ribavirin backbone drugs. In addition, adverse events will be more frequent, and some novel ones will require special attention.

REFERENCES

1. Alter MJ, Kruszon-Moran D, Nainan OV, et al. The prevalence of hepatitis C virus infection in the United States, 1988 through 1994. N Engl J Med 1999;341(8): 556–62.
2. WHO. Hepatitis C—global prevalence. Wkly Epidemiol Rec 1999;49:425–7.
3. Lauer MG, Walker DB. Hepatitis C virus infection. N Engl J Med 2001;345(1): 41–52.
4. Leevy CB. Consensus interferon and ribavirin in patients with chronic hepatitis C who were nonresponders to pegylated interferon alfa-2b and ribavirin. Dig Dis Sci 2008;53:1961–6.
5. Saracco G, Rizzetto M. Predictors of response to interferon therapy. Dig Dis Sci 1996;41:115S–20S.
6. Moreno L, Quereda C, Moreno A, et al. Pegylated interferon alpha2b plus ribavirin for the treatment of chronic hepatitis C in HIV infected patients. AIDS 2004;18:67–73.

7. Kasahara A, Hayashi N, Mochizuki K, et al. Risk factors for hepatocellular carcinoma and its incidence after interferon treatment in patients with chronic hepatitis C. Hepatology 1998;27:1394–402.
8. Yoshida H, Shiratori Y, Moriyama M, et al. Interferon therapy reduces the risk for hepatocellular carcinoma: national surveillance program of cirrhotic and noncirrhotic patients with chronic hepatitis C in Japan. Ann Intern Med 1999;131: 174–81.
9. Bacon BR, Shiffman ML, Mendes F, et al. Retreating chronic hepatitis C with daily interferon Alfacon-1/ribavirin after nonresponse to pegylated interferon/ribavirin: direct results. Hepatology 2009;49:1838–46.
10. Fried MW, Hadziyannis SJ, Shiffman ML, et al. Rapid virological response is the most important predictor of sustained virological response across genotypes in patients with chronic hepatitis C virus infection. J Hepatol 2011. [Epub ahead of print].
11. Hoofnagle JH. A step forward in therapy for hepatitis C. N Engl J Med 2009; 360(18):1899–901.
12. Fried MW, Shiffman ML, Reddy KR, et al. Peginterferon alfa-2a plus ribavirin for chronic hepatitis C virus infection. N Engl J Med 2002;347:975–82.
13. Manns MP, McHutchison JG, Gordon SC, et al. Peginterferon alfa-2b plus ribavirin compared with interferon alfa-2b plus ribavirin for initial treatment of chronic hepatitis C: a randomized trial. Lancet 2001;358:958–65.
14. Hadziyannis SJ, Sette H Jr, Morgan TR, et al. Peginterferon alfa-2a (40 kilodaltons) and ribavirin combination therapy in chronic hepatitis C: a randomized study of the effect of treatment duration and ribavirin dose. Ann Intern Med 2004;140:346–55.
15. Conjeevaram HS, Fried MW, Jeffers LJ, et al. Peginterferon and ribavirin treatment in African American and Caucasian American patients with hepatitis C genotype 1. Gastroenterology 2006;131:470–7.
16. Rodriguez-Torres M, Jeffers LJ, Sheikh MY, et al. Peginterferon alfa-2a and ribavirin in Latino and non-Latino whites with hepatitis C. N Engl J Med 2009;360:257–67.
17. Ghany GM, Strader BD, Thomas LD, et al. Diagnosis, management, and treatment of hepatitis C: an update. Hepatology 2009;49(4):1335–74.
18. Poynard T, Colombo M, Bruix J, et al. Peginterferon alfa-2b and ribavirin: effective in patients with hepatitis C who failed interferon alfa/ribavirin therapy. Gastroenterology 2009;136:1618–28.
19. Jensen DM, Marcellin P, Freilich B, et al. Re-treatment of patients with chronic hepatitis C who do not respond to peginterferon-alfa2b. Ann Intern Med 2009; 150:528–40.
20. Kaiser S, Lutze B, Sauter B, et al. Retreatment of HCV genotype 1 relapse patients to peginterferon/ribavirin therapy with an extended treatment regimen of 72 weeks with consensus interferon/ribavirin versus peginterferon alpha/ribavirin. Hepatology 2007;46(4 Suppl 1):819.
21. Thompson AJ, Muir AJ, Sulkowski MS, et al. Interleukin-28B polymorphism improves viral kinetics and is the strongest pretreatment predictor of sustained virologic response in the genotype 1 hepatitis C virus. Gastroenterology 2010; 139:120–9.
22. Poordad F, Bronowicki JP, Gordon SC, et al. IL28B polymorphism predicts virologic response in patients with hepatitis C genotype 1 treated with boceprevir (BOC) combination therapy. J Hepatol 2011;54:S6.
23. Kwo PY, Lawitz EJ, McCone J, et al. Efficacy of boceprevir, an NS3 protease inhibitor, in combination with peginterferon alfa-2b and ribavirin in treatment-

naive patients with genotype 1 hepatitis C infection (SPRINT-1): an open-label, randomised, multicentre phase 2 trial. Lancet 2010;376(9742):705–16.
24. Berman K, Kwo PY. Boceprevir, an NS3 protease inhibitor of HCV. Clin Liver Dis 2009;13(3):429–39.
25. McHutchison JG, Everson GT, Gordon SC, et al. Telaprevir with peginterferon and ribavirin for chronic HCV genotype 1 infection. N Engl J Med 2009;360:1827–38.
26. Hézode C, Forestier N, Dusheiko G, et al. Telaprevir and peginterferon with or without ribavirin for chronic HCV infection. N Engl J Med 2009;360:1839–50.
27. Sherman KE, Flamm SL, Afdhal NH. Telaprevir in combination with peginterferon alfa2a and ribavirin for 24 or 48 weeks in treatment-naive genotype 1 HCV patients who achieved an extended rapid viral response: final results of phase 3 ILLUMINATE study. 61st AASLD; Boston (MA), October 29 to November 2010. Hepatology 2010;52:106A.
28. Jacobson IM, McHutchison GJ, Dusheiko MG. Telaprevir in combination with peginterferon and ribavirin in genotype 1 HCV treatment-naive patients: final results of phase 3 ADVANCE study. 61st AASLD; Boston (MA), October 29 to November 2010. Hepatology 2010;52:427A.
29. McHutchison JG, Manns MP, Muir AJ, et al. Telaprevir for previously treated chronic HCV infection. N Engl J Med 2010;362:1292–303.
30. Poordad F, McCone J Jr, Bacon BR, et al. Boceprevir with peginterferon/ribavirin for untreated chronic hepatitis C. N Engl J Med 2011;54:1195–206.
31. Bacon BR, Gordon SC, Lawitz E, et al. Boceprevir for treatment of chronic hepatitis C genotype 1 nonresponders. N Engl J Med 2011;54:1207–17.
32. Foster GW, Zeuzem S, Andreone P, et al. Telaprevir-based therapy in genotype 1 hepatitis C virus-infected patients with prior null response, partial response or relapse to peginterferon/ribavirin: REALIZE Trial Final Results. Oral presentation, Asia Pacific Association for the Study of Liver, Bangkok (Thailand), February 18, 2011.
33. Poordad F. Big changes are coming in hepatitis C. Curr Gastroenterol Rep 2011; 13(1):72–7.

The HIV/HCV-Coinfected Patient and New Treatment Options

Marie-Louise C. Vachon, MD, MSc[a,b], Douglas T. Dieterich, MD[b,*]

KEYWORDS

- HIV • Hepatitis C • Coinfection • Treatment
- Direct-acting antivirals

Hepatitis C treatment is on the cusp of change with the approval of the first direct-acting antivirals (DAAs) by the Food and Drug Administration. The addition of a hepatitis C virus (HCV) protease inhibitor (PI) to the combination of peginterferon (pegIFN) and ribavirin (RBV) will increase the proportion of patients achieving sustained virological response (SVR) while allowing shorter treatment durations with response-guided therapy (RGT) in HCV–monoinfected patients. In human immunodeficiency virus (HIV)/HCV-coinfected patients, the first clinical trials evaluating safety and efficacy of HCV PIs are under way. Drug-drug interactions (DDIs) with HIV antiretrovirals (ARVs), increased toxicity, and rapid selection of HCV-resistant mutants are among the treatment complexities expected in this difficult-to-treat population. The results of these trials should be available in 2011. Meanwhile, focus should be on strategies to optimize management of HIV/HCV-coinfected patients with currently available options. Successful management depends primarily on identification of patients in need of treatment. When possible, clinicians should attempt to correct factors affecting response to HCV treatment before initiating state-of-the-art HCV treatment, and preemptively treat potential side effects; for example, starting antidepressants in anticipation of treatment in patients who previously required antidepressants.

Marie-Louise C. Vachon has nothing to disclose.
Douglas T. Dieterich has received grants, contracts and honoraria for consulting and speaking from Boehringer Ingelheim, Idenix, Pharmasset, Merck, Vertex, Tibotec, Gilead, and BMS.
[a] Division of Infectious Diseases, Mount Sinai School of Medicine, 1, Gustave L. Levy Place, New York, NY 10029, USA
[b] Division of Liver Diseases, Mount Sinai School of Medicine, 1, Gustave L. Levy Place, New York, NY 10029, USA
* Corresponding author.
E-mail address: Douglas.dieterich@mountsinai.org

Clin Liver Dis 15 (2011) 585–596
doi:10.1016/j.cld.2011.05.006 liver.theclinics.com
1089-3261/11/$ – see front matter

HCV AND MORTALITY IN HIV/HCV-COINFECTED PATIENTS

HIV infection negatively affects the natural history of chronic hepatitis C, increasing the rate of progression to cirrhosis, end-stage liver disease, hepatocellular carcinoma (HCC), and death compared with HCV–monoinfected individuals.[1–3] Data concerning the impact of HCV on the natural history of HIV disease are conflicting.[4–6] Since the introduction of combination antiretroviral therapy (cART), morbidity and mortality caused by liver diseases, mostly chronic hepatitis C, are rising in the aging HIV population.[7,8] In a recent meta-analysis of studies performed in the cART era, HIV/HCV-coinfected patients had a 35% increased overall mortality (relative risk 1.35; 95% confidence interval 1.11–1.63) compared with HIV–monoinfected patients and this was unrelated to HIV disease progression.[9] Efforts should focus on primary prevention of HCV transmission and on secondary prevention by aggressively treating HCV in HIV-infected individuals. Treating acute HCV in HIV-infected men who have sex with men (MSM) is an excellent opportunity for secondary prevention. SVR, defined as undetectable HCV RNA 24 weeks after HCV treatment completion, reduces liver-related complications and mortality in HIV/HCV-coinfected patients. **Table 1** defines commonly used terms related to HCV treatment.[10]

CURRENT STANDARD OF CARE

The current standard of care in coinfected patients is pegIFN-alfa + RBV for 48 weeks, for all genotypes.[11] The 2 formulations of pegIFN (α-2-a and α-2-b) have comparable efficacy and safety in coinfected patients.[12] The combination of pegIFN and RBV leads to SVR in 14% to 38% of patients with HCV genotype 1 and in 44% to 73% of patients with HCV genotypes 2 and 3 with an overall SVR rate of 27% to 44% (**Table 2**).[13–17] Weight-based RBV (1000 mg for patients <75 kg and 1200 mg for those ≥75 kg) led to high rates of SVR in patients of all genotypes in the nonrandomized PRESCO trial.[18] However, the randomized clinical trial PARADIGM did not find a significant advantage of weight-based RBV in terms of SVR in patients with HCV genotype 1, except in subgroup analyses where African American and Latino patients benefited from it.[17]

Table 1
Definitions of commonly used acronyms related to treatment of hepatitis C

Acronym	Definition
RVR	Rapid Virological Response; Undetectable hepatitis C virus (HCV) RNA at treatment week 4
EVR	Early Virological Response
pEVR	Partial EVR; 2 $\log_{10}$ drop of HCV RNA at treatment week 12 compared with baseline
cEVR	Complete EVR; Undetectable HCV RNA at treatment week 12 compared with baseline
eRVR	Extended Rapid Virological Response; Undetectable HCV RNA at treatment week 4 that remains undetectable at week 12
EOT	End of treatment; Undetectable HCV RNA at the end of the treatment period
SVR	Sustained Virological Response; Undetectable HCV RNA 24 weeks after treatment completion
RGT	Response-Guided Therapy; In trials of direct-acting antivirals, individualization of HCV treatment duration according to virological response

Table 2
Summary of results from pioneer trials in HIV/HCV coinfected patients

Study	N	Treatment	SVR (%) All	SVR (%) Gt-1	SVR (%) Non Gt-1
RIBAVIC[16]	412	PegIFN-α-2b + RBV 800 mg versus	27	17	44
		IFN-α-2b + RBV 800 mg	20	6	43
ACTG[14]	133	PegIFN-α-2a + RBV 600 mg[a] versus	27	14	73
		IFN-α-2a + RBV 600 mg[a]	12	6	33
APRICOT[13]	860	PegIFN-α-2a + RBV 800 mg versus	40	29	62
		IFN-α-2a + RBV 800 mg	12	7	20
LAGUNO[15]	93	PegIFN-α-2b + W/B RBV	44	38	53
		IFN-α-2b + W/B RBV	21	7	47
PRESCO[18]	389	PegIFN-α-2a + W/B RBV Gt-1: 48W versus 72W Non Gt-1: 24W versus 48W	50	36	72

Abbreviations: GT-1, HCV genotype 1; non Gt-1, genotypes 2 and 3; HCV, hepatitis C virus; HIV, human immunodeficiency virus; IFN, interferon; N, number of patients; pegIFN, pegylated interferon; RBV, ribavirin; SVR, sustained virological response; W, weeks; W/B, weight-based.

[a] Dose-escalation schedule, 600 mg × 4 weeks, 800 mg × 4 weeks, 1000 mg thereafter.

Most experts still recommend weight-based RBV to treat patients with HCV genotype 1. Several factors can affect response to HCV treatment in HIV/HCV-coinfected patients and explain the wide range of SVR from one clinical trial to the other. With the current standard of care, identifying these factors can (1) better guide clinicians and patients in the decision to initiate/reinitiate HCV treatment and (2) point to an individual patient's potentially modifiable negative predictors that, when corrected, can make the difference between treatment success and treatment failure.

FACTORS AFFECTING RESPONSE TO HCV TREATMENT

Because of the relatively low SVR with interferon-based therapy and the significant side-effect profile, several baseline and on-treatment factors have been identified to explain differences in response and better target patients most likely to respond to treatment. Various host and viral baseline factors have been consistently associated with SVR, such as HCV genotypes 2 and 3 as opposed to HCV genotypes 1 and 4, low baseline viral load (HCV RNA threshold varies among studies), no prior HCV treatment, non-Hispanic white as opposed to black patients, low fibrosis stage, younger age, female sex, lower weight, and others. The cumulative dosage of drugs taken (both pegIFN and RBV) and achievement of rapid virological response (RVR) are examples of well-recognized on-treatment factors associated with higher SVR rates. The effects of these factors are discussed in detail elsewhere[11] and will not be reviewed here but, instead, a review of the latest possible predictive factors of response to treatment is presented (**Box 1**).

GENETIC DETERMINANTS OF RESPONSE

Genome-wide association studies have recently identified interleukin 28B (IL28B) gene polymorphisms as strong predictors of response to pegIFN and RBV therapy in both HCV–monoinfected and HIV/HCV-coinfected patients.[19,20] HIV-coinfected patients with HCV genotype 1 infection having the homozygous C/C genotype at the single nucleotide polymorphism (SNP) rs12979860 near the IL28B gene are significantly

Box 1
How to improve SVR in 2011

- Control the HIV first; improve the CD4^{+} T-cell count to as high as possible
- Rule out other causes of liver disease so they can be treated
  - Sometimes liver biopsy is the best way to do that
- For acute HCV, diagnose early and treat early
- Be aware of the effect of steatosis and steatohepatitis on response to treatment and attempt to correct insulin resistance
- Assess 25 (OH)D status and replete if insufficient (<30 ng/mL)
- Watch for drug-drug interactions with pegIFN/RBV: didanosine, stavudine, zidovudine, and abacavir
- Maximize doses of pegIFN and RBV
- Be aware of IL28B status
- Use longer treatment durations when possible
- Follow-up regularly and at close intervals during HCV treatment; identify and treat side effects to increase adherence

Abbreviations: HCV, hepatitis C virus; IL28B, interleukin 28B; pegIFN, pegylated interferon; RBV, ribavirin; SVR, sustained virological response; 25 (OH)D, 25-hydroxyvitamin D.

more likely to achieve SVR with standard of care than those with the C/T or T/T genotype (65% vs 30%, respectively; *P*<.001).[19] Among these 164 HIV/HCV-coinfected patients undergoing HCV treatment, 46% had the CC genotype versus 44% with the CT genotype and 10% with the unfavorable TT genotype. IL28B genotype in patients with HCV genotypes 3 and 4 was not significantly associated with SVR in this study although there was a trend for the HCV genotype 4 alone. The C allele is most commonly found in patients of Asian and European ancestries and is uncommon in those of African ancestry. This finding only partly explains the lower treatment response rate among HCV-infected patients of black race. Other genetic determinants of response likely exist, as reported recently. For example, an SNP (rs4242392) of the tumor necrosis factor–related apoptosis-inducing ligand receptor 1 gene predicted poor outcome to HCV therapy in 53 HIV/HCV-coinfected individuals undergoing interferon-based therapy.[21]

VITAMIN D STATUS

Vitamin D is an immune modulator. Patients with chronic HCV infection have a higher incidence of vitamin D deficiency compared with healthy controls matched for age and sex.[22,23] Among HCV–monoinfected patients, low 25-hydroxyvitamin D (25[OH]D) levels have been related to severe liver fibrosis and a low likelihood of response to HCV treatment.[22,23] In this last study, a CYP27B1-1260 promoter polymorphism significantly affected 1,25-dihydroxyvitamin D serum levels and SVR rates in patients with HCV genotype 1 infection. Vitamin D supplementation was also shown to improve response to HCV treatment in patients with HCV genotype 1 infection[24] and in post-transplant recurrent hepatitis C.[25] Vitamin D deficiency (25[OH]D <10 ng/mL) is common among HIV-infected individuals and patients of black race.[26,27] Both HIV-coinfection and black race are predictive of a low likelihood of response to HCV treatment. There is a clear need for studies of the influence of vitamin D deficiency on HCV treatment response in HIV/HCV-coinfected patients of all races and ethnicities as well as studies of the impact of vitamin D supplementation on treatment response. Although there is no official recommendation, we test 25(OH)D levels on every HIV/HCV-coinfected patient and we attempt to replete those who have insufficient levels (<30 ng/mL) before undergoing HCV treatment.

INSULIN RESISTANCE

HCV is associated with insulin resistance (IR) in HIV-infected patients.[28] IR has been associated with liver steatosis and advanced liver fibrosis both in HCV–monoinfected patients[29,30] and HIV/HCV-coinfected patients.[31,32] Several studies have identified IR as independent negative predictor of SVR in HCV mono-infection.[33,34] Its association with SVR in coinfection has been recognized more recently both at the time of initial HCV treatment[35,36] and at retreatment of HIV/HCV-coinfected patients.[37] One study did not find IR to be a significant predictor of SVR.[38] IR is a host factor potentially modifiable with dieting, weight loss, and use of insulin-sensitizing agents. Whether improving insulin sensitivity before initiating HCV treatment might affect SVR rates is not clear. Although it is logical to assume that it would, the results of studies in HCV–monoinfected patients have not clearly demonstrated a benefit.[39–41] A study in HIV/HCV-coinfected patients is under way (ACTG 5239).

CD4$^+$ T-CELL COUNT

The baseline CD4$^+$ T-cell count might influence SVR rates, although its importance as a predictor of response is inconsistent from one study to another. In a recent study, patients infected with HCV genotype 1 tended to achieve higher SVR rates at higher baseline CD4$^+$ T-cell counts.[42] No such association was found in patients infected with HCV genotypes 2 and 3. When HCV treatment is considered, clinicians should attempt to increase the CD4$^+$ T-cell count before starting HCV treatment, without deferring treatment when the expected rise does not occur. When HIV is controlled, there is no CD4$^+$ T-cell threshold under which HCV treatment has been shown to be ineffective or unsafe, although data on HCV treatment outcomes in HIV-infected patients with low CD4$^+$ T-cell count are scarce.

TREATMENT DURATION

The standard duration of HCV treatment in HIV-infected patients is 48 weeks. An option often considered for slow responders or relapsers to prior HCV treatment is to extend treatment duration. For patients infected with HCV genotype 1, evidence shows that extending treatment duration from 48 to 72 weeks can improve SVR.[43] In HIV/HCV-coinfected patients, the question as to whether treatment extension is beneficial is still being debated. In the nonrandomized PRESCO trial, patients infected with HCV genotype 1 treated for 72 weeks had a significantly higher SVR rate than those treated for 48 weeks, but with a high drop-out rate of 80% (36/45) in the extended treatment duration arm.[18] In a recent report from Spain, extending treatment from 12 to 15 months significantly improved the chance of SVR in HIV/HCV-coinfected patients not achieving RVR.[44] In a Brazilian randomized multicenter trial of 180 HIV/HCV-coinfected patients, extension of treatment to 72 weeks was significantly associated with SVR by per-protocol analysis (31 [39%] vs 19 [25%], $P = .04$).[45] It did not reach significance by intention-to-treat analysis, although there was a trend (31 [37%] vs 19 [24%], $P = .54$). In this study, extending treatment duration from 48 to 72 weeks reduced relapse rate, as expected.[46] Among patients with end-of-treatment (EOT) response who completed 48 weeks of therapy, 47.4% achieved SVR compared with 75.7% of those who completed 72 weeks of therapy ($P = .02$). We have completed a randomized study in the United States comparing 48 to 72 weeks of treatment for patients achieving HCV RNA undetectability at week 24.[47] In this study, there was no difference in SVR between 48 and 72 weeks of treatment because of a high drop-out rate in the 72-week treatment group. Based on these preliminary results, it seems that treatment extension can be beneficial for the minority of patients who are able to adhere to 72 weeks of treatment.

ACUTE HCV IN HIV

In the past decade, reports of increasing incidence of acute HCV among HIV-infected MSM have come from Europe, the United States, and Australia.[48] Patients at risk are MSM who report unprotected anal intercourse and traumatic sexual practices with or without concomitant ulcerative sexually transmitted infections (STIs). HIV-infected patients are less likely to spontaneously clear acute HCV compared with patients who are not infected with HIV, and once the infection becomes chronic, they are also less likely to respond to HCV treatment. In patients who do not spontaneously clear, early initiation of HCV treatment leads to higher SVR rates. Thus, the recommendations are to monitor HCV RNA at presentation and every 4 weeks thereafter in patients presenting with acute HCV. In the cases where HCV RNA has not decreased 2 $\log_{10}$ by week 4 or in the cases where HCV RNA is still detectable at week 12, it is recommended to promptly initiate HCV treatment. In the latest recommendations, the combination of pegIFN and RBV is recommended for the treatment of acute HCV.[48] Treatment duration depends on achievement of RVR. Patients who achieve RVR should be treated for 24 weeks, whereas those not achieving RVR should be considered for 48 weeks of therapy. The same stopping rules apply as in the treatment of chronic HCV.

NEW HCV TREATMENT OPTIONS

The first data on the use of DAAs in HIV/HCV-coinfected individuals will soon be published. Currently, 2 phase II trials are under way in the United States to test safety and efficacy of the 2 HCV PIs, telaprevir and boceprevir, in combination with pegIFN and RBV in HIV/HCV-coinfected patients. No clinical data have been published yet, and many questions still remain to be answered. Potential DDIs between HIV ARVs and HCV PIs are challenging (**Fig. 1**).[49] Certain DDIs have been recognized between ARVs and the current standard of care, pegIFN and RBV. Didanosine and, to a lesser extent, stavudine are known to increase the risk of mitochondrial toxicity with concomitant RBV use.[50] The combination of zidovudine with pegIFN and RBV is associated with severe anemia. Abacavir (ABC)-based regimens have been reported to be associated with lower SVR rates as compared with tenofovir-based regimens.[51,52] RBV and ABC are both guanosine analogs. Intracellular inhibitory competition for phosphorylation is the most likely explanation. Telaprevir and boceprevir can be enhanced by co-dosing or "boosting" with low-dose ritonavir, a potent cytochrome P-450 CYP3A inhibitor,[53] although it seems that telaprevir concentrations are increased only after the first doses are given and is lost thereafter.[54] Like in treatment of HIV, this effect can be used to the patient's advantage to improve efficacy and dosing intervals, and/or to reduce toxicity of HCV PIs. Two HCV PIs (danoprevir [aka R05190591] and ABT-450) are currently being studied in combination with low-dose ritonavir in HCV–monoinfected patients. Several commonly used drugs metabolized by CYP3A will potentially interact with HCV PIs, such as other HIV PIs, HIV non-nucleoside reverse transcriptase inhibitors, ketoconazole, erythromycin, and others.

Antiretrovirals		Anti-HCV drugs			
		Standard of care for HIV/HCV co-infected patients		Protease inhibitors approved by the FDA for treatment of HCV	
		pegIFN	ribavirin	boceprevir (BOC)	telaprevir (TVR)
PIs	atazanavir/ ritonavir	No clinically significant interaction	Potentially increased hyperbili-rubinemia		TVR AUC ↓ 20% ATZ AUC ↑ 17%
	darunavir/ ritonavir				TVR AUC ↓ 35% DRV AUC ↓ 40%
	fosamprenavir/ ritonavir				TVR AUC ↓ 32% fAPV AUC ↓ 47%
	lopinavir/ ritonavir				TVR AUC ↓ 54% LPV AUC unchanged
	ritonavir			BOC AUC ↓ 19%	TVR AUC increased on day 1 only
NNRTIs	efavirenz			BOC AUC ↓ 19% EFV AUC ↑ 20%	TVR AUC ↓ 18%[a] EFV AUC ↓ 18%
NRTIs	abacavir		Possible decrease in SVR rates[c]		
	emtricitabine		No clinically significant interaction		
	didanosine		Increased risk of lactic acidosis		
	lamivudine		No clinically significant interaction		
	stavudine		Increased risk of lactic acidosis		
	tenofovir			BOC AUC unchanged TDF AUC unchanged	TVR AUC ↓ 18%[a,b] TDF AUC ↑ 10%[a,b]
	zidovudine		Increased risk of anemia	Potentially increased risk of anemia	Potentially increased risk of anemia

[a] Telaprevir administered at 1125 mg every 8 hours instead of 750 mg every 8 hours.
[b] Tenofovir and efavirenz administered in combination.
[c] Potential competition for metabolic pathway since both are guanosine analogs.

Fig. 1. Known drug-drug interactions between HIV antiretrovirals, pegylated interferon and ribavirin, and the newly-approved HCV protease inhibitors boceprevir and telaprevir. ATZ, atazanavir; AUC, area under the curve; BOC, boceprevir; DRV, darunavir; EFV, efavirenz; fAPR, fosamprenavir; FDA, food and drug administration; HCV, hepatitis C virus; HIV, human immunodeficiency virus; LPV, lopinavir; NNRTIs, non nucleoside reverse transcriptase inhibitors; NRTIs, nucleos (t) ide reverse transcriptase inhibitors; PIs, protease inhibitors; SVR, sustained virological response; TDF, tenofovir disoproxil fumarate; TVR, telaprevir. (*From* Seden K, Back D, Khoo S. New directly acting antivirals for hepatitis C: potential for interaction with antiretrovirals. J Antimicrob Chemother 2010;65:1082; with permission; Garg V, Luo X, McNair L, et al. Low-dose RTV and the Pharmacokinetics of the Investigational HCV Protease Inhibitor TVR in Healthy Volunteers. CROI 2011 [abstract: #629]; Kassera C, Hughes E, Treitel M, et al. Clinical pharmacology of BOC: metabolism, excretion, and drug-drug interactions. CROI 2011 [abstract: #118]; Van Heeswijk R, Vandevoorde A, Boogaerts G, et al. Pharmacokinetic interactions between ARV agents and the investigational HCV protease inhibitor TVR in healthy volunteers. CROI 2011 [abstract: #119].)

Other HCV DAA classes, such as polymerase inhibitors and cyclophilin inhibitors, that might eventually undergo testing in HIV/HCV-coinfected patients have distinct potential interactions with ARVs.[49]

Because HIV and HCV PIs have some structural resemblances (although different protein targets), it has been suggested that HIV PIs might induce changes in the HCV protease. In a study of 28 HIV/HCV-coinfected patients in whom the HCV NS3 gene was sequenced before and after HIV PI use, there was no evidence of selection of resistance mutations after HIV PI use.[55]

HCV–monoinfected patients naïve to HCV treatment harbor anti-HCV drug-resistance mutations at baseline.[56,57] This is because of a rapid replication rate of the HCV virus (10^{12} virions daily) and a highly error-prone NS5B polymerase. Although no data are currently available on the prevalence of baseline resistance mutants in HIV/HCV-coinfected patients, it is expected to be more important than in HCV–monoinfected patients at least because of the higher HCV viral load. This raises the question of which and how many drugs will be needed to rapidly suppress HCV RNA and prevent the emergence of resistance in these patients. The role pegIFN and RBV play in preventing emergence of resistance mutations during treatment with DAAs may turn out to be more important in HIV/HCV-coinfected patients in whom a higher HCV viral load and a slower viral decline in response to treatment predispose to emergence of HCV resistance.

SUMMARY

With the introduction of the first 2 HCV PIs, the year 2011 for HCV is analogous to 1995 for HIV: 2011 will usher in the new era of DAAs for HCV and offer great hope for curing HCV in the vast majority of patients, instead of in a vanishingly small minority of patients with HIV. There will be many more DAAs arriving on the scene in the next few years, offering the possibility of combinations of HCV DAAs with different mechanisms of action and quite possibly excluding interferon from the mixture. The role for RBV in interferon-free combinations is under study, but so far the data are in favor of RBV. The complexity of HIV regimens is immense and the potential permutations for combining HCV DAA drugs is nearly incomprehensible. The combination of HCV DAAs and HIV ARVs will be challenging to manage, but the arrival of DAAs for HCV offers the opportunity to cure the number 1 killer of patients with HIV today: hepatitis C.

REFERENCES

1. Giordano TP, Kramer JR, Souchek J, et al. Cirrhosis and hepatocellular carcinoma in HIV-infected veterans with and without the hepatitis C virus: a cohort study, 1992-2001. Arch Intern Med 2004;164(21):2349–54.
2. Martinez-Sierra C, Arizcorreta A, Diaz F, et al. Progression of chronic hepatitis C to liver fibrosis and cirrhosis in patients coinfected with hepatitis C virus and human immunodeficiency virus. Clin Infect Dis 2003;36(4):491–8.
3. Merchante N, Giron-Gonzalez JA, Gonzalez-Serrano M, et al. Survival and prognostic factors of HIV-infected patients with HCV-related end-stage liver disease. AIDS 2006;20(1):49–57.
4. Potter M, Odueyungbo A, Yang H, et al. Impact of hepatitis C viral replication on CD4+ T-lymphocyte progression in HIV-HCV coinfection before and after antiretroviral therapy. AIDS 2010;24(12):1857–65.
5. Sulkowski MS, Moore RD, Mehta SH, et al. Hepatitis C and progression of HIV disease. JAMA 2002;288(2):199–206.

6. Peters L, Mocroft A, Soriano V, et al. Hepatitis C virus coinfection does not influence the CD4 cell recovery in HIV-1-infected patients with maximum virologic suppression. J Acquir Immune Defic Syndr 2009;50(5):457–63.
7. Data Collection on Adverse Events of Anti-HIV drugs (D:A:D) Study Group, Smith C, Sabin CA, et al. Factors associated with specific causes of death amongst HIV-positive individuals in the D:A:D Study. AIDS 2010;24(10):1537–48.
8. Weber R, Sabin CA, Friis-Moller N, et al. Liver-related deaths in persons infected with the human immunodeficiency virus: the D:A:D study. Arch Intern Med 2006; 166(15):1632–41.
9. Chen TY, Ding EL, Seage GR III, et al. Meta-analysis: increased mortality associated with hepatitis C in HIV-infected persons is unrelated to HIV disease progression. Clin Infect Dis 2009;49(10):1605–15.
10. Berenguer J, Alvarez-Pellicer J, Martin PM, et al. Sustained virological response to interferon plus ribavirin reduces liver-related complications and mortality in patients coinfected with human immunodeficiency virus and hepatitis C virus. Hepatology 2009;50(2):407–13.
11. Soriano V, Puoti M, Sulkowski M, et al. Care of patients coinfected with HIV and hepatitis C virus: 2007 updated recommendations from the HCV-HIV International Panel. AIDS 2007;21(9):1073–89.
12. Berenguer J, Gonzalez-Garcia J, Lopez-Aldeguer J, et al. Pegylated interferon {alpha}2a plus ribavirin versus pegylated interferon {alpha}2b plus ribavirin for the treatment of chronic hepatitis C in HIV-infected patients. J Antimicrob Chemothor 2009;63(6):1256–63.
13. Torriani FJ, Rodriguez-Torres M, Rockstroh JK, et al. Peginterferon Alfa-2a plus ribavirin for chronic hepatitis C virus infection in HIV-infected patients. N Engl J Med 2004;351(5):438–50.
14. Chung RT, Andersen J, Volberding P, et al. Peginterferon Alfa-2a plus ribavirin versus interferon alfa-2a plus ribavirin for chronic hepatitis C in HIV-coinfected persons. N Engl J Med 2004;351(5):451–9.
15. Laguno M, Murillas J, Blanco JL, et al. Peginterferon alfa-2b plus ribavirin compared with interferon alfa-2b plus ribavirin for treatment of HIV/HCV co-infected patients. AIDS 2004;18(13):F27–36.
16. Carrat F, Bani-Sadr F, Pol S, et al. Pegylated interferon alfa-2b vs standard interferon alfa-2b, plus ribavirin, for chronic hepatitis C in HIV-infected patients: a randomized controlled trial. JAMA 2004;292(23):2839–48.
17. Rodriguez-Torres M, Slim J, Lea B. Standard versus high dose ribavirin in combination with peginterferon alfa-2a (40KD) in genotype 1 (G1) HCV patients coinfected with HIV: final results of the PARADIGM study. An Oral Presentation AASLD 60th Meeting, 2009 [abstract: 1561].
18. Nunez M, Miralles C, Berdun MA, et al. Role of weight-based ribavirin dosing and extended duration of therapy in chronic hepatitis C in HIV-infected patients: the PRESCO trial. AIDS Res Hum Retroviruses 2007;23(8):972–82.
19. Rallon NI, Naggie S, Benito JM, et al. Association of a single nucleotide polymorphism near the interleukin-28B gene with response to hepatitis C therapy in HIV/hepatitis C virus-coinfected patients. AIDS 2010;24(8):F23–9.
20. Ge D, Fellay J, Thompson AJ, et al. Genetic variation in IL28B predicts hepatitis C treatment-induced viral clearance. Nature 2009;461(7262):399–401.
21. Rizza SA, Cummins NW, Rider DN, et al. Polymorphism in tumor necrosis factor-related apoptosis-inducing ligand receptor 1 is associated with poor viral response to interferon-based hepatitis C virus therapy in HIV/hepatitis C virus-coinfected individuals. AIDS 2010;24(17):2639–44.

22. Petta S, Camma C, Scazzone C, et al. Low vitamin D serum level is related to severe fibrosis and low responsiveness to interferon-based therapy in genotype 1 chronic hepatitis C. Hepatology 2010;51(4):1158–67.
23. Lange CM, Bojunga J, Ramos-Lopez E, et al. Vitamin D deficiency and a CYP27B1-1260 promoter polymorphism are associated with chronic hepatitis C and poor response to interferon-alfa based therapy. J Hepatol 2011;54(5):887–93.
24. Mouch SA, Fireman Z, Jarchovsky J, et al. Vitamin D supplement improves SVR in chronic hepatitis C (genotype 1) naive patients treated with pegInterferon and ribavirin. J Hepatol 2010;52(Suppl 1):S26.
25. Bitetto D, Fabris C, Fornasiere E, et al. Vitamin D supplementation improves response to antiviral treatment for recurrent hepatitis C. Transpl Int 2011;24(1):43–50.
26. Mueller NJ, Fux CA, Ledergerber B, et al. High prevalence of severe vitamin D deficiency in combined antiretroviral therapy-naive and successfully treated Swiss HIV patients. AIDS 2010;24(8):1127–34.
27. Childs KE, Fishman SL, Constable C, et al. Short communication: inadequate vitamin D exacerbates parathyroid hormone elevations in tenofovir users. AIDS Res Hum Retroviruses 2010;26(8):855–9.
28. Howard AA, Lo Y, Floris-Moore M, et al. Hepatitis C virus infection is associated with insulin resistance among older adults with or at risk of HIV infection. AIDS 2007;21(5):633–41.
29. Hui JM, Sud A, Farrell GC, et al. Insulin resistance is associated with chronic hepatitis C virus infection and fibrosis progression [corrected]. Gastroenterology 2003;125(6):1695–704.
30. Camma C, Bruno S, Di Marco V, et al. Insulin resistance is associated with steatosis in nondiabetic patients with genotype 1 chronic hepatitis C. Hepatology 2006;43(1):64–71.
31. Sterling RK, Contos MJ, Smith PG, et al. Steatohepatitis: risk factors and impact on disease severity in human immunodeficiency virus/hepatitis C virus coinfection. Hepatology 2008;47(4):1118–27.
32. Ryan P, Berenguer J, Michelaud D, et al. Insulin resistance is associated with advanced liver fibrosis and high body mass index in HIV/HCV-coinfected patients. J Acquir Immune Defic Syndr 2009;50(1):109–10.
33. Romero-Gomez M, Del Mar Viloria M, Andrade RJ, et al. Insulin resistance impairs sustained response rate to peginterferon plus ribavirin in chronic hepatitis C patients. Gastroenterology 2005;128(3):636–41.
34. D'Souza R, Sabin CA, Foster GR. Insulin resistance plays a significant role in liver fibrosis in chronic hepatitis C and in the response to antiviral therapy. Am J Gastroenterol 2005;100(7):1509–15.
35. Cacoub P, Carrat F, Bedossa P, et al. Insulin resistance impairs sustained virological response rate to pegylated interferon plus ribavirin in HIV-hepatitis C virus-coinfected patients: HOMAVIC-ANRS HC02 Study. Antivir Ther 2009;14(6):839–45.
36. Ryan P, Resino S, Miralles P, et al. Insulin resistance impairs response to interferon plus ribavirin in patients coinfected with HIV and hepatitis C virus. J Acquir Immune Defic Syndr 2010;55(2):176–81.
37. Vachon ML, Factor SH, Branch AD, et al. Insulin resistance predicts re-treatment failure in an efficacy study of peginterferon-alpha-2a and ribavirin in HIV/HCV co-infected patients. J Hepatol 2011;54(1):41–7.
38. Merchante N, de los Santos-Gil I, Merino D, et al. Insulin resistance is not a relevant predictor of sustained virological response to pegylated interferon plus ribavirin in HIV/HCV co-infected patients. J Hepatol 2009;50(4):684–92.

39. Romero-Gomez M, Diago M, Andrade RJ, et al. Treatment of insulin resistance with metformin in naive genotype 1 chronic hepatitis C patients receiving peginterferon alfa-2a plus ribavirin. Hepatology 2009;50(6):1702–8.
40. Khattab M, Emad M, Abdelaleem A, et al. Pioglitazone improves virological response to peginterferon alpha-2b/ribavirin combination therapy in hepatitis C genotype 4 patients with insulin resistance. Liver Int 2009;30(3):447–54.
41. Overbeck K, Genne D, Golay A, et al. Pioglitazone in chronic hepatitis C not responding to pegylated interferon-alpha and ribavirin. J Hepatol 2008;49(2):295–8.
42. Opravil M, Sasadeusz J, Cooper DA, et al. Effect of baseline CD4 cell count on the efficacy and safety of peginterferon Alfa-2a (40KD) plus ribavirin in patients with HIV/hepatitis C virus coinfection. J Acquir Immune Defic Syndr 2008;47(1):36–49.
43. Farnik H, Lange CM, Sarrazin C, et al. Meta-analysis shows extended therapy improves response of patients with chronic hepatitis C virus genotype 1 infection. Clin Gastroenterol Hepatol 2010;8(10):884–90.
44. Barreiro P, Tuma P, Rivero A, et al. Length of peginterferon-ribavirin therapy according to HCV genotype and rapid virological response in HIV/HCV coinfected patients: the EXTENT trial. Hepatology 2010;52(Suppl 4):753A.
45. Barone AA, Cheinquer H, Brandao-Mello CE, et al. HCV treatment duration in HIV/HCV genotype 1 co-infected patients. Results of a multicenter randomized trial. Hepatology 2010;52(Suppl 4):82A.
46. Brandao-Mello CE, Cheinquer H, Barone AA, et al. 72 weeks treatment duration reduces relapse rate in HCV/HIV co-infected patients with end of treatment response. Hepatology 2010;52(Suppl 4):785A.
47. Vachon ML, Factor S, Sterling RK, et al. Peginterferon-a-2b plus weight-based ribavirin for 48 vs 72 weeks in HIV/HCV co-infected patients: a randomized trial. A Poster Presentation CROI 18th, Meeting. Boston, February 27–March 2, 2011 [abstract: # Q-205].
48. The European AIDS Treatment Network (NEAT) Acute Hepatitis C Infection Consensus Panel. Acute hepatitis C in HIV-infected individuals: recommendations from the European AIDS Treatment Network (NEAT) consensus conference. AIDS 2011;25(4):399–409.
49. Seden K, Back D, Khoo S. New directly acting antivirals for hepatitis C: potential for interaction with antiretrovirals. J Antimicrob Chemother 2010;65(6):1079–85.
50. Bani-Sadr F, Carrat F, Pol S, et al. Risk factors for symptomatic mitochondrial toxicity in HIV/hepatitis C virus-coinfected patients during interferon plus ribavirin-based therapy. J Acquir Immune Defic Syndr 2005;40(1):47–52.
51. Pineda JA, Mira JA, Gil Ide L, et al. Influence of concomitant antiretroviral therapy on the rate of sustained virological response to pegylated interferon plus ribavirin in hepatitis C virus/HIV-coinfected patients. J Antimicrob Chemother 2007;60(6):1347–54.
52. Vispo E, Barreiro P, Pineda JA, et al. Low response to pegylated interferon plus ribavirin in HIV-infected patients with chronic hepatitis C treated with abacavir. Antivir Ther 2008;13(3):429–37.
53. Kempf DJ, Klein C, Chen HJ, et al. Pharmacokinetic enhancement of the hepatitis C virus protease inhibitors VX-950 and SCH 503034 by co-dosing with ritonavir. Antivir Chem Chemother 2007;18(3):163–7.
54. Garg V, Luo X, McNair L, et al. Low-dose RTV and the pharmacokinetics of the investigational HCV protease inhibitor TVR in healthy volunteers. CROI 2011 [abstract: 629].

55. Bottecchia M, Madejon A, Sanchez-Carillo M, et al. Naturally occurring drug resistance mutations in the hepatitis C virus NS3 protease in HIV/HCV coinfected patients treated with HIV protease inhibitors. J Hepatol 2010;52(Suppl 1): S289.
56. Bartels DJ, Zhou Y, Zhang EZ, et al. Natural prevalence of hepatitis C virus variants with decreased sensitivity to NS3.4A protease inhibitors in treatment-naive subjects. J Infect Dis 2008;198(6):800–7.
57. Kuntzen T, Timm J, Berical A, et al. Naturally occurring dominant resistance mutations to hepatitis C virus protease and polymerase inhibitors in treatment-naive patients. Hepatology 2008;48(6):1769–78.

Second-wave Protease Inhibitors: Choosing an Heir

Sandra Ciesek, MD[a,b], Thomas von Hahn, MD[a], Michael P. Manns, MD[a,*]

KEYWORDS

• Protease inhibitor • Second wave • Hepatitis C virus
• Antiviral therapy

Infection with the hepatitis C virus (HCV) is a major cause of chronic liver disease and the leading indication of liver transplantations worldwide. Around 130 million people are chronically infected with HCV, representing 2.2% of the world's population.[1] The local prevalence of HCV infection ranges from 0.1% to 20% of the population. The highest rates have been reported from Egypt.[2,3] Because of sequence diversity, the virus can be divided into 7 different genotypes (1–7), which differ from each other by 31% to 33% on the nucleotide level.[4] Among the different genotypes further subtypes (a, b, c, and so forth) have been described, which show sequence differences between 20% and 25%. The most common genotype is genotype 1. This high diversity is a result of both the error-prone NS5B RNA-dependent RNA polymerase lacking a proof-reading function, and the high replication rate of HCV, thus leading to a high mutation rate.[4]

Acute infection with HCV is usually mild, with only 20% to 30% of all patients developing any clinical symptoms. However, up to 80% of acute HCV infections turn chronic, and may then lead to chronic hepatitis, liver cirrhosis (10%–20%), and hepatocellular carcinoma (HCC; 1%–4%).[5,6] The current standard of care (SOC) for chronic hepatitis C is a nonspecific combination of pegylated interferon-α and ribavirin that is effective in slightly more than half of cases in selected clinical trial populations, and is associated with significant side effects.[7,8] The first directly acting antivirals (DAA; ie, drugs blocking viral enzymes) are expected to reach the US market in summer 2011 (Q 03) and in Europe in fall 2011 (Q 04). These antivirals will be the 2 first-wave/wave HCV protease inhibitors (PIs) telaprevir (TPV) and boceprevir (BOC). However, these compounds will at least initially complement rather than replace the current

[a] Klinik für Gastroenterologie, Hepatologie und Endokrinologie, Medizinische Hochschule Hannover, Carl-Neuberg-Straße 1, 30625 Hannover, Germany
[b] Abteilung für Experimentelle Virologie, Twincore, Zentrum für Experimentelle und Klinische Infektionsforschung GmbH, Feodor-Lynen-Straße 7, 30625 Hannover, Germany
* Corresponding author.
E-mail address: manns.michael@mh-hannover.de

Clin Liver Dis 15 (2011) 597–609
doi:10.1016/j.cld.2011.05.014
liver.theclinics.com

SOC.[9] Moreover, as outlined later, first-wave PIs will have several shortcomings that will hopefully be overcome by the next generation (second wave) of PIs that is already in clinical development. This article gives an overview of the compounds that will succeed TPV and BOC in the near future.

MOLECULAR BIOLOGY OF HCV

The viral RNA genome, 9.6 kb in size, encodes for at least 10 proteins. These proteins reside in a single open reading frame (3000 amino acids) that is enclosed by nontranslated regions (NTR) at the 5′ and 3′ ends.[10] An internal ribosomal entry site (IRES) is located in the highly conserved 5′ NTR, mediating the initial interaction with the ribosome and resulting in translation of a polyprotein. Subsequently, processing of the polyprotein precursor is essential for viral replication to occur. It is mediated by cellular and viral proteases that cleave the polyprotein into the individual structural proteins (core, E1, E2), the ion channel p7, and the nonstructural proteins (NS2, NS3, NS4A, NS4B, NS5A, NS5B).[10] Cleavage sites from the N-terminus to the p7/NS2 junction are substrates for cellular proteases. Cleavage between NS2 and NS3 is mediated by the viral cysteine autoprotease NS2, whereas the remaining downstream sites are cleaved by the viral NS3/NS4A serine protease (**Fig. 1**). The viral replication complex is made up of NS3, NS4A, NS4B, NS5A, and NS5B, and likely an assortment of host factors.[11] The critical RNA-dependent RNA polymerase (RdRp) activity resides in NS5B. Of the structural proteins, core (C) forms the nucleocapsid, whereas E1 and E2 are glycosylated type-I transmembrane proteins that are C-terminally anchored in the lipid bilayer of the viral envelope.[1] The viroporin, p7, is an integral membrane protein, functioning as an ion channel, and is crucial for assembly and release of infectious particles.[12,13]

HCV NS3/4A SERINE PROTEASE AS AN ANTIVIRAL TARGET

The NS3 protein has an N-terminal serine protease domain (amino acids 1–181) that requires NS4A as a cofactor as well as a C-terminal RNA-helicase/NTPase domain. It catalyzes *cis*-cleavage at the NS3-NS4A junction and *trans*-cleavage at all further downstream junctions (NS3/4A, NS4A/4B, NS4B/5A, and NS5A/5B) and is essential for genome replication in vitro and in vivo.[14] In addition to its critical role in the liberation of the final viral gene products and hence formation of the replication complex,

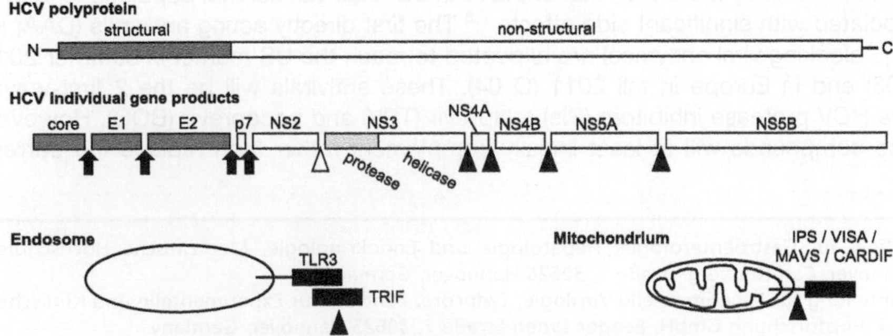

Fig. 1. Functions of the HCV NS3/4A protease. The HCV polyprotein (*top*) is cleaved into 10 individual gene products by host proteases (*filled arrows*), the NS2/3 cysteine autoprotease (*open arrowhead*) and the NS3/4A serine protease (*filled arrowheads*). In addition to its function in polyprotein processing, NS3/4A also recognizes and degrades the innate immunity signaling molecules TRIF and IPS/VISA/MAVS/CARDIF.

the NS3/4A protease promotes evasion of cellular antiviral defenses by degrading TRIF and MAVS, 2 key mediators of innate immune processes.[15] Thus, inhibition of NS3/4A is believed to simultaneously restrict viral replication and restore cellular antiviral capabilities.

The NS3/4A protease has long been seen as a highly promising target.[16,17] It is considered a member of the chymotrypsin family based on structural and functional similarities, notable for a shallow substrate binding site that slowly releases cleavage products and can be inhibited by certain peptide cleavage products.[18] This trait has been extensively exploited for the generation of therapeutic lead compounds and all NS3/4A PIs currently in clinical testing target the enzyme's active site and are based on peptide cleavage products.

Broadly, NS3/4A PIs can be divided into 2 groups: linear peptide mimetics with a ketoamide group that covalently, but reversibly, reacts with a serine in the catalytic triad and noncovalent peptide mimetic inhibitors that have a macrocyclic structure.[14] In 2002, the first DAA against HCV showing a profound effect in humans was the macrocyclic NS3/4A PI BILN2061 (ciluprevir).[19] BILN2061 has high antiviral activity in genotype 1 and a variable antiviral activity in patients infected with genotype 2/3. Its development has since been abandoned because of safety concerns, but structural derivatives of it are still being developed.

FIRST-WAVE NS3/4A SERINE PIS: BOCEPREVIR AND TELAPREVIR

PIs are currently the most advanced DAAs for the treatment of HCV infection: 2 linear peptidomimetic NS3/4A PIs, TPV (Vertex/Tibotec) and BOC (Schering-Plough, now Merck) have received regulatory approval for these compounds as an addition to current SOC seems feasible within 2011, so that TPV and BOC can be viewed as the first wave of PIs to reach the market.[20–22]

The addition of first-wave HCV PIs to SOC does improve HCV therapies in treatment-naïve patients with genotype 1 by raising expected sustained virologic response (SVR) rates from between 38% and 44% to between 63% and 75%. The addition of TPV or BOC also reduces duration of therapy for a significant proportion of patients. Triple therapy including SOC plus either TPV or BOC is also promising for previous treatment failures. However, the outcome differs whether patients are previous relapsers, partial responders, or nonresponders to a previous course of SOC. However, TPV and BOC have several shortcomings that may be overcome by second-wave HCV PIs. These shortcomings include 3-times-a-day dosing, early development of resistance with resistance patterns between subgenotypes 1a and 1b, limited efficacy against non-1 genotypes, and side effects (mostly rash and mild anemia for TPV and anemia and dysgeusia for BOC). Viral resistance to HCV DAAs is a major novel challenge.[23] First-wave PIs have only a moderate genetic barrier to resistance and selection of resistant variants occurs rapidly: during monotherapy for individuals infected with genotype 1 for 14 days emergence of multiple viral variants with resistance mutations has been detected. Important changes within the NS3 protease conferring resistance include V36A/M, T54S/A, V55A, R155K/T/Q, A156S/T, and V170A/T, occurring either alone or in combination (eg, 36 plus 155 or 156).[24] However, the degree of cross-resistance between BOC and TPV seems to be high. An obvious countermeasure to meet this threat is to combine PIs with other classes of drugs. In addition, different PIs are needed with a higher genetic barrier to resistance and/or without cross-resistance.[25] Moreover, first-wave PIs are highly effective only in patients infected by genotype 1, and have a suboptimal pharmacokinetic profile that necessitates administration of the drug 3 times daily. To reach the long-term goal of an interferon-free and ribavirin-free therapeutic regimen that achieves SVR in a high percentage of patients, even better PIs, as well as DAAs targeting other viral factors (eg, NS5A, NS5B) or drugs targeting host factors essential for viral replication (eg, cyclophilins), are needed.[14,24] Distinction between HCV subtypes 1 a and 1 b has become particularly relevant in the era of HCV PI–based therapies because the resistance pattern and antiviral potency varies between the different HCV PIs and, this will be a criterion for differentiation of the various first-wave and second-wave HCV PIs.

SECOND-WAVE NS3/4A SERINE PIS

To meet the needs described earlier, several companies have developed second-wave PIs that promise 1 or more advantages, including a higher barrier to resistance, activity at concentrations in the low nanomolar range, better activity against multiple HCV genotypes, more convenient dosing schedules, and improved safety and tolerability.[17,25] In contrast with BOC and TPV, many second-wave PIs are macrocyclic inhibitors and have a more favorable resistance profile with mutations mainly in position R155K/T/Q and D168A/V/T/H. By second-wave PIs, we refer to all HCV NS3/4A PIs potentially to be approved following BOC and TPV. Thus, we reserve the term second generation for substances that are broadly active against viral isolates carrying resistance mutations associated with BOC and TPV, which is not generally the case for the second-wave PIs discussed later.

Most of the many second-wave HCV PIs (**Table 1**) are in early stages of development and have to prove whether they offer advantages compared with data on the antiviral potency of the first-generation HCV PIs as indicated by log10 decline by week 4, resistance pattern, and week-4 HCV undetectability (RVR). Studies with TPV and BOC have shown that RVR best predicts SVR results. Moreover, it has to be established whether a lower level of quantification (LLQ; usually <25 IU/mL) or a lower level of detection (LLD; usually <10 IU/mL) was chosen, and the appropriate technology has to be used; usually a real-time TaqMan polymerase chain reaction with an LLQ of less than 25 IU/mL and an LLD of less than 10 IU/mL. In addition, it is of interest whether the PI has activity against non-1 HCV genotypes (ie, 2, 3, 4, 5 and 6). Furthermore, for further use in special patient populations, it is important to know whether the PI is metabolized by enzymes of the cytochrome P450 (eg, CYP 3A4) or uridine 5′-diphospho-glucuronosyltransferase (UGT) supergene families. This article reviews the present daily changing knowledge on the numerous members of the second-wave HCV PIs published as scientific publications in peer-reviewed journals, meeting reports, or press releases. The peer-reviewed scientific publications for HCV second-generation PIs until now have been rare. This article summarizes the knowledge on antiviral potency, resistance pattern, safety profile, pharmacokinetics, and genotype specificity as far as the information is available. However, in these early days of HCV DAA drug development, the only outcome that counts is SVR and long-term safety. Most of the other criteria are surrogate markers that cannot decide which drug will eventually be able to replace TPV and BOC in the addition of SOC, or be candidates for all oral interferon-free therapy for the future, or whether they will not successfully complete the process of drug development.

TMC-435 (TMC-435,350)

TMC435 is a macrocyclic second-wave NS3/4A PI developed by Tibotec and Johnson & Johnson.[26] One advantage is that the compound has a 40-hour half-life, which makes it amenable to once-a-day dosing. It is active against multiple genotypes, but clinical development has focused on genotype 1. An interim 24-week analysis of the

Table 1
Overview of second-wave PIs

Inhibitor	Company	Current Clinical Phase	Doses Per Day	Chemical Structure and Mode of Action	Addition of
TMC-435 (TMC-435,350)	Tibotec/Medevir/Johnson	3	1	Macrocyclic, noncovalent	(Evavirenz/raltegravir)[a]
Danoprevir (ITMN-191, RG7227)	Roche (formally Intermune)	2	2	Macrocyclic, noncovalent	Ritonavir
ABT-450	Abbott/Enanta	2	1	Acylsulfonamide	Ritonavir
BI 201,335	Boehringer Ingelheim	3	1/2	Macrocyclic	None
Vaniprevir (MK-7009)	Merck	2	2	Macrocyclic	None
BMS-650,032	Bristol-Myers Squibb	2	2	Active site	None
Narlaprevir (SCH900518)	Schering-Plough/Merck	2	1	Linear, reversible	Ritonavir
ACH-1625 (ACH-0,141,625)	Achillion	2	1	Linear, reversible	None
GS-9256	Gilead	2	2	linear, reversible	None
MK-5172	Merck	1	1	?	None
ACH-2684	Achillion	Preclinical	n.d.	?	None
IDX320	Idenix	1	n.d.	Macrocyclic, noncovalent	None
AVL-181	Avila	Preclinical	n.d.	Covalent, irreversible	None
AVL-192	Avila	Preclinical	n.d.	Covalent, irreversible	None

Abbreviations: n.d., not determined; ?, unknown.
[a] Under investigation in another trial.

ongoing phase 2b study was presented at the Liver Meeting of the American Association for the Study of Liver Diseases (AASLD) in autumn 2010, the PI TMC435 trial assessing the optimal dose and duration as a once-daily antiviral regimen (PILLAR).[27] In this study, all 386 patients received a backbone SOC regimen for 24 weeks, and were then randomized to add either 75 mg or 150 mg oral TMC435 once daily for 12 or 24 weeks. The fifth group received SOC only for 48 weeks. All patients included in this study and assigned to a TMC-435 arm had a rapid and steep decline in HCV RNA during the first 4 weeks (RVR) of treatment that was maintained throughout the 12-week or 24-week dosing period. In contrast, the control group showed a much slower slope of decline, needing about 8 weeks to achieve a 4 log decline, and it never achieved the same depth of decline in HCV RNA as the TMC-435 groups. The proportion of patients with very low or undetectable HCV RNA (<25 IU/mL) at week 4 ranged from 88% to 96% in the TMC435 groups, compared with 16% in the control group. At week 12 (early virologic response [EVR]), undetectable HCV RNA was recorded in 91% of those randomized to 12 weeks of TMC435 treatment, 97% in those randomized to 24 weeks of TMC435, and 69% in those randomized to the control group, respectively. Viral breakthrough by week 24 occurred in 2.5% to 7.8% of the TMC435 groups, compared with 3.9% of the control group. There was no correlation between dose of drug and breakthrough, although patients on the longer course of treatment did have lower rates of breakthrough. Resistance was most often found at positions 80 and 155, as well as some unique ones at 168 residues of the HCV genotype 1. Rates of discontinuation and adverse events with TMC435 were similar to those seen with SOC alone. There were increases in bilirubin, particularly with the higher dose of TMC435. The company is currently preparing for a phase 3 trial.

Danoprevir (ITMN-191, RG7227)

Danoprevir, formerly referred to as ITMN-191 or R7227, is a new noncovalent macrocyclic acyl sulfonamide–containing PI initially developed by Intermune and now licensed by Roche. Danoprevir has shown potent activity in vitro, both in biochemical assays with recombinant HCV NS3 proteases, and in the HCV replicon model, and seems to be effective against several HCV genotypes.[28] At the AASLD Liver Meeting 2010 in Boston (MA), Roche presented data of the ongoing phase 2 study in treatment-naive patients in combination with SOC.[29] At week 12, 88% of those taking 300 mg danoprevir plus SOC, 89% taking 600 mg danoprevir plus SOC, and 92% taking 900 mg danoprevir plus SOC achieved undetectable viral load compared with 43% taking SOC alone. Danoprevir can be boosted with low doses of the CYP3A inhibitor ritonavir to achieve a more favorable pharmacokinetic profile, and this option is now being moved forward in ongoing studies to avoid the alanine aminotransferase (ALT) increases seen in some patients treated with danoprevir. Increases were reported to be asymptomatic, occurring between 6 and 12 weeks of dosing, and being reversible on discontinuation of danoprevir. Ritonavir boosting may allow for the use of lower doses of danoprevir not be expected to result in ALT increases. Otherwise, danoprevir was well tolerated.

The INFORM-1 study has evaluated the combination of danoprevir with a nucleoside inhibitor of the HCV NS5B RNA polymerase (RG7128) without concomitant administration of interferon or ribavirin. Around 5 log reductions of plasma HCV RNA levels within 14 days were achieved, whereas treatment was overall well tolerated and undetectable HCV RNA was achieved in some cases. There was no viral breakthrough detected during 4 weeks of treatment.

ABT-450

ABT-450 is an acylsulfonamide PI developed by an alliance of Abbott and Enanta and intended for the treatment of HCV genotype 1 infection. Recently, first data of an ongoing placebo controlled phase 2 study were presented where ritonavir-boosted ABT-450 at 50 to 200 mg daily was given as monotherapy for 3 days followed by 12 weeks of ABT-450/ritonavir plus SOC and another 36 weeks of SOC alone.[30] Ritonavir boosting allowed once-daily administration of the study drug. First 3-day and 4-week results suggested that ritonavir-boosted ABT-450 has potent antiviral activity in genotype 1 treatment-naïve adults. An impressive 91.3% of patients (21 of 23) on the study drug achieved HCV RNA levels of less than 25 IU/mL after 4 weeks of treatment compared with 1 of 8 (12.5%) of those who received the placebo. Overall, the regime appeared safe and well tolerated.

BI 201,335

BI 201,335 is a linear second-wave PI with an optimized chemical structure believed to improve interactions with the NS3 substrate binding site.[31] It features a C-terminal carboxylic acid, which is the same functional group found in natural cleavage products.

Data from a phase 1b study (SOUND-C1) were presented at the AASLD Liver Meeting 2010 in Boston, MA.[32] It assessed an interferon-free triple therapy consisting of BI 201,335 (PI) plus BI 207,127 (an NS5B polymerase inhibitor) and ribavirin to treat HCV genotype 1 treatment-naïve patients. Thirty-two treatment-naive patients with genotype 1 HCV received BI 207,127 in either 400-mg or 600-mg doses 3 times a day, BI 201,335 120 mg once daily and ribavirin (1000/1200 mg daily in 2 doses) for 28 days. All patients had a rapid and sharp decline in HCV viral load during the first 2 days, followed by a slower second-phase decline. In the lower and higher dose groups, 73% and 100% of patients achieved a rapid virologic response (ie, HCV RNA less than the lower limit of quantification after 4 weeks of treatment). One patient experienced a viral breakthrough (increase by >1 LOG10 from nadir during treatment) and 1 other patient experienced a 0.7 log10 increase in viral load. Both were in the lower dose group of BI 207,127 and were patients with high baseline viral load. On day 29, all patients were switched to treatment with BI 201,335 and PegIFN/ribavirin for an additional 44 weeks per the defined study protocol, and will be followed to evaluate SVR. This work may be an important step toward a viable treatment option for the large number of patients with contraindications or intolerance to interferon. Recently, data about safety and pharmacokinetics of BI 201,335 in 43 treatment-naïve patients were published. Although BI 201,335 induced strong antiviral responses in most patients with a viral load decline similar to other potent PIs in clinical development, a dose-dependent but asymptomatic unconjugated hyperbilirubinemia could be observed.[31]

Vaniprevir (MK-7009)

MK-7009, also named vaniprevir, is a macrocyclic inhibitor of HCV NS3/4A protease with an HCV replicon EC50 of 3.5 nM in clinical development by Merck and currently in phase 2 trials.[33] A study of 45 HCV genotype 1 treatment-naïve noncirrhotic patients who were administered 1 of 5 regimens (SOC plus either placebo, 300 mg twice daily, 600 mg twice daily, 600 mg daily, or 800 mg daily) for 4 weeks followed by an additional 44 weeks of SOC alone resulted in SVR rates of 84% in the highest dose arm compared with 63% in the placebo arm.[34] The unexpectedly high SVR rate in the placebo group is believed to be caused by the small (19 individuals) cohort size.

Overall, vaniprevir was well tolerated when given in combination with SOC and no dose-limiting toxicity was observed. The incidence of vomiting with MK-7009 600 mg twice daily was higher than in the placebo group. A phase 2B study of vaniprevir in combination with SOC in treatment-experienced patients is ongoing.

BMS-650,032

Currently, BMS has 2 PIs and also an NS5A inhibitor in clinical development. The combination of the PI BMS-650,032, active against genotypes 1a and 1b, and an NS5A inhibitor BMS-790,052 was evaluated in genotype 1 null responders to a prior course of SOC therapy.[35] The interim results at 12 weeks (total study duration is 24 weeks) showed antiviral activity, but 6 of the 11 people treated had viral breakthrough, indicating that this combination does not represent an interferon-free option. When BMS-650,032 plus BMS-790,052 was combined with SOC, 9 of 10 genotype 1 former null responders to SOC became HCV RNA undetectable by week 12. The trial is still underway to study SVR as well as safety, tolerability, and dose ranging.

Narlaprevir (SCH900518)

Narlaprevir (SCH 900,518) is a potent linear inhibitor of the NS3/4A protease developed by Schering-Plough as an improvement on BOC suitable for once-daily dosing.[36] In the NEXT-1 study (phase 2), ritonavir-boosted narlaprevir is used in combination with SOC with previously untreated patients with genotype 1 chronic hepatitis C. The study compares SOC alone with 6 experimental arms containing 200 to 400 mg narlaprevir with or without a 4-week SOC lead-in phase.

Week-4 rapid virologic response (RVR) and week-12 EVR data were reported at the Liver Meeting 2009.[37] After 12 weeks, 65% to 87% of patients in the experimental arms achieved undetectable HCV RNA levels, compared with 17% with SOC alone. No treatment-limiting adverse events were observed during this timeframe. The in vitro resistance profile is similar to that of BOC and PIs. After the merger between Merck and Schering-Plough, clinical development of narlaprevir was suspended for priority reasons because the New Merck then had 3 HCV PIs in clinical development (narlaprevir, MK-7009/vaniprevir and MK-5172).

ACH-1625 (ACH-0,141,625)

ACH-1625 is a potent NS3 PI that was discovered and is being advanced by Achillion.[38] In earlier studies, ACH-1625 displayed good human metabolic stability and high human hepatoselectivity in vitro. ACH-1625 is well tolerated after administration of single and multiple doses of up to 2000 mg in healthy volunteers, and displays a mean maximal viral load reduction of 4.25 log10 after administration of 500 mg twice daily in patients infected with HCV genotype 1. A phase 2 trial was initiated to evaluate ACH-1625 in conjunction with SOC in patients infected with chronic HCV genotype 1. Although results from the 4-week study are expected in the first quarter of 2011, the 12-week study results are anticipated by the end of 2011. Recently, Achillon presented data of the ongoing study at the APASL 2011 meeting in Bangkok showing that ACH-1625 resulted in rapid and near-complete clearance of HCV.

GS-9256

GS-9256 is a PI from Gilead. Data from a phase IIa study show that GS-9256 plus tegobuvir (GS-9190), a polymerase inhibitor, used in conjunction with SOC, produced substantial suppression of HCV within 28 days of treatment.[39] Treatment-naive adults with chronic HCV genotype 1 infection were enrolled and, in the group that was given quadruple therapy for 4 weeks followed by 44 weeks of SOC alone, 14 of 14 patients were HCV RNA negative by day 28. Overall, GS-9190 and GS-9256 were generally well tolerated, with the most adverse events being grade 1 or 2 and resolving with continued treatment. However, Gilead reported in a press release on its homepage in January 2011 that data from clinical studies may not warrant further development of these product candidates, including the clinical studies evaluating GS-9256 for the treatment of hepatitis C.

MK-5172

MK-5172, developed by Merck, is a promising NS3/4A PI with potent in vitro activity against a broad range of HCV genotypes and viral variants and with known resistance mutations against other PIs. In vitro, NS3/4A enzymes from genotypes 1b, 2a, 2b, and 3a are all inhibited, with similar inhibitory constant (Ki) values in the subnanomolar range and both genotype 1b and 2a replicons are potently inhibited. Moreover, MK-5172 exhibits excellent selectivity for other serine proteases such as elastase and trypsin and shows only modest inhibitory potency with chymotrypsin. At the AASLD meeting in November 2010, data on a phase 1 trial of MK-5172 monotherapy (400 mg daily for 7 days) in patients infected with HCV genotype 1 or 3 was reported.[40] The mean maximum reductions from baseline of HCV viral RNA were 5.4 and 3.98 log10 IU/mL for genotypes 1 and 3, respectively, and 5 patients with genotype 1 had decreases in HCV RNA to levels less than the lower limit of detection during the study period. Currently, a phase 1 study of MK-5172 is still recruiting patients.

ACH-2684

ACH-2684 is a PI from Achillion with potency in the picomolar range. ACH-2684 shows good pharmacokinetic and safety profiles in preclinical studies and the compound reportedly has potent activity against all genotypes (1–6) and against strains of HCV resistant to other NS3/4a PIs.[41] Thus, it is hoped that ACH-2684 may provide a rescue treatment option for emerging resistant variants. The compound is currently in phase I studies, and patient data have yet to be reported.

IDX320

IDX320 is a noncovalent NS3/4A HCV PI from Idenix. In vitro data show that IDX320 inhibits the protease of HCV genotypes 1a, 1b, 2a, and 4a, as well as 3a at a higher concentration. In contrast, it did not interfere with 9 human cellular proteases. The NS3 mutation D168V was the signature resistance mutation for IDX320, but HCV with these mutations remained fully susceptible to interferon/ribavirin and different classes of direct-acting antiviral agents. First results a 3-day proof-of-concept study were presented at AASLD in 2010 in Boston (MA) and showed a potent, dose-dependent antiviral activity in treatment-naive patients infected with HCV genotype 1.[42] However, in September 2010, the IDX320 program was placed on hold by the US Food and Drug Administration because of 3 serious adverse events involving increased liver function tests in healthy volunteers taking IDX320 in combination with the nucleotide analogue IDX184.

AVL-181 and AVL-192

AVL-181 and AVL-192 are highly selective, small-molecule HCV PIs being developed by Avila.[43,44] Both drugs inhibit NS3/4A irreversibly by covalent binding to NS3 cysteine residue 159 and are reportedly active against all genotypes. In vitro, AVL-181 was curative as monotherapy in the genotype 1b replicon clearance assay at very low concentrations (24 nM) and durably inhibited the HCV protease, including drug resistant mutants, for more than 24 hours after a single exposure; this contrasts with the need for nearly continuous exposure to the reversible HCV PIs currently in late-stage clinical trials.

DISCUSSION

There are many NS3/4A PIs being developed that may remedy some or all of the foreseeable shortcomings of the first-wave PIs, BOC and TPV.

Although BOC and TPV have to be taken orally 3 times a day, the second-wave PIs only have to be taken twice or even once a day (see **Table 1**). This difference is an important improvement in pharmacokinetics and will help to maximize compliance.

Another important difference between BOC and TPV and some of the second-wave PIs is the activity against different HCV genotypes: BOC and TPV will be marketed exclusively for the treatment of HCV genotype 1 infection, MK-5172 and TMC435 have been shown to be active against all genotypes (MK-5172) or all genotypes other than 3 (TMC-435) (**Table 2**). Thus, these second-wave PIs will provide a new therapeutic option to a larger number of patients and, most importantly, close the gap in the treatment of patients with genotype 4. In addition, some second-wave PIs (eg, MK-5172, ACH-2684) are active against viral isolates carrying certain resistance mutations, so that these compounds could be considered to be true second-generation PIs.

Major side effects observed in patients treated with first-wave PIs are mainly anemia (BOC, TPV), rash (TPV), dysgeusia (BOC), and pruritus (TPV). Although some of the second-wave PIs also have rash as a side effect (BI 201,335), others seem to have a different profile of adverse events including gastrointestinal problems (danoprevir, vaniprevir, BI 201,335), increases in bilirubin (TMC435, BI 201,335) or ALT (danoprevir), and blood count changes like neutropenia (danoprevir) (see **Table 2**).

In particular, hyperbilirubinemia during treatment with second-wave PIs has raised some concern; however, it has been asymptomatic and reversible in all cases and has not been linked to overt liver injury because no concomitant ALT increases were observed.[31] A possible underlying mechanism is an inhibition of UGT1A1. Discontinuation rates because of adverse events are reported to be in the order of 10% to 14% for first-wave PIs and less than 10% for second-wave PIs. Nonetheless, in direct

Table 2
Clinical characteristics of some second-wave PIs

Inhibitor	RVR (%)	EVR (%)	SVR (%)	Active Against HCV Genotype	Side Effects
TMC-435 (TMC-435,350)	—	—	91–93 SVR4	1, 2, 4, 5, 6	Bilirubinemia
Danoprevir (ITMN-191, RG7227)	73–86	88–92		1, 2 ?	Nausea, diarrhea, neutropenia, ALT increase
BI 201,335	62–69	54–59		1, 2 ?	Jaundice, rash, gastrointestinal
Vaniprevir (MK-7009)	67–84	74–85	62–84	1, 2 ?	Vomiting
MK-5172	n.a.	n.a.	n.a.	1, 2, 3, 4, 5, 6	n.a.

Abbreviations: EVR, early virologic response (week 12 of therapy); n.a., not applicable; RVR, rapid virologic response (week 4 of therapy); SVR, sustained virologic response (6 months after therapy); ?, effect on other genotypes is unknown.

comparison with other drugs in clinical development for HCV treatment, such as NS5B polymerase inhibitors or cyclophilin inhibitors, the frequency and severity of serious adverse events may be a disadvantage for the application of these drugs in the future.

Although long-term data are still missing, first results of phase II studies indicate that the second-wave PIs will achieve comparable or even increased EVR or SVR rates. In the long run, the treatment choices for chronic hepatitis C can be expected to expand rapidly. Thus, therapy will become both more powerful and more complex, and continuously determining the best choice for any given patient will pose a formidable challenge to clinicians for years to come.

REFERENCES

1. von Hahn T, Steinmann E, Ciesek S, et al. Know your enemy: translating insights about the molecular biology of hepatitis C virus into novel therapeutic approaches. Expert Rev Gastroenterol Hepatol 2010;4(1):63–79.
2. Wasley A, Alter MJ. Epidemiology of hepatitis C: geographic differences and temporal trends. Semin Liver Dis 2000;20(1):1–16.
3. Shepard CW, Finelli L, Alter MJ. Global epidemiology of hepatitis C virus infection. Lancet Infect Dis 2005;5(9):558–67.
4. Simmonds P. Genetic diversity and evolution of hepatitis C virus–15 years on. J Gen Virol 2004;85(Pt 11):3173–88.
5. Ghany MG, Strader DB, Thomas DL, et al. Diagnosis, management, and treatment of hepatitis C: an update. Hepatology 2009;49(4):1335–74.
6. Ascione A, Tartaglione T, Di Costanzo GG. Natural history of chronic hepatitis C virus infection. Dig Liver Dis 2007;39(Suppl 1):S4–7.
7. Fried MW, Shiffman ML, Reddy KR, et al. Peginterferon alfa-2a plus ribavirin for chronic hepatitis C virus infection. N Engl J Med 2002;347(13):975–82.
8. Manns MP, McHutchison JG, Gordon SC, et al. Peginterferon alfa-2b plus ribavirin compared with interferon alfa-2b plus ribavirin for initial treatment of chronic hepatitis C: a randomised trial. Lancet 2001;358(9286):958–65.
9. Ciesek S, Manns MP. Hepatitis in 2010: the dawn of a new era in HCV therapy. Nat Rev Gastroenterol Hepatol 2011;8(2):69–71.
10. Bartenschlager R, Frese M, Pietschmann T. Novel insights into hepatitis C virus replication and persistence. Adv Virus Res 2004;63:71–180.
11. Lohmann V, Körner F, Koch J, et al. Replication of subgenomic hepatitis C virus RNAs in a hepatoma cell line. Science 1999;285(5424):110–3.
12. Steinmann E, Penin F, Kallis S, et al. Hepatitis C virus p7 protein is crucial for assembly and release of infectious virions. PLoS Pathog 2007;3(7):e103.
13. Jones CT, Murray CL, Eastman DK, et al. Hepatitis C virus p7 and NS2 proteins are essential for production of infectious virus. J Virol 2007;81(16):8374–83.
14. Lin C, Tan SL, editor. Hepatitis C viruses: genomes and molecular biology. Norfolk (UK): Horizon Bioscience; 2006. Chapter 6.
15. Dustin LB, Rice CM. Flying under the radar: the immunobiology of hepatitis C. Annu Rev Immunol 2007;25:71–99.
16. Manns MP, Foster GR, Rockstroh JK, et al. The way forward in HCV treatment–finding the right path. Nat Rev Drug Discov 2007;6(12):991–1000.
17. Fusco DN, Chung RT. New protease inhibitors for HCV - Help is on the way. J Hepatol 2011;54(6):1087–9.
18. Steinkuhler C, Biasiol G, Brunetti M, et al. Product inhibition of the hepatitis C virus NS3 protease. Biochemistry 1998;37(25):8899–905.

19. Lamarre D, Anderson PC, Bailey M, et al. An NS3 protease inhibitor with antiviral effects in humans infected with hepatitis C virus. Nature 2003;426(6963):186–9.
20. McHutchison JG, Manns MP, Muir AJ, et al. Telaprevir for previously treated chronic HCV infection. N Engl J Med 2010;362(14):1292–303.
21. Poordad F, McCone J Jr, Bacon BR, et al. Boceprevir with peginterferon/ribavirin for untreated chronic hepatitis C. N Engl J Med 2011;54:1195–206.
22. Jacobson IM, McHutchison GJ, Dusheiko MG. Telaprevir in combination with peginterferon and ribavirin in genotype 1 HCV treatment-naive patients: final results of phase 3 ADVANCE study. 61st AASLD. Boston (MA), October 29 to November 2010.
23. Rong L, Dahari H, Ribeiro RM, et al. Rapid emergence of protease inhibitor resistance in hepatitis C virus. Sci Transl Med 2010;2(30):30ra32.
24. Sarrazin C, Zeuzem S. Resistance to direct antiviral agents in patients with hepatitis C virus infection. Gastroenterology 2010;138(2):447–62.
25. Asselah T, Marcellin P. New direct-acting antivirals' combination for the treatment of chronic hepatitis C. Liver Int 2011;31(Suppl 1):68–77.
26. Reesink HW, Fanning GC, Farha KA, et al. Rapid HCV-RNA decline with once daily TMC435: a phase I study in healthy volunteers and hepatitis C patients. Gastroenterology 2010;138(3):913–21.
27. Fried MW, Buti M, Dore GJ, et al. Efficacy and safety of TMC 435 in combination with peginterferon-2a and ribavirin in treatment-naive genotype-1 HCV patients: 24-week interim results from the PILLAR study. Hepatology 2010; 52(Suppl S1):LB-5.
28. Gane EJ, Rouzier R, Stedman C, et al. Antiviral activity, safety, and pharmacokinetics of danoprevir/ritonavir plus PEG-IFN alpha-2a/RBV in hepatitis C patients. J Hepatol 2011. [Epub ahead of print].
29. Terrault N, Cooper C, Balart LA, et al. Phase II randomised, partially-blind, parallel-group study of oral danoprevir (RG7227) with PEGIFNa-2A (Pegasys) plus ribavirin in treatment-naive genotype 1 patients in treatment-naive genotype 1 patients with CHC: results of planned week 12 interim analysis of the ATLAS study. Hepatology 2010;52(S1):335A–6A.
30. Lawitz E, Gaultier I, Poordad F, et al. 4-week virologic response and safety of ABT-450 given with low-dose ritonavir (ABT-450/r) in combination with pegylated interferon alpha-2A and ribavirin (SOC) after 3-day monotherapy in genotype 1 HCV-infected treatment-naive subjects. Hepatology 2010;52(S1):[abstract 1885].
31. Manns MP, Bourliere M, Benhamou Y, et al. Potency, safety, and pharmacokinetics of the NS3/4A protease inhibitor BI201335 in patients with chronic HCV genotype-1 infection. J Hepatol 2011;54(6):1114–22.
32. Zeuzem S, Asselah T, Angus PW, et al. Strong antiviral activity and safety of IFN-sparing treatment with the protease inhibitor BI201335, the HCV polymerase inhibitor BI207127 and ribavirin in patients with chronic hepatitis C. Hepatology 2010;52(S1):223A.
33. McCauley JA, McIntyre CJ, Rudd MT, et al. Discovery of vaniprevir (MK-7009), a macrocyclic hepatitis C virus NS3/4a protease inhibitor. J Med Chem 2010; 53(6):2443–63.
34. Manns MP, Gane EJ, Rodriguez-Torres M, et al. Sustained viral response (SVR) rates in genotype 1 treatment-naive patients with chronic hepatitis C (CHC) infection treated with Vaniprevir (MK-7009), a NS3/4A protease inhibitor, in combination with pegylated interferon alfa-2A and ribavirin for 28 days. Hepatology 2010;52(S1):361A.

35. Lok AS, Gardiner E, Lawitz E, et al. Combination therapy with BMS-790052 and BMS-650032 alone or with pegIFN/RBV results in undetectable HCV RNA trough 12 weeks of therapy in HCV genotype 1 null responders. Hepatology 2010; 52(S1):LB-8.
36. de Bruijne J, Bergmann JF, Reesink HW, et al. Antiviral activity of narlaprevir combined with ritonavir and pegylated interferon in chronic hepatitis C patients. Hepatology 2010;52(5):1590–9.
37. Vierling JM, Poordad F, Lawitz E, et al. Once daily narlaprevir (SCH 900518) in combination with PEGIntron/Ribavirin for treatment-naive subjects with genotype-1 CHC: interim results from NEXT-1, a phase 2A study. Hepatology 2009;50(S4):90A.
38. Huang M, Agarwal A, Stauber KL. ACH-1625 demonstrates sustained viral suppression in presence of uncommon drug resistant HCV variants: pharmacokinetic, pharmacodynamic and clinical virology analysis of phase I study. Hepatology 2010;52(S1).
39. Zeuzem S, Buggisch P, Agarwal K, et al. Dual, triple, and quadruple combination treatment with a protease inhibitor (GS-9256) and a polymerase inhibitor (GS-9190) alone and in combination with ribavirin (RBV) or PEGIFN/RBV for up to 28 days in treatment naive genotype 1 HCV subjects. Hepatology 2010; 52(S1):400A–1A.
40. Brainard DM, Petry A, Van Dyk K, et al. Safety and antiviral activity of MK-5172, a novel HCV NS3/4A protease inhibitor with potent activity against known resistance mutants, in genotype 1 and 3 HCV-infected patients. Hepatology 2010; 52(S1):182A.
41. Huang M, Podos S, Patel D, et al. ACH-2684: HCV NS3 protease inhibitor with potent activity against multiple genotypes and known resistant variants. Hepatol ogy 2010;52(S1):299A.
42. Reesink H, van Vliet AA, Mühr F, et al. Antiviral activity, safety and pharmacokinetics of IDX-320, a novel macrocyclic HCV protease inhibitor, in a 3-day proof-of-concept study in patients with chronic hepatitis C. Hepatology 2010; 52(S1):224A.
43. Hagel M, Niu D, St Martin T, et al. Next generation of covalent irreversible inhibitors have superior potency across genotypes and drug resistant mutants. Hepatology 2010;52(S1):301A.
44. Niu D, Hagel M, Qiao T, et al. AVL-181, a potent and selective irreversible HCV protease inhibitor, requires a helper amino acid in the binding microenvironment to form a covalent bond with cys-159. J Hepatol 2010;52(S1):S297.

The HCV NS5B Nucleoside and Non-Nucleoside Inhibitors

Fernando E. Membreno, MD, MSc, Eric J. Lawitz, MD, CPI*

KEYWORDS

- Hepatitis C virus • NS5B nucleoside inhibitors
- Non-nucleoside inhibitors • Polymerase inhibitors

In the world, approximately 130 to 170 million people are chronically infected with hepatitis C virus (HCV) and it is estimated that more than 350,000 people die from this infection each year.[1] Since its discovery in 1989, there has been a slow evolution of therapies for this disease, which currently are still marked by marginal effectiveness and significant toxicities. For approximately 20 years there have not been had any major breakthroughs in the development of therapies except for the addition of ribavirin (RVB) and the pegylation of interferon alfa, which have boosted genotype 1 (GT-1) sustained viral response (SVR) rates to a disappointing 40% to 41%.[2] The inability to cure this virus has led to the accumulation of nonresponder patients who are at continued risk of progressive liver disease, liver decompensation, and consequently liver transplantation.

A new era of direct-acting antivirals (DAAs) is beginning. Unlike the current standard of care (SOC) therapy, pegylated interferon (PegIFN) and RBV, these new molecules target specific sites that disrupt the function of viral proteases and polymerases that are vital for the virus life cycle. During the past 10 years, a profound understanding of the molecular structure of HCV, which is an enveloped, single-stranded-RNA virus that encodes a polyprotein of approximately 3300 amino acids that lead to the formation of 4 structural proteins (core, E1, E2, and p7) and 6 nonstructural proteins (NS2, NS3, NS4A, NS4B, NS5A, and NS5B), has been acquired.[3] This polypeptide chain is proteolytically processed by host proteases to release proteins involved in packaging of progeny virions and viral proteases cleave the rest of the polyprotein. This article focuses on the NS5B, the RNA-dependent RNA polymerase that is essential for viral replication.[4] After the structure of the NS5B polymerase was solved in 1999, laboratory developments in biochemical enzymatic assays and cell-based HCV replicon systems[5] built a framework for an explosion of new molecules targeting various sites of the HCV polymerase.

Alamo Medical Research, 621 Camden Street, San Antonio, TX 78215, USA
* Corresponding author.
E-mail address: lawitz@alamomedicalresearch.com

Clin Liver Dis 15 (2011) 611–626
doi:10.1016/j.cld.2011.05.003 liver.theclinics.com
1089-3261/11/$ – see front matter

Similar to other viral polymerases, NS5B has a right-hand motif consisting of a thumb domain and a finger domain, both encircling the active site located within the palm domain.[6] The active site includes a highly conserved GDD motif,[6,7] less prone to mutations. The NS5B inhibitors are classified into nucleoside/nucleotide inhibitors (NIs) and non-nucleoside inhibitors (NNIs).[8–10] The NIs mimic natural polymerase substrates and bind to the NS5B active site, causing chain termination and/or an increased number of errors when incorporated into a growing RNA chain. They tend to have similar efficacy across all HCV genotypes, because the NS5B's active site is well conserved among genotypes.[11] NNIs bind to 1 of the 4, less conserved, allosteric sites inhibiting important conformational changes in the polyprotein replication complex necessary for the catalytic efficiency of the enzyme's active site.[4] In contrast to NIs, these molecules have shown a restricted spectrum of activity against the various HCV genotypes. So far, NNIs have targeted 4 main allosteric sites in the NS5B polymerase, thumb domains 1 and 2 and palm domains 1 and 2 (depicted in **Fig. 1**).[11] Because there are 5 targets of antivirals in this class (4 allosteric and 1 active), it is likely that combinations of agents with different targets in this class would be complementary to each other. Both intraclass and interclass combinations are expected in the future.

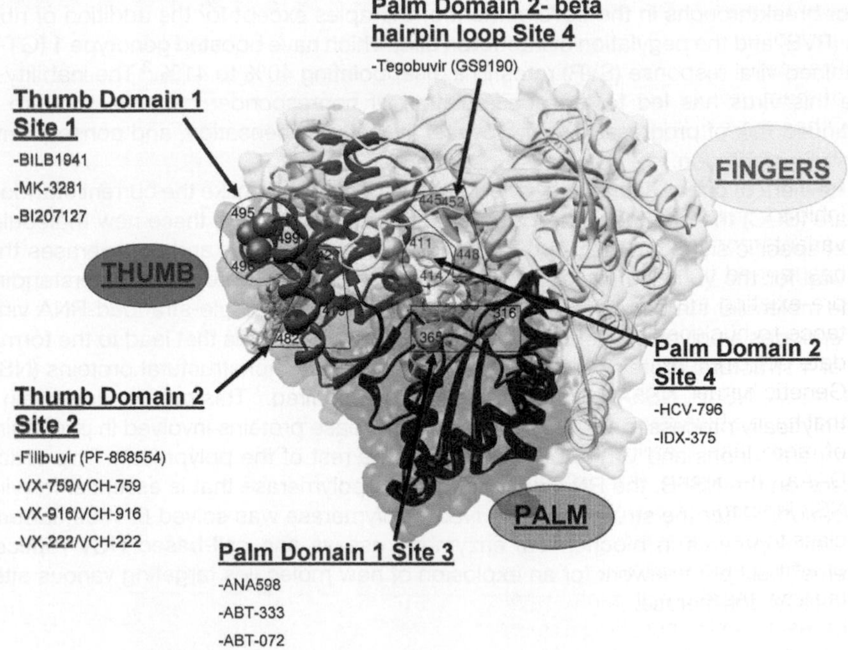

Fig. 1. Binding sites for non-nucleoside HCV NS5B polymerase inhibitors. The palm, fingers, and thumb domains are colored blue, yellow, and red respectively. Mutations in different regions have a different color: salmon for residues P495, P496, V499 in thumb domain 1; magenta for L419, M423, I482 in thumb domain 2; gold for N411, M414 in palm domain 1; cyan for C316, S365 in palm domain 2; and green for C445, Y448, Y452 in the β-hairpin loop. (*Adapted from* Delang L, Coelmont L, Neyts J. Antiviral therapy for hepatitis C virus: beyond the standard of care. Viruses 2010;2:826–66.)

FACTORS THAT AFFECT VIRAL CLEARANCE

HCV has a high rate of replication, with a half-life of only 2 to 5 hours, with the production and elimination of an estimated 10^{10} and 10^{12} virions per day.[12,13] In order for DAAs to be effective in obtaining an SVR, they must be able to completely eliminate the replication of both wild-type and pre-existent resistant variants to reach a state of sustained viral elimination.[4] NS5B is responsible for the replication of the viral genome; due to the lack of proofreading, this process leads to a high error rate that results in the formation of multiple variant strains, classified into the 6 genotypes (1–6) with several subtypes (a, b, c, and so forth).[14] This issue becomes even more complex because each individual infected with HCV also harbors different variants or quasispecies that could be resistant to the NS5B inhibitors even before drug exposure.[15]

The issue of resistance in DAA drug development is complex and for non-nucleoside NS5B inhibitors the barrier of resistance seems low, but the intrinsic potency of these compounds is high.[16] Resistance can vary according to genotype/subtype, pre-existing variants, genetic barrier, pharmokinetics, and compliance issues.

1. Genotype/subtype. The NIs that bind to the highly conserved active site seem to have a similar activity against different HCV genotypes and subtypes, 1a, 1b, 2, and 3, as reported for NM283, R1626, and R7128.[17–20] Some NNIs, alternatively, seem to be less active against GT-1a than GT-1b, as reported for agents such as BI 207127 and BILB 1941.[21,22] An example of this is seen during therapy with a protease inhibitor (telaprevir); to generate the resistant mutation, only a single nucleotide change is required in GT-1a, whereas 2 are required in GT-1b.[23,24]
2. Pre-existing mutation. Multiple HCV mutants are generated on a daily basis; most of them are not fit enough to replicate and are eliminated from the population.[25] Other pre-existing mutants containing the drug-resistant mutations may already exist as the dominant or minority quasispecies. This subpopulation grows exponentially under drug pressure and diminishes the antiviral activity of an NS5B inhibitor.[26] Increasing numbers of studies have looked at baseline frequency of variants conferring resistance to NNIs. The baseline frequency of these variants has ranged from 0.6% to 2.8% when direct sequencing has demonstrated these pre-existing major variants.[27–31] Pre-existing mutations that confer in vitro resistance to nucleoside analogs that inhibit NS5B (S96T, S282T, and N142T) have to date not been detected in patients with HCV GT-1 infections.[26]
3. Genetic barrier. Experience with hepatitis B and HIV has led to knowledge of drugs that have a high genetic barrier due to a flexible binding pattern[32] or the requirement of more than 1 amino acid exchange to confer resistance.[33] In evaluation of the DAAs, the agents with the lowest genetic barrier of resistance are the NNIs and NS3 inhibitors. Conversely, the NIs have the highest barrier of resistance than any class to date. In the case of NNIs, the allosteric binding sites may undergo a series of amino acid exchanges without affecting the overall function of the NS5B polymerase; therefore, it is intrinsically difficult to design an inhibitor with a high genetic barrier to resistance. Furthermore, it is likely that variants with low sensitivity to these inhibitors are pre-existing at baseline in many patients. On the contrary, NIs are less prone to encounter resistance, because the active site is highly preserved and, therefore, naturally occurring resistant variants are unlikely to exist.[26]
4. Pharmacokinetics and compliance. These factors, like in HIV, are particularly important in DAA drugs that have a short half-life and need to be dosed up to 3 times per day, such as the first-generation protease inhibitors, telaprevir and boceprevir. It has been shown that keeping adequate drug plasma trough levels is

associated with less viral breakthrough and resistance.[34] That is why, recently, there have been clinical trials with the addition of ritonavir (CYP3A-mediated inhibitor) to DAA drug regimens in an effort to raise trough level concentrations that allow prolongation of dosing intervals and increase compliance. The real impact of ritonavir boosting will not be known until these agents are used in a large cohort of patients.[26]

DAA monotherapy's high association with the emergence of resistance is the basis for multidrug combinations targeting different mechanisms of actions. This review focuses on clinically relevant NS5B polymerase inhibitors that have shown promise and are being developed in clinical trials (**Table 1**).

NUCLEOSIDE ANALOG NS5B POLYMERASE INHIBITORS

Nucleoside analog NS5B polymerase inhibitors share characteristics with the natural nucleoside substrates found in cells and, once phosphorylated to the nucleoside-triphosphate, cause termination of the newly encoded viral genome.

RG7128

RG7128 is a prodrug of PSI-6130, an oral cytidine nucleoside analog (pyrimidine), and is currently the most advanced nucleoside polymerase inhibitor in clinical development. An interim analysis of the ongoing phase 2b PROPEL trial was reported by Jenson and colleagues.[43] A total of 408 GT-1 and GT-4 subjects were randomized to one of five treatment arms: Arm 1: RG7128 500 mg BID+PEG-Interferon and Ribavirin (SOC) for 12 weeks followed by SOC for 12/36 weeks [response guided therapy (RGT)], Arm 2: RG7128 1000 mg BID+SOC for 8 weeks followed by SOC for 16/40 weeks (RGT), Arm 3: 1000 mg BID+SOC for 12 weeks followed by SOC for 12/36 weeks (RGT), Arm 4: 1000 mg BID+SOC for 12 weeks followed by SOC for 36 weeks (fixed duration), Arm 5: Control arm of PEG-Interferon and Ribavirin for 48 weeks. The rapid viral response (RVR) rates were 39% in the 500-mg twice-a-day arm and 62% in all three 1000-mg twice-a-day arms compared with 18% in the SOC control arm. Complete early viral response rates occurred in 83% in the 500-mg twice-a-day arm, 68% in the 1000-mg twice-a-day for 8 weeks arm, and 80% and 88% in the 2 1000-mg twice-a-day for 12-weeks arms compared with the SOC control arm complete early viral response of 49%. Subjects who were cirrhotic had a decrement in rates of RVR of 8% to 25% compared with noncirrhotics across all treatment groups. There was no significant difference in complete early viral response rates when comparing GT-1a, GT-1b, and GT-4. Treatment-emergent laboratory and serious and nonserious adverse events were evenly distributed across both active and control treatment groups. The most frequent adverse events were headache (48%–52%), fatigue (35%–49%), and nausea (27%–40%). Resistance testing in 11 subjects with viral loads greater than1000 IU/mL at the end of RG7128 treatment did not show evidence of the signature S282T variant.[44]

RG7128, like all nucleoside polymerase inhibitors, has preserved potency across HCV genotypes due to the consistent mechanism of action of chain termination. Gane and colleagues[20] presented the results of 20 GT-2 and GT-3 previous nonsustained responders to interferon-based therapy. Subjects were treated with 4 weeks of RG7128 (1500 mg twice a day) in combination with SOC. RVR rates were 95% and SVR was seen in 65% of these previous nonsustained responders. This trial demonstrated the effectiveness of RG7128 in GT-2 and GT-3 subjects who previously failed SOC.

A phase 3 program in GT-1 and phase 2 studies in GT-2 and GT-3 are planned for 2011.[39]

Table 1
Hepatitis C NS5B nucleoside and non-nucleoside inhibitors

Agent	Company	Status
Nucleoside analog NS5B polymerase inhibitors		
Valopicitabine	Idenix	Halted
R1626	Roche	Halted
R7128/PSI-6130	Roche/Pharmasset	Phase 2b
PSI-7977	Pharmasset	Phase 2b
IDX184	Idenix	Phase 2a
PSI-938	Pharmasset	Phase 1
INX 189	Inhibitex	Phase 1
PSI-661	Pharmasset	Preclinical
Non-nucleoside NS5B polymerase inhibitors		
NNI-Site 1 (Thumb 1)		
BILB 1941	Boehringer Ingelheim	Halted
MK-3281	Merck	Halted
BI 207127	Boehringer Ingelheim	Phase 2a
NNI-Site 2 (Thumb 2)		
Filibuvir (PF-00868554)	Pfizer	Phase 2b
VX-759/VCH-759	Vertex/Virochem Pharma	Phase 1
VX-916/VCH-916	Vertex/Virochem Pharma	Phase 1
VX-222/ VCH-222	Vertex/Virochem Pharma	Phase 2a
NNI-Site 3 (Palm 1)		
ANA598	Anadys	Phase 2b
ABT-333	Abbott	Phase 2a
ABT-072	Abbott	Phase 2a
NNI-Site 4 (Palm 2)		
HCV-796	ViroPharma/Wyeth	Halted
Tegobuvir (GS9190)	Gilead	Phase 2b
IDX375	Idenix	Phase 1
Oral NS5B-based direct antiviral combination trials, without interferon (NS5B component in bold)		
GS 9256 + **tegobuvir** ± RBV[35]		
BI 201335 + **BI 207127** + RBV[36]		
ABT-450/ritonavir + **ABT-072** + RBV[37]		
Telaprevir + **VX-222**[38]		
PSI-938 + PSI-7977[39]		
Danoprevir + **RG7128**[40]		
Danoprevir/ritonavir + **RG7128** ± RBV[41]		
PSI-7977 + BMS-790052[42]		

PSI-7977

PSI-7977 is an investigational uridine nucleotide analog (pyrimidine). PSI-7977 is a phosphoramidate prodrug of β-D-2'-deoxy-2'-fluoro-2'-*C*-methyluridine 5'-monophosphate (PSI-6206 monophosphate). PSI-7977 is currently in stage 2b. The phase 2b trial includes 125 treatment-naive subjects with HCV GT-1 who were randomized

2:2:1 into 1 of 3 arms. Patients randomized to each arm receive SOC together with PSI-7977 (200 mg), PSI-7977 (400 mg), or matching placebo for 12 weeks. HCV GT-1 patients who receive PSI-7977 and achieve an extended RVR (eRVR) receive an additional 12 weeks of SOC. Subjects who receive PSI-7977 who do not achieve an eRVR and all subjects randomized to receive placebo plus SOC receive an additional 36 weeks of SOC. In addition, 25 treatment-naive subjects with HCV GT-2 or GT-3 receive a total of 12 weeks of therapy with PSI-7977 (400 mg every day) with SOC.[45] To date, results have only been reported for the GT-2 and GT-3 cohort, RVR was seen in 96% (24/25) of subjects, and all 24 continued to be HCV RNA undetectable at the end of therapy (week 12). One patient was lost to follow-up after the first dose. No interim results have been reported for the GT-1 subjects.[39] The phase 2a[46] trial enrolled 63 GT-1 subjects who were randomized to PSI-7977 (100 mg), PSI-7977 (200 mg), PSI-7977 (400 mg), or placebo in combination with SOC for 28 days followed by 44 weeks of SOC. RVR (<15 IU/mL) were seen in 88%, 94%, and 93% respectively for PSI-7977–treated subjects compared with 21% in the SOC control group. Adverse events were seen at similar rates across all PSI-7977 and SOC groups. There has been no detection of the signature variant S282T to date.

SVR results in the phase 2b GT-2 and GT-3 subjects and interim on-therapy results in the GT-1 subjects should be reported in 2011.

IDX184

IDX184 is a prodrug of 2'-methylguanosine monophosphate (purine).[47] The phase 2a trial enrolled 81 subjects in a 2-week trial of IDX184 at 50 mg every day or twice a day, 100 mg every day or twice a day, 150 mg every day, and 200 mg every day in combination with SOC compared with an SOC control arm. At the end of 14 days of therapy, HCV RNA was undetectable (<15 IU/mL) at rates of 13% and 50% in the 50-mg everyday and twice-a-day groups, respectively; 50% and 29% in the 100-mg everyday and twice-a-day groups, respectively; 40% in the 150-mg everyday group; and 25% in 200-mg everyday group. Mean viral loads were 1.2 to 2.8 logs lower at 14 days (range 2.7 to 4.3 log) compared with the SOC control (1.5 log). Adverse events were seen at similar rates across all IDX184 and SOC groups. There has been no detection of the signature variant S282T variant to date.[48] On September 3, 2010, the Food and Drug Administration placed the IDX184 and IDX320 programs on clinical hold. This decision was made after Idenix notified the Food and Drug Administration of 3 serious adverse events that occurred during a drug-drug interaction study of the combination of IDX184 and IDX320 in healthy volunteers. These observed serious adverse events were elevated liver function tests detected in 3 subjects during post-exposure safety visits. The liver function tests returned to nearly normal levels in all 3 subjects during follow-up.[49]

PSI-938

PSI-938 is an investigational guanine nucleotide analog polymerase inhibitor (purine). In a phase 1 trial, PSI-938 administered once daily or twice daily for 7 days (doses of 100 mg every day) or twice a day (200 mg every day or 300 mg every day) versus placebo with mean viral load declines at day 8 in the active groups of 3.94 to 4.64.[39] In an additional phase 1 trial, PSI-938 (300 mg every day) was administered for 14 days as monotherapy. Evaluation at the end of therapy revealed 50% (4/8) of subjects became HCV RNA undetectable (<15 IU/mL) with a mean viral decline of 5.23 log at day 14.[39]

PSI-938 (purine) is active against the S282T-resistant variant selected in vitro by the pyrimidine analogs; the purines are metabolized to the active triphosphate through a different phosphorylation pathway than the pyrimidines. Given these characteristics, purine and pyrimidine analogs have the potential to be used in combination. This strategy is currently being evaluated in a clinical trial (see **Table 1**).

INX-189

INX-189 is an investigational phosphoramide analog of the nucleoside 2'-*C*-methyl-guanosine analog (purine). In November 2010, a phase 1b trial was initiated in hepatitis C subjects.[42] Its signature variant, like other nucleos(t)ide inhibitors, is the S282T variant.[50]

PSI-661

PSI-661 uses a different prodrug strategy than PSI-938 but is metabolized to the same active guanine triphosphate (purine) as PSI-938 and retains activity against hepatitis C with an S282T mutation. Phase 1 trials are planned in 2011.[39]

NON-NUCLEOSIDE NS5B POLYMERASE INHIBITORS

In contrast to NIs, the heterogeneous class of NNIs binds to different allosteric enzyme sites, which results in conformational protein change before the elongation complex is formed.[51] NS5B is structurally organized in a characteristic right-hand motif (see **Fig. 1**) containing finger, palm, and thumb domains and offers at least 4 NNI-binding sites: a benzimidazole (thumb 1, site 1) binding, thiophene (thumb 2, site 2) binding, benzothiadiazine (palm 1, site 3) binding, and benzofuran (palm 2, site 4) binding.[6,51]

NNI-Site 1 (Thumb 1/Benzimidazole Site)

BI 207127 is an orally bioavailable, reversible, thumb 1 allosteric inhibitor of the HCV RNA-dependent polymerase in vitro. A phase 2a trial by Larrey and colleagues[52] treated 57 HCV GT-1 subjects for 28 days with 400-mg, 600-mg, or 800-mg BI 207127 or placebo 3 times a day in combination with SOC. Treatment-naive patients (n = 27) were randomized in a 2:2:2:3 ratio to 1 of the 3 BI 207127 doses or placebo and treatment-experienced patients (all PegIFN/RBV nonresponders; n = 30) in a 1:1:1 ratio to the 3 BI 207127 doses. In treatment-naive patients, RVR (<10 IU/mL) was achieved in 50% (3/6) at 400 mg, 57% (4/7) at 600 mg, and 50% (3/6) at 800 mg compared with 0/8 in the SOC control arm. In treatment-experienced patients, RVR was achieved in 0/10 at 400 mg, 22% (2/9) at 600 mg, and 18% (2/11) at 800 mg. There was no evidence of viral breakthrough in the treatment-naive patients; however, 9% to 22% of treatment experienced subjects developed viral breakthrough. Adverse events of nausea, vomiting, diarrhea, and rash were more common in BI 207127–treated subjects compared with placebo.

NNI-Site 2 Inhibitors (Thumb 2/Thiophene Site)

Filibuvir (PF-00868554)

Filibuvir (PF-00868554) is an allosteric inhibitor of the thumb 2 HCV RNA-dependent polymerase in vitro. A phase 2a trial by Jacobson and colleagues[53] treated 35 HCV GT-1 subjects for 28 days with 200 mg, 300 mg, or 500 mg of filibuvir or placebo twice a day in combination with SOC. All subjects completed an additional 44 weeks of SOC. RVR was seen in 60% (6/10) at 200 mg, 75% (6/8) at 300 mg, 63% (5/8) at 500 mg, and 0% (0/8) in placebo. End-of-therapy response at week 48 was seen in 60% (6/10) at 200 mg, 75% (6/8) at 300 mg, 63% (5/8) at 500 mg, and 50% (4/8) in placebo. Week 12 sustained virological response (SVR12) was seen in 30% (3/10) at 200 mg, 50% (4/8) at 300 mg, 50% (4/8) at 500 mg, and 50% (4/8) in placebo.

Relapse rates were 20% to 50% in filibuvir-treated subjects and 0% in placebo subjects. The most frequent adverse events were fatigue, nausea, and headache. Nine of 26 (35%) filibuvir-treated subjects did not achieve an RVR. Six of these 9 (67%) had mutations at position 423. Five of the 6 (83%) had a null response on week 12 analysis.

VX-222/VCH-222

VX-222 is an NNI, thiophene-2-carboxylic acid that acts as a noncompetitive allosteric inhibitor of the NS5B thumb domain, site 2. VX-222 has low micromolar (90% inhibitory concentration [IC90] = 0.03–0.06 μM) antiviral activity against HCV GT-1a and GT-1b in the replicon assay. This inhibitor was evaluated in a phase 1 trial by Rodriguez-Torres and colleagues[54] in naive GT-1 patients. The trial included 4 dosing arms (250 mg twice a day, 500 mg twice a day, 750 mg twice a day, and 1500 mg every day) for 3 days. At day 4, VX-222 achieved a mean HCV RNA reduction of 3.2 $\log_{10}$ after 3 days of monotherapy. The majority of adverse events were mild: diarrhea (25%), headache (20%), and nausea (12%); no serious adverse events were observed. The impressive viral drop and acceptable overall profile seen with this molecule makes it a suitable candidate for further development. Studies evaluating VX-222 in combination with PegIFN and RBV and with telaprevir with or without PegIFN and RBV are ongoing (phase 2a).

VX-916/VCH-916

VX-916 has a chemical structure, mechanism, and site of action similar to VX-222. VCH-916 is equipotent against HCV GT-1a and GT-1b replicons. This drug was evaluated in a phase 1 study by Lawitz and colleagues[55] in naive HCV GT-1 patients. The study included 4 dosing arms (100 mg 3 times a day for 15 days, 200 mg 3 times a day for 15 days, 300 mg twice a day for 4 days, and 400 mg twice a day for 4 days). VCH-916 achieved a mean maximal HCV RNA reduction of 1.5 $\log_{10}$ after 3 day of monotherapy (200 mg 3 times a day 300 and 400 mg twice a day). In the 100-mg and 200-mg 3-times-a-day 14-day cohorts, VCH-916 was well tolerated with the most frequently reported adverse events: gastrointestinal (35%), central nervous system symptoms (25%), and throat irritation (20%). In the 300-mg and 400-mg twice-a-day 3-day cohorts, throat irritation and nausea were reported by 50% and 33% of subjects, respectively.[54] The viral load drop with this drug is not as impressive as that seen for VX-222; therefore, VX-916 will likely remain as an acceptable backup drug. At this time the authors are not aware of any future clinical trials planned for this NNI.

VX-759/VCH-759

VX-759 is another NNI similar in structure, mechanism, and site of action to both VX-222 and VX-916. A phase 1 study was conducted by Cooper and colleagues[56] in HCV treatment- naive GT-1 patients. Three dosing cohorts were evaluated—400 mg 3 times a day, 800 mg twice a day, and 800 mg 3 times a day—each arm received 10 days of therapy. The mean maximal decrease in HCV RNA $\log_{10}$ was 1.97, 2.30, and 2.46 for the 400-mg 3-times-a-day, 800-mg twice-a-day, and 800-mg 3-times-a-day groups, respectively. The antiviral activity seemed similar for both GT-1a and GT-1b. Is was reported that a patient harboring GT-6 who received 10 days of VX-759 (400 mg 3 times a day) did not have a significant change in HCV RNA level from baseline during or after dosing. This is further proof that NNIs are genotype specific. Resistant variants, identified through genotypic and phenotypic analysis, most likely originated from pre-existing minor populations. Through in vitro drug-resistant studies, it was demonstrated that these variants remain sensitive to interferon alfa-2a and RBV.[57] The compound was well tolerated and no serious adverse events were reported. The most common mild and moderate adverse reported were diarrhea (79% vs 56% [placebo]), headache (30%), flatulence (24%), dyspepsia (19%), and fatigue (22%). The investigators believed that the predominance of gastrointestinal side effects could have been related to the vehicle formulation (an aqueous mixture of polyethylene glycol 400 and Solutol HS15) used in the compound. Overall, this drug has been shown safe and virologically potent over a short period of time. The authors believe this drug may also remain as a backup drug to VX-222 in the future.

NNI-Site 3 Inhibitors (Palm 1/Benzothiadiazine Site)

ANA598

ANA598 is an allosteric inhibitor of the palm 1 HCV RNA-dependent polymerase in vitro. A phase 2 trial by Lawitz and colleagues[58] treated 95 HCV GT-1 subjects with 200 mg or 400 mg twice a day with ANA598 (loading dose of 800 mg twice a day on day 1) or placebo twice a day in combination with SOC for 12 weeks followed by an additional 12 to 24 weeks of SOC. The duration of SOC was response guided with total therapy of 24 weeks for those who achieved an eRVR, defined as HCV RNA negative at weeks 4 and 12, or 48 weeks of therapy for those without an eRVR. The addition of ANA598 to SOC enhanced antiviral response in all patients. Evaluation of results based on IL28B polymorphism showed CC patients had an accelerated rate of achieving undetectable virus and CT/TT patients had a decreased percentage of nonresponders. RVR was seen in 56% and 42% in ANA598-treated subjects (200 mg and 400 mg) compared with 13% in placebo subjects. HCV RNA was undetectable at weeks 12 in 73% and 75% (200 mg and 400 mg) compared with 63% in placebo treated subjects. Adverse events in ANA598-treated subjects (200 mg) were similar to placebo. ANA598 (400-mg dose) had a higher frequency and severity of rash. Variants seen on therapy were G554D, Y448H, and M414T. Sixty-five percent of subjects with variants proceeded to achieve undetectable levels of HCV RNA on SOC. A phase 2b trial is ongoing.

ABT-333

ABT-333 is an NNI that binds to the palm domain 1, site 3. This drug seems active against GT-1a and GT-1b. Rodríguez-Torres and colleagues[59] conducted a phase 2a study in HCV-naive patients with GT-1. ABT-333 (300 mg twice a day for 2 days, 600 mg twice a day for 2 days and 1200 mg daily for 2 days) in conjunction with 26 days of PegIFN/RBV compared to placebo for 28 days, showed an HCV RNA mean change from baseline of −3.65, −3.68 and −3.55 $\log_{10}$ in the 3 treatment arms, respectively, compared with only −1.42 $\log_{10}$ in the placebo arm. A total of 10/24 (41.7%) in all treatment arms achieved an HCV RNA of less than 25 IU/mL at day 28. The most frequent mutation seen S556G but did not lead to virologic rebound in the presence of PegIFN/RBV. ABT-333 proved safe and well tolerated. Currently, there is an ongoing phase 2b trial of ABT-033-based triple therapy for 12 weeks followed by PegIFN and RBV to complete 48 weeks of therapy.[60]

ABT-072

ABT-072 is an NNI that also targets the palm domain 1, site 3. It has selective activity against GT-1a and GT-1b. When administered at a dose of 160 mg for 2 days, the HCV mean viral decline was 1.5 $\log_{10}$ IU/mL compared with 0.3 $\log_{10}$ in the placebo group. The drug was well tolerated in single and multiple doses up to 320 mg in healthy volunteers.[60] Currently, there is an ongoing phase 2 trial of ABT-072 based triple therapy for 12 weeks followed by PegIFN and RBV to complete 48 weeks of therapy.[61]

NNI-Site 4 Inhibitors (Palm 2/Benzofuran Site)

Tegobuvir (GS9190)

Tegobuvir (GS9190) is a class of imidazopyridine that acts as an NNI at the palm domain 2, site 4. It targets the NS5B allosteric site located within the β-hairpin loop. This site is located in close proximity to the active site and is thought to be involved in primer independent initiation of RNA replication.[11,62] In the replicon system, it has shown higher activity in GT-1 compared with GT-2.[5,62] This compound underwent a phase 1 study[63] in HCV-naive GT-1a and GT-1b patients who received ascending doses (40 mg twice a day, 120 mg twice a day, and 240 mg every day and twice a day) of the NNI for 8 days. After 24 hours, the median viral load decline was between 0.46 and 1.49 log across cohorts. After 8 days of dosing (40 mg twice a day and 120 mg twice a day) the maximal mean viral load reductions were 1.61 and 1.95 log, respectively. Sequence analysis showed the Y448H NS5B polymerase mutation in 58% of subjects in the multidose cohorts. Levels of Y448H declined after stopping therapy, suggesting impaired replication of this mutant. Phenotypic analysis showed that Y448H alone or in combination with Y452H showed reduced susceptibility to GS-9190. These mutations remained sensitive to interferon alfa, RBV, and HCV protease inhibitors telaprevir and boceprevir. This lack of cross-resistance supports the use of GS-9190 in combination with these DAA.[64] There were no serious treatment-limiting side effects. The results of a phase IIa, randomized, open-label trial evaluating GS 9190 and GS 9256, an oral protease inhibitor, in combination and with RBV or with RBV/PegIFN were recently reported (discussed later). A phase 2b trial was initiated in 2008 to compare triple therapy with a response-guided duration (24 vs 48 weeks) versus a fixed 48-week duration of therapy compared with a control arm of SOC. Final SVR results will be presented at the European Association for the Study of Liver International Liver Congress 2011. There is also an ongoing phase 2 trial of quadruple therapy with GS9190 and GS9256 in combination with PegIFN and RBV to study response-guided therapy with durations as short as 16 weeks for some GT-1 subjects.[65]

IDX375

IDX375 is NNI that targets the palm domain 2, site 4 of the NS5B polymerase. The phase I study of IDX375 evaluated sequential, single ascending doses in healthy volunteers and a single 200-mg twice-a-day dose for 1 day in 3 HCV GT-1–infected patients. For the 3 HCV GT-1a–infected patients, anti-HCV activity with a decline in viral load was associated with IDX375 concentrations of greater than 1 μg/mL. At doses of 200 mg every day and twice a day, the drug was generally well tolerated and achieved pharmacologically relevant drug concentrations. Adverse events were mild and the most common side effect was diarrhea (3/30). A 3-day proof-of-concept study with IDX375 in treatment-naive, GT-1 HCV–infected patients is ongoing.[66]

NS5B COMBINATION TRIALS

There are currently several trials under way using combinations of DAAs for the treatment of hepatitis C. NS5B inhibitors play a key role in many of these combination trials. These trials are evaluating the effectiveness of these regimens in addition to monitoring for evidence of viral breakthrough. Results are awaited from these trials to determine if DAA without an immune modulator can result in SVRs. The trial that demonstrated proof of principle for this approach was the INFORM-1 trial,[40] in which subjects were treated with RG7128 (nucleoside polymerase inhibitor) in combination with danoprevir (protease inhibitor) twice daily for 14 days. In the cohort with the highest doses studied (1000-mg twice-a-day RG7128 and 900-mg twice-a-day danoprevir), mean viral declines were 4.9 log and 5.1 log in previous null responders and naive subjects, respectively. There was no evidence of viral breakthrough during the 14 days of therapy. In null responders, 25% (2/8), and in treatment-naive patients 63% (5/8) achieved HCV RNA results below the level of detection.

There were 3 DAA combination trials presented at the annual meeting of the American Association for the Study of Liver Diseases in 2010 and additional trials are planned or ongoing (see **Table 1**). Two of the 3 trials involved an NS5B component in the treatment regimen. Zeuzem and colleagues[35] presented data on the treatment of 46 subjects with a combination of GS-9256 (75 mg twice a day) (protease inhibitor) and tegobuvir (40 mg twice a day) (dual therapy), in combination with RBV (triple therapy), and in combination with PegIFN and RBV (quadruple therapy) for 28 days. Dual therapy produced early and frequent breakthroughs; the addition of RBV (triple therapy) resulted in breakthroughs developing later in time and less frequent in occurrence; and the quadruple therapy produced robust viral suppression with 100% (14/14) having HCV RNA less than 25 IU/mL and 93% (13/14) with HCV RNA less than 10 IU/mL after 28 days. The most frequent adverse events on dual therapy were headache, nausea, and diarrhea. A second trial also presented by Zeuzem and colleagues[36] treated 32 subjects with a combination of BI 201335 (protease inhibitor) (120 mg daily) and BI 207127 (400 mg or 600 mg 3 times a day) in combination with weight-based RBV (1000–1200 mg for 4 weeks). Loading doses were used on day 1 (1200 mg of BI 207127 and 240 mg of BI 201335). After 4 weeks of combination therapy, the 400-mg 3-times-a-day group of BI 207127, BI 201335, and RBV 73% (11/15) patients were below of HCV RNA detection (<25 IU/mL). The same combination, except with 600 mg 3 times a day of BI 207127, resulted in 100% (17/17) of subjects below the limit of detection. At the higher dose there was no difference between GT-1a and GT-1b; however, at the lower dose of BI 207127, GT-1a had lower response rates than the GT-1b subjects. Most frequent adverse events were gastrointestinal (nausea, vomiting, and diarrhea) and skin reactions (rash and/or photosensitivity). Virologic breakthrough (1 log rise) occurred in 1 subject.

There are 5 additional combination trials planned or under way (see **Table 1**).

SUMMARY

The treatment paradigm of for chronic hepatitis C is in a dynamic state as the first few DAAs enter the market and many other compounds move through development. The optimal combination still needs to be investigated and clinical trials are needed to determine the optimal treatment regimens and durations of therapy. There are many NS5B agents in development and these agents are now aligning as key components of combination trials. The nucleoside inhibitors with a high barrier of resistance are a potential backbone of future combination trials. The NNIs having complementary resistance profiles to protease inhibitors and NS5A agents are also positioned to become important components in combination trials. Future studies are needed to fully understand efficacy, safety, and resistance profiles of most of the agents in this class. Ultimately the most successful combination therapy will be the regimen that provides the highest efficacy but minimizes toxicity and breakthrough. The future looks bright for the treatment of hepatitis C, and the NS5B agents will be a key component of new therapeutic regimens.

REFERENCES

1. Viral Hepatitis. Sixty-Third World Health Assembly. Provisional agenda item 11.12. World Health Organization; 2010. A63/15. Available at: http://apps.who.int/gb/ebwha/pdf_files/WHA63/A63_15-en.pdf. Accessed May 19, 2011.
2. McHutchison JG, Lawitz EJ, Shiffman ML, et al. Peginterferon alfa-2b or alfa-2a with ribavirin for treatment of hepatitis C infection. N Engl J Med 2009;361(6):580–93.
3. Pauwels F, Mostmans W, Quirynen LM, et al. Binding-site identification and genotypic profiling of hepatitis C virus polymerase inhibitors. J Virol 2007;81(13): 6909–19.
4. Kwong AD, McNair L, Jacobson I, et al. Recent progress in the development of selected hepatitis C virus NS3.4A protease and NS5B polymerase inhibitors. Curr Opin Pharmacol 2008;8(5):522–31.
5. Burton JR Jr, Everson GT. HCV NS5B polymerase inhibitors. Clin Liver Dis 2009; 13(3):453–65.
6. Lesburg CA, Cable MB, Ferrari E, et al. Crystal structure of the RNA-dependent RNA polymerase from hepatitis C virus reveals a fully encircled active site. Nat Struct Biol 1999;6(10):937–43.
7. Miller RH, Purcell RH. Hepatitis C virus shares amino acid sequence similarity with pestiviruses and flaviviruses as well as members of two plant virus supergroups. Proc Natl Acad Sci U S A 1990;87(6):2057–61.
8. Ma H, Leveque V, De Witte A, et al. Inhibition of native hepatitis C virus replicase by nucleotide and non-nucleoside inhibitors. Virology 2005;332(1):8–15.
9. Sarisky RT. Non-nucleoside inhibitors of the HCV polymerase. J Antimicrob Chemother 2004;54(1):14–6.
10. Tomei L, Altamura S, Paonessa G, et al. HCV antiviral resistance: the impact of in vitro studies on the development of antiviral agents targeting the viral NS5B polymerase. Antivir Chem Chemother 2005;16(4):225–45.
11. Delang L, Coelmont L, Neyts J. Antiviral therapy for hepatitis C virus: beyond the standard of care. Viruses 2010;2(4):826–66.
12. Herrmann E, Neumann AU, Schmidt JM, et al. Hepatitis C virus kinetics. Antivir Ther 2000;5(2):85–90.
13. Neumann AU, Lam NP, Dahari H, et al. Hepatitis C viral dynamics in vivo and the antiviral efficacy of interferon-alpha therapy. Science 1998;282(5386):103–7.
14. Simmonds P, Bukh J, Combet C, et al. Consensus proposals for a unified system of nomenclature of hepatitis C virus genotypes. Hepatology 2005;42(4): 962–73.
15. Gomez J, Martell M, Quer J, et al. Hepatitis C viral quasispecies. J Viral Hepat 1999;6(1):3–16.
16. Gao M, Nettles RE, Belema M, et al. Chemical genetics strategy identifies an HCV NS5A inhibitor with a potent clinical effect. Nature 2010;465(7294):96–100.
17. Afdhal N, Godofsky E, Dienstag J. Final phase I/II trial results for NM283, a new polymerase inhibitor for hepatitis C: antiviral efficacy and tolerance in patients with HCV-1 infection, including previous interferon failures. Hepatology 2004; 40(Suppl 1):726A.
18. Roberts SK, Cooksley G, Dore GJ, et al. Robust antiviral activity of R1626, a novel nucleoside analog: a randomized, placebo-controlled study in patients with chronic hepatitis C. Hepatology 2008;48(2):398–406.
19. Lalezari J, Gane E, Rodriguez-Torres M. Potent antiviral activity of the HCV nucleoside polymerase inhibitor R7128 with PEG-IFN and ribavirin: interim results of R7128 500mg BID for 28 days. J Hepatol 2008;40(Suppl 2):29A.

20. Gane E, Rodriguez-Torres M, Nelson DE. Sustained virologic response (SVR) following RG7128 1500mg BID/peg-IFN/RBV for 28 days in HCV genotype 2/3 prior non-responders. 45th Annual Meeting of the European Association for the Study of the Liver (EASL 2010). Vienna (Austria), April 14–18, 2010.
21. Larrey D, Benhamou Y, Lohse A, et al. Safety, pharmacokinetics and antiviral effect of BI 207127, a novel HCV RNA polymerase inhibitor, after 5 days oral treatment in patients with chronic hepatitis C. J Hepatol 2009;50(Suppl 1):S383–4.
22. Erhardt A, Deterding K, Benhamou Y, et al. Safety, pharmacokinetics and antiviral effect of BILB 1941, a novel hepatitis C virus RNA polymerase inhibitor, after 5 days oral treatment. Antivir Ther 2009;14:23–32.
23. Zhou Y, Muh U, Hanzelka BL, et al. Phenotypic and structural analyses of hepatitis C virus NS3 protease Arg155 variants: sensitivity to telaprevir (VX-950) and interferon alpha. J Biol Chem 2007;282(31):22619–28.
24. McHutchison JG, Everson GT, Gordon SC, et al. Telaprevir with peginterferon and ribavirin for chronic HCV genotype 1 infection. N Engl J Med 2009;360(18): 1827–38.
25. Duffy S, Shackelton LA, Holmes EC. Rates of evolutionary change in viruses: patterns and determinants. Nat Rev Genet 2008;9(4):267–76.
26. Sarrazin C, Zeuzem S. Resistance to direct antiviral agents in patients with hepatitis C virus infection. Gastroenterology 2010;138(2):447–62.
27. Gaudieri S, Rauch A, Pfafferott K, et al. Hepatitis C virus drug resistance and immune-driven adaptations: relevance to new antiviral therapy. Hepatology 2009;49(4):1069–82.
28. Troke P, Lewis M, Simpson P, et al. Genotypic characterisation of HCV NS5B following 8-day monotherapy with the polymerase inhibitor PF 00868554 in HCV-infected subjects. J Hepatol 2009;50:S351.
29. Kuntzen T, Timm J, Berical A, et al. Naturally occurring dominant resistance mutations to hepatitis C virus protease and polymerase inhibitors in treatment-naive patients. Hepatology 2008;48(6):1769–78.
30. Le Pogam S, Seshaadri A, Kosaka A, et al. Existence of hepatitis C virus NS5B variants naturally resistant to non-nucleoside, but not to nucleoside, polymerase inhibitors among untreated patients. J Antimicrob Chemother 2008;61(6):1205–16.
31. Marquis M, Deterding K, Erhardt A, et al. Genotypic and phenotypic analysis of hepatitis C virus NS5B polymerase variants to BILB1941 inhibition. Hepatology 2008;48(Suppl):1159A.
32. McKeage K, Perry CM, Keam SJ. Darunavir: a review of its use in the management of HIV infection in adults. Drugs 2009;69(4):477–503.
33. Ghany MG, Doo EC. Antiviral resistance and hepatitis B therapy. Hepatology 2009;49(5 Suppl):S174–84.
34. Sarrazin C, Kieffer TL, Bartels D, et al. Dynamic hepatitis C virus genotypic and phenotypic changes in patients treated with the protease inhibitor telaprevir. Gastroenterology 2007;132(5):1767–77.
35. Zeuzem S, Buggisch P, Agarwal K, et al. Dual, Triple, and Quadruple Combination Treatment with a Protease Inhibitor (GS-9256) and a Polymerase Inhibitor (GS-9190) alone and in Combination with Ribavirin (RBV) or PegIFN/RBV for up to 28 days in Treatment Naïve, Genotype 1 HCV Subjects. 61st Annual Meeting of the American Association for the Study of Liver Diseases (AASLD 2010). Boston (MA), October 29 to November 2, 2010. p. LB-1.
36. Zeuzem S, Asselah T, Angus PW, et al. Strong antiviral activity and safety of IFN-sparing treatment with the protease inhibitor BI 201335, the HCV polymerase inhibitor BI 207127 and ribavirin in patients with chronic hepatitis C. 61st Annual

Meeting of the American Association for the Study of Liver Disease. Boston (MA), October 29 to November 2, 2010. p. LB-7.
37. Available at: http://www.clinicaltrials.gov/ct2/show/NCT01221298. Accessed January 8, 2011.
38. Available at: http://www.clinicaltrials.gov/ct2/show/NCT01080222. Accessed January 8, 2011.
39. Available at: http://investor.pharmasset.com/releasedetail.cfm?ReleaseID=542051. Accessed January 8, 2011.
40. Gane EJ, Roberts SK, Stedman CA, et al. Oral combination therapy with a nucleoside polymerase inhibitor (RG7128) and danoprevir for chronic hepatitis C genotype 1 infection (INFORM-1): a randomised, double-blind, placebo-controlled, dose-escalation trial. Lancet 2010;376(9751):1467–75.
41. Available at: http://www.clinicaltrials.gov/ct2/show/NCT01278134. Accessed January 21, 2011.
42. Available at: http://markets.financialcontent.com/ir/?Module=MediaViewer&GUID=15373203&Ticker=INHX. Accessed January 12, 2011.
43. Jensen DM, Wedemeye RH, Herring RW, et al. High rates of early viral response, promising safety profile and lack resistance-related breakthrough in HCV GT1/4 patients treated with RG7128 plus pegIFN alfa-2a (40KD)/RBV: planned week 12 interim analysis from the PROPEL study. Program and abstracts of the 61st Annual Meeting of the American Association for the Study of Liver Diseases. Boston (MA), October 29 to November 2, 2010. p. A81.
44. Le Pogam S, Yan JM, Kosaka A, et al. No evidence of drug resistance or baseline S282T resistance mutation among GT1 and GT4 HCV infected patients on nucleoside polymerase inhibitor RG7128 and peg-IFN/RBV combination treatment for up to 12 weeks: interim analysis from the PROPEL study. Program and abstracts of the 61st Annual Meeting of the American Association for the Study of Liver Diseases. Boston (MA), October 29 to November 2, 2010:799.
45. Available at: http://www.clinicaltrials.gov/ct2/show/NCT01188772?term=NCT01188772&;rank=1. Accessed January 8, 2011.
46. Lalezari JP, O'Riordan W, Poordad F, et al. A Phase IIa Study of IDX184 in Combination with Pegylated Interferon (pegIFN) and Ribavirin (RBV) in Treatment-Naïve HCV Genotype 1-Infected Subjects. Program and abstracts of the 61st Annual Meeting of the American Association for the Study of Liver Diseases. Boston (MA), October 29 to November 2, 2010. p. A34.
47. Available at: http://www.ihlpress.com/pdf%20files/hepdart09_presentations/pharmacology/IDX184%20DNStandring%20HepDart%202009%20FINAL%2012.6.09.pdf. Accessed January 8, 2011.
48. Lawitz EJ, Lalezari J, Rodriguez-Torres M, et al. High Rapid Virologic Response (RVR) with PSI-7977 daily dosing plus PEG-IFN/RBV in a 28-day Phase 2a trial. Program and abstracts of the 61st Annual Meeting of the American Association for the Study of Liver Diseases. Boston (MA), October 29 to November 2, 2010. p. A806.
49. Available at: http://ir.idenix.com/phoenix.zhtml?c=131556&p=irol-newsArticle&ID=1467491&highlight=. Accessed January 8, 2011.
50. Kolykhalov A, Liu Y, Bleiman B, et-al. Characterization of the in vitro selected Hepatitis C virus replicon Mutants Resistant to the Phosphoramidate analog of 2'-C-Methyl-Guanosine, INX-189. Program and abstracts of the 61st Annual Meeting of the American Association for the Study of Liver Diseases. Boston (MA), October 29 to November 2, 2010. p. A1888.

51. Beaulieu PL. Non-nucleoside inhibitors of the HCV NS5B polymerase: progress in the discovery and development of novel agents for the treatment of HCV infections. Curr Opin Investig Drugs 2007;8(8):614–34.
52. Larrey D, Lohse A, De Ledinghen V, et al. 4 week therapy with the non-nucleosidic polymerase inhibitor BI 207127 in combination with peginterferon alfa2A and ribavirin in treatment naïve and treatment experienced chronic HCV GT1 patients. 45th Annual Meeting of the European Association for the Study of the Liver (EASL). Vienna (Austria), April 14–18, 2010.
53. Jacobson I, Pockros PJ, Lalezari J, et al. Virologic Response Rates Following 4 Weeks of Filibuvir in Combination with Pegylated Interferon Alfa-2a and Ribavirin in Chronically-Infected HCV Genotype-1 Patients. 45th Annual Meeting of the European Association for the Study of the Liver (EASL). Vienna (Austria), April 14–18, 2010.
54. Rodriguez-Torres M, Lawitz EJ, Conway B, et al. Safety and antiviral activity of the HCV non-nucleoside polymerase inhibitor VX-222 in treatment-naïve genotype 1 HCV-infected patients. J Hepatol 2010;52(Suppl 1):A31.
55. Lawitz EJ, Cooper C, Rodriguez-Torres M, et al. Safety, tolerability and antiviral activity of VCH-916, a novel non-nucleoside HCV polymerase inhibitor in patients with chronic HCV genotype-1 infection. J Hepatol 2009;50(Suppl 1):A92.
56. Cooper C, Lawitz EJ, Ghali P, et al. Evaluation of VCH-759 monotherapy in hepatitis C infection. J Hepatol 2009;51(1):39–46.
57. David M, Nicolas O, Fex P, et al. Combinations studies of VCH-916, a novel allostoric inhibitor of HCV NS5B polymerase, with interferon-alfa-2a. 15th International Symposium on Hepatitis C Virus and Related Viruses. San Antonio (TX), October 5–9, 2008.
58. Lawitz EJ, Rodriguez-Torres M, Rustg VK, et al. Safety and antiviral activity of ANA600 in combination with pegylated interferon Alfa 2A plus ribavirin in treatment-naive genotype-1 chronic HCV patients. Program and abstracts of the 61st Annual Meeting of the American Association for the Study of Liver Diseases. Boston (MA), October 29 to November 2, 2010. p. A31.
59. Rodríguez-Torres M, Lawitz E, Cohen D, et al. Treatment-naïve, genotype-1 HCVinfected subjects show significantly greater HCV RNA decreases when treated with 28 days of ABT-333 plus peginterferon and ribavirin compared to peginterferon and ribavirin alone. Hepatology 2009;50(Suppl 4):LB6.
60. Klein CE, Cohen D, Menon RM, et al. Safety, tolerability, pharmacokinetics and antiviral activity of the HCV polymerase inhibitor ABT-072 following single and multiple dosing in healthy adult volunteers and two days of dosing in treatment-naïve HCV genotype 1-infected subjects. Kohala Coast (HI): HepDART; 2009. Poster #56.
61. Available at: http://clinicaltrials.gov/ct2/show/NCT01074008. Accessed January 8, 2011.
62. Shih I, Vliegen I, Peng B, et al. Mechanistic characterization of GS-9190, a novel non-nucleoside inhibitor of HCV NS5B polymerase with potent antiviral activity and a unique mechanism of action. Hepatology 2007;46(Suppl 1):859A.
63. Bavisotto L, Wang C, Jacobson I, et al. Antiviral Pharmakinetic and safety datafFor GS-9190, a non-nucleoside HCV NS5B polymerase inhibitor, in a phase-1 trial in HCV genotype 1 infected subjects. Hepatology 2007;46(Suppl 1):A49.
64. Harris J, Bae S, Sun S, et al. Antiviral response and resistanve analysis of treatment-naive HCV infected subjects receiving single and multi doses of GS-9190. 61st Annual Meeting of the American Association for the Study of Liver Diseases. Boston (MA), October 29 to November 2, 2010. Poster #833.

65. Available at: http://clinicaltrials.gov/ct2/show/NCT00743795. Accessed January 8, 2011.
66. De Bruijne J, Van de Wetering de Rooij J, Van Vliet A, et al. Phase I study in healthy volunteers and patients with IDX375, a novel non-nucleoside HCV polymerase inhibitor. Hepatology 2010;52(Suppl S1):A1891.

The NS5A Replication Complex Inhibitors: Difference Makers?

Robert G. Gish, MD[a,*], Nicholas A. Meanwell, PhD[b]

KEYWORDS

• Hepatitis C • NS5A • Replication • Inhibitor

The seroprevalence of hepatitis C virus (HCV) infection in the United States is 1.3% to 1.9%, infecting 4.1 to 5.0 million individuals.[1,2] Worldwide, at least 170 million persons are infected.[3] A total of 75% to 85% of primary infections become chronic, making hepatitis C one of the leading causes of chronic liver disease, cirrhosis, liver transplantation, and hepatocellular carcinoma globally and in the United States.[4,5]

Response to currently available therapy is strongly influenced by the viral genotype. Genotype 1 HCV, which predominates in North America and Europe, is associated with a poor sustained virologic response (SVR); cure rates are approximately 40% to 45% among patients who are treatment naïve and much lower (≈10%) for previous nonresponders who did not experience a greater than or equal to 2 $\log_{10}$ reduction in viral load during therapy with pegylated interferon-α and ribavirin.[6–8] In contrast, SVR rates for patients infected with HCV genotypes 2 and 3 are considerably higher (approximately 80%).[6] However, as a result of contraindications to treatment, individual circumstances, or intolerance, a large patient population exists who require improved treatment regimens. These patients include incarcerated persons, intravenous drug users, individuals with medical and psychiatric contraindications to interferon, and the substantial proportion of patients who have previously failed to respond to a course of pegylated interferon-α with ribavirin who together comprise a population that may currently exceed 2 million in the United States.

New direct-acting antiviral agents in development that target specific HCV enzymes and proteins are beginning to address these unmet needs. Two inhibitors of the HCV nonstructural (NS) 3/4A protease enzyme, telaprevir and boceprevir, are expected to

Author disclosures: Robert Gish was not reimbursed for this article. All funds are donated to research and education. Nicholas A. Meanwell is an employee and shareholder of Bristol-Myers Squibb.

[a] Division of Gastroenterology, University of California at San Diego, 200 West Arbor Drive, MC8413 (mail code), San Diego, CA 92103-8413, USA

[b] Department of Medicinal Chemistry, Bristol-Myers Squibb Research and Development, 5 Research Parkway, Wallingford, CT 06492, USA

* Corresponding author.

E-mail address: rgish@ucsd.edu

Clin Liver Dis 15 (2011) 627–639

doi:10.1016/j.cld.2011.05.010

1089-3261/11/$ – see front matter

be approved by mid 2011.[9–11] Used together with the current optimal therapy, pegylated interferon-α and ribavirin, these agents have achieved increased SVR rates of 67% to 75% among genotype 1 treatment-naïve patients, and have also demonstrated that treatment duration may be reduced to 24 to 28 weeks for patients who suppress HCV RNA early in therapy.[12–14] Response rates in previous nonresponders for regimens including these new agents were also improved over the current optimal therapy, but duration of therapy for these patients will likely continue to extend to 48 weeks.[15]

Although telaprevir and boceprevir will make it possible to achieve higher rates of SVR, the risks associated with their use, such as the emergence of resistance and the occurrence of systemic adverse effects, may require careful attention and individualized decision making by clinicians. In addition, many patients cannot undergo interferon- or ribavirin-based therapy because of underlying medical or psychiatric issues. HCV resistance to protease inhibitors is caused by variants that are either present before therapy or may emerge on treatment, with resistance rates of up to 20% observed after only 2 days of monotherapy with these agents.[16] In terms of tolerability, telaprevir treatment has been associated with anemia, rash, and diarrhea, and boceprevir has been associated with anemia that requires a reduction of ribavirin doses or the addition of erythropoietin.[12–14] Rates of treatment discontinuation or dose modifications were also higher in trials of these agents when compared with current treatment regimens.[12–14]

Beyond the development of telaprevir and boceprevir, a new wave of advances in HCV treatment options is progressing. Other direct-acting antivirals in development include compounds that inhibit the NS5B RNA-dependent RNA polymerase; second generation protease inhibitors, with once-daily dosing schedules[17,18]; and replacements for pegylated interferon-α, such as pegylated interferon-λ.[19] Novel agents that inhibit the HCV NS5A protein are also in development and have been shown to interact in an additive/synergistic fashion with other classes of direct-acting antiviral agents, including protease and polymerase inhibitors. The HCV NS5A protein and its role in viral replication is described here, along with the discovery and development of the first NS5A replication complex inhibitors to demonstrate a clinical effect. This development process allows us to predict the future possibility of interferon- and ribavirin-free treatment regimens using agents, such as the NS5A replication complex inhibitors, that would form the basis for high-potency, low-resistance combination protocols.

THE DISCOVERY AND DEVELOPMENT OF INHIBITORS OF HCV NS5A

Following the characterization of HCV as the cause of non-A, non-B hepatitis, the development of HCV inhibitors presented several challenges to a pharmaceutical industry focused on identifying direct-acting antiviral agents with the potential to replace pegylated interferon-α and ribavirin as the preferred therapy.[20] An important early limitation was the absence of virus replication systems that could assess compound activity in cell-based assays, a circumstance only resolved in 1999 with the description of the first subgenomic replicon.[21] This limitation restricted therapeutic targets to those enzymes for which biochemical assays could readily be recapitulated in vitro, leading to a focus on the identification of inhibitors of HCV NS3/4A protease and the NS5B RNA-dependent RNA polymerase. These initiatives were aided significantly by the solving of x-ray crystallographic structures of both proteins that facilitated structure-based drug design campaigns. A second deficiency was the lack of convenient and inexpensive animal models of HCV infection that could be employed to characterize the efficacy of test compounds in vivo, with only the chimpanzee model and, more recently, mice transplanted with chimeric human livers available. As a consequence, most pharmaceutical houses chose to assess compound efficacy in humans based on the convenience of measuring viral load as a rapid, responsive, and effective biomarker. Preclinical compound profiling was based on achieving acceptable pharmacokinetic properties in animal species that allowed predictive scaling to humans coupled with the demonstration of adequate liver exposure to a candidate compound. Although the latter is an important consideration, it has not presented a significant issue because the physical properties of many HCV inhibitors are such that the liver is a natural destination following oral administration.

The potential for the emergence of resistance to direct-acting antiviral inhibitors of HCV, a function of fundamental aspects of virus biochemistry, was also a consideration of considerable importance. The HCV NS5B RNA-dependent RNA polymerase possesses poor proofreading capacity, leading to the error-prone replication of viral RNA.[22] The rate of incorporation of errant bases has been estimated to be between 10^{-5} and 10^{-4} per nucleotide, a frequency that predicts an average number of changes per RNA genome synthesized of between 0.1 and 1.0 base. Taken together with the high replication rate of the virus, estimated to be 10^{12} virions per day (a figure that is 10- to 100-fold higher than that estimated for HIV), and the small genome size ($\approx$9600 bases), these data can be used to predict the probability of generating HCV variants incorporating nucleotide changes. The estimates reveal that even at the conservative error rate of 10^{-5} per nucleotide, 9% of virions produced in an infected individual per day will incorporate at least 1 nucleotide change, which translates to a daily production rate of 87×10^{10} particles incorporating a single change and as many as 4.2×10^{9} virions that incorporate 2 base changes. These numbers are in excess of the total number of possible single and double HCV mutants, 2.9×10^{4} and 4.1×10^{8}, respectively, predicting that every possible single and double mutant is generated multiple times on a daily basis.[22] The life span of HCV virions in plasma has been estimated to be approximately 4 hours, based on viral decay rates in the presence of interferon-α therapy, suggesting that any mutant virus produced more than 6 times per day will have a persistent presence. Taken together, these data predict the rapid emergence of preexisting or (less likely) de novo variants that are resistant to the use of direct-acting antiviral agents as a monotherapy[16] and anticipate the importance of combination therapy.[23–25]

With this information as the backdrop, pharmaceutical companies have generally adopted an aggressive approach by pursuing the identification and development of drug candidates designed to interfere with mechanistically distinct HCV targets that can be used in combination with other oral or injection therapies. Although the identification of potent inhibitors of the HCV NS3/4A protease and the NS5B polymerase initially presented significant challenges, considerable progress has been made over the last 15 years, and potent and selective inhibitors of both enzymes have advanced into clinical trials, where efficacy has been demonstrated in short-term clinical studies. Protease inhibitor design has been based on inhibitors that interact with the enzyme active site either by a reversible covalent (telaprevir and boceprevir) or noncovalent (vaniprevir, MK-5172, BMS-650032, TMC-435350, and BI-201335) binding mechanism. Inhibitors of the polymerase are based on nucleoside analogs, represented by R-7128, PSI-7977, IDX-184, and INX-189, or agents that bind to the thumb (filibuvir, BI-207127 and MK-3281) or palm (ANA-598, GS-9190 and IDX-375) domains of the enzyme and that function by an allosteric inhibitory mechanism.[26]

The advent of HCV subgenomic replicons and, subsequently, replicating virus, provided an opportunity to conduct mechanistically unbiased, high-throughput screening campaigns designed to identify inhibitors acting by novel and unanticipated modes of action.[27] This kind of approach is particularly useful and effective for generating novel antiviral agents because the identification of the target is facilitated by the sequencing of the virus that has developed resistance to a lead inhibitor. It was this kind of strategy, typically referred to as a chemical genetics approach to lead inhibitor generation, that was employed by a group at Bristol-Myers Squibb to identify the first documented inhibitors of HCV NS5A. HCV NS5A is a critically important viral protein of enigmatic function in replication that does not exhibit any known enzymatic function. The successful screening campaign relied upon a dual replicon assay format that simultaneously characterized compounds as inhibitors of HCV genotype 1b and bovine viral diarrhea virus (BVDV) replicons, while also assessing cytotoxicity to the host HuH-7 hepatocyte cell line.[28] Taking advantage of orthogonal reporters of viral replication and cell viability, compounds were rapidly triaged for specificity toward HCV compared with the closely related BVDV, resulting in the identification of BMS-858 as a lead inhibitor (**Fig. 1**).[29] Resistance to BMS-858 was mapped to changes in the amino terminus of the NS5A protein, specifically a Y93H variant or the dual L31V/Q54L mutant.[29] However, this lead structure proved to be somewhat cryptic in nature. This circumstance was a function of an intrinsic chemical instability under the assay conditions that resulted in a radical-mediated dimerization of BMS-858 to compounds characterized to possess highly potent inhibitory activity in replicons.[30] Simplification of the dimer to a palindromic stilbene derivative elucidated the NS5A-inhibiting pharmacophore, triggering a drug discovery campaign focused on enhancing potency, broadening genotype coverage to encompass the 1a subtype prevalent in the United States, and optimizing pharmacokinetic properties to promote plasma and liver exposure that was sustained following oral dosing to animals.[30,31] Following extensive study, BMS-790052 was identified as a candidate NS5A replication complex inhibitor with properties suitable for clinical evaluation (see **Fig. 1**).[31] This molecule potently inhibits replicons representative of all of the 6 major HCV genotypes with 50% effective concentrations (EC_{50}) of less than 1 nM without overt cytotoxicity to host cells (**Table 1**). The discovery of this compound represents a significant advance because the majority of

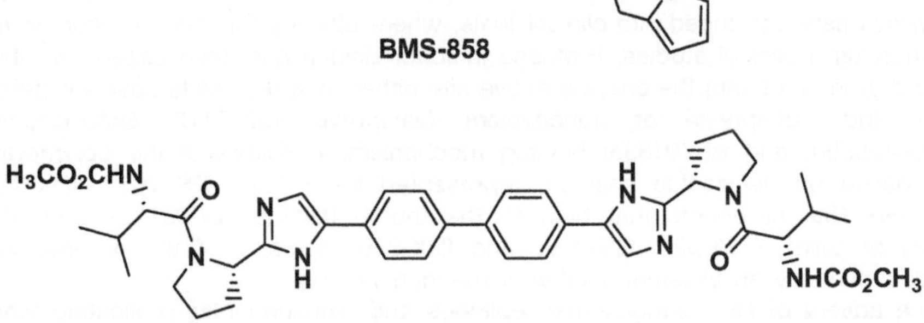

BMS-858

BMS-790052

Fig. 1. Chemical structures of BMS-858 and BMS-790052.

Table 1
In vitro inhibition of HCV replicons by BMS-790052

Assay	EC_{50}
HCV replicon genotype 1a, H77	50 ± 13 pM
HCV replicon genotype 1b, Con1	9 ± 4 pM
HCV replicon genotype 2a, JFH	71 ± 17 pM
HCV replicon genotype 2a, JFH[a]	103 ± 36 pM
HCV replicon genotype 3a[a]	146 ± 34 pM
HCV replicon genotype 4a[a]	12 ± 4 pM
HCV replicon genotype 5a[a]	33 ± 10 pM
Cytotoxicity HuH−7cells	17 ± 1 μM

[a] Data derived from hybrid replicons.
Data from Gao M, Nettles RE, Belema M, et al. Chemical genetics strategy identifies an HCV NS5A inhibitor with a potent clinical effect. Nature 2010;465:97.

direct-acting antiviral agents, other than nucleoside analogs, exhibit a restricted genotype focus. Importantly, BMS-790052 was shown to inhibit the genotype 2a virus designated JFH with an EC_{50} of 28 pM. Portending the potential to be used in combination therapy, BMS-790052 interacted synergistically with interferon-α2b (Intron A) and additively to synergistically with a representative NS3/4A protease inhibitor, a non-nucleoside NS5B polymerase inhibitor targeting the thumb domain, and the nucleoside-based NS5B polymerase inhibitor NM-107 to inhibit HCV replication in subgenomic replicons.

HCV NS5A AND ITS ROLE IN VIRAL REPLICATION

HCV NS5A is a 447 amino acid phosphoprotein comprising amino acids 1973 to 2419 of the genomic polyprotein, which has been classified into 3 distinct domains based on the occurrence of sequences of low complexity (**Fig. 2**).[32–34] Domain I comprises residues 1 to 213 and incorporates an amphipathic α-helix domain (residues 5–25) that anchors the protein in the membrane. A Zn^{2+}-binding element has been identified by x-ray crystallographic analysis of a portion of domain I.[35,36] This portion is composed of the 4 cysteine residues (Cys39, Cys57, Cys59, and Cys80) and contributes an important stabilizing element to the protein. Domain II, residues 250 to 342, contains a putative interferon sensitivity-determining region, residues 237 to 276, whose existence is controversial.[37] This domain also contains a binding site for cyclophilin, the cis-trans proline isomerase that is an important regulator of HCV replication, which provides a basis for the antiviral activity of cyclosporine and the related nonimmunosuppressive analogs NIM-811, SCY-635, and DEBIO-25.[38] Domain III is composed of the C-terminal residues 356 to 447 and has been identified as playing an important role in virus assembly.[39,40] The NS5A protein is basally phosphorylated at the conserved Ser222, with Ser225, Ser229, and Ser232 as the sites where hyperphosphorylation occurs. Binding sites for the viral proteins NS4A and NS5B have been mapped to domain I with an additional NS5B binding site located in domain II, and NS5A is an important component of the replication complex.[41] All 3 domains of HCV NS5A have been shown to be important to viral replication. The effect of HCV NS5A on host cell signaling pathways and its interaction with host cell proteins has been extensively explored. These studies demonstrate the pleiotropic nature of the protein and reveal considerable complexity, a circumstance that has prevented the

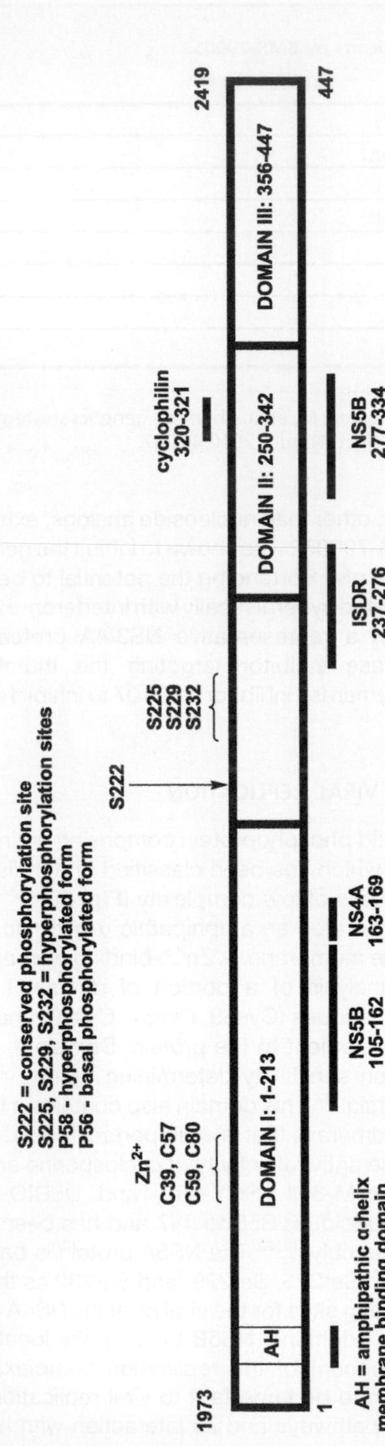

Fig. 2. Map of the HCV NS5A protein. ISDR, interferon sensitivity determining region.

development of a coherent picture of function in viral replication and host cell modulation.

Inhibitors of NS5A that interact with domain I have been solved, based on resistance mapping studies and x-ray crystallographic structures of the protein.[35,36] Residues 36 to 198 and 33 to 191 of domain I each revealed a dimeric species with a similar topography, although the interfacial sites were quite different. The solid-state form of residues 36 to 191 formed a dimer that relied on contacts near the amino terminus, with residues 36 to 38 contributing to the interfacial recognition to adopt a U-shaped topology. This spatial arrangement forms a groove lined with basic amino acids and is postulated to bind viral RNA. The monomers of residues 33 to 191 presented a very similar structure to residues 36 to 198; however, the dimer interface relied upon interactions between residues 92 to 99, 112 to 116, 139 to 143, 146 to 149, and 160 to 161 from each monomer in contrast to the structure of 36 to 198. Taken together, the x-ray structures anticipate an oligomeric form of the protein that can bind viral RNA. NS5A may function to sequester the viral RNA, thereby protecting it from chemical and enzymatic degradation while being able to present a template to the replication machinery.[42] Oligomerization of HCV NS5A has been observed biochemically,[43] and domain I of HCV NS5A has been shown to associate with RNA, although domains II and III also contribute.[44–46]

The palindromic topology of BMS-790052 complements the dimeric solid-state structure of domain I residues 36 to 198, and the mapping of resistance mutations suggest a binding interaction with NS5A in which the inhibitor interacts across the dimer interface, close to the amino terminus and on the side of the protein opposite the RNA binding domain. The high potency of HCV NS5A inhibitors in HCV replicons may be caused by a distortion of the dimer association or function in the context of the higher-order oligomer or the consequence of interference with multiple functions of NS5A that combine synergistically to inhibit virus replication.

CLINICAL STUDIES WITH BMS-790052

BMS-790052 was advanced into phase 1 clinical trials where initial studies demonstrated a dose-related exposure in the plasma of normal healthy volunteers following the administration of single oral doses of the drug ranging from 1 to 200 mg. The drug concentration in plasma at 24 hours after administration surpassed the protein binding-adjusted EC_{90} for both genotypes 1a (383 pM) and 1b (49 pM) at all of the doses studied. When patients infected with HCV were administered single doses of 1, 10, and 100 mg of BMS-790052, rapid and profound reductions in viremia were readily apparent. Viral load diminished by a maximum of 3.6 $\log_{10}$ at the 100-mg dose, which was sustained for 144 hours postdose in 2 patients infected with genotype 1b virus (**Fig. 3**). This trial provided the first clinical validation for inhibition of HCV NS5A as a therapeutic modality for the treatment of HCV infection, highlighting the potency of this mechanistic approach and representing an advance in treatment options.

Subsequent clinical studies have evaluated BMS-790052 in conjunction with the combination of pegylated interferon-α and ribavirin in a treatment-naïve population. Following 12 weeks of triple combination therapy, 75% of patients in the 60-mg cohort and 83% in the 10-mg dose group achieved early rapid virologic response, defined as undetectable levels of viremia (limit of detection, HCV RNA <10 IU/mL) at weeks 4 and 12 following the initiation of therapy (**Table 2**).[47] In a second phase 2a study, a combination of BMS-790052 and the NS3/4A protease inhibitor BMS-650032, administered with and without pegylated interferon-α and ribavirin, was studied in genotype 1 null

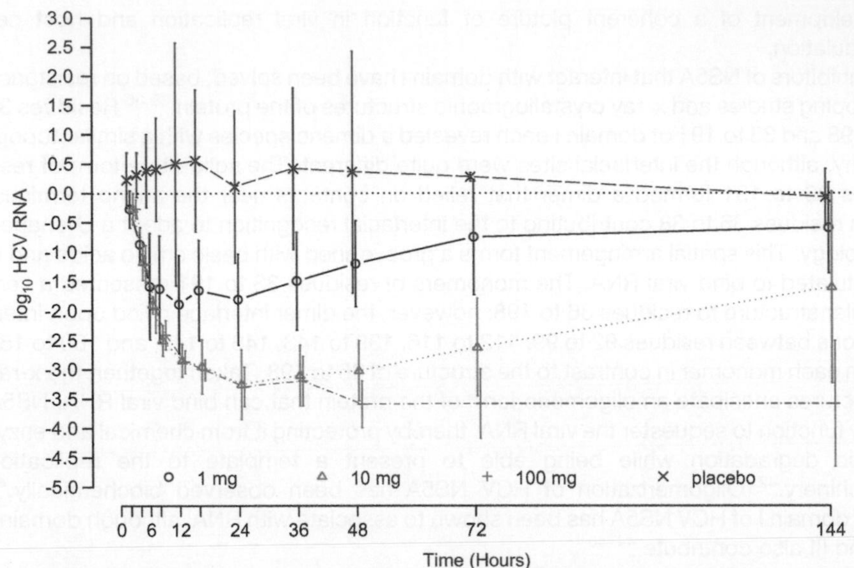

Fig. 3. Mean change in $\log_{10}$ HCV RNA with 90% confidence intervals following administration of single oral doses of BMS-790052 to patients infected with HCV. (*From* Gao M, Nettles RE, Belema M, et al. Chemical genetics strategy identifies an HCV NS5A inhibitor with a potent clinical effect. Nature 2010;465:99. *Reprinted from* Macmillan Publishers Ltd, copyright 2010; with permission.)

responders. All patients treated with quadruple therapy and 2 genotype 1b patients receiving only a combination of the direct-acting antiviral drugs maintained viral suppression. However, 6 patients infected with genotype 1a experienced a virologic breakthrough that occurred as early as week 3 of therapy and as late as week 12. Pegylated interferon-α and ribavirin were added to their regimens, and all patients exhibited a positive response.[48]

The disclosure of the potent clinical effect of BMS-790052 has stimulated considerable interest in HCV NS5A replication complex inhibition as a target for therapy, and several additional inhibitors have been either advanced into clinical trials or identified as candidates for preclinical toxicology studies. Those compounds that are currently in development are summarized in **Table 3**.

Table 2
Antiviral activity of BMS-790052 in a phase 2a clinical trial after 12 weeks of therapy

QD dose with P/R (all n = 12)	PBO (%)	3 mg (%)	10 mg (%)	60 mg (%)
RVR (week 4 undetectable)	8	42	92	83
cEVR (week 12 undetectable)	42	58	83	83
eRVR (weeks 4 & 12 undetectable)	8	42	83[a]	75
Achieved undetectable RNA	42	58	92	100

Abbreviations: cEVR, complete early virologic response; eRVR, early virologic; PBO, placebo; P/R, pegylated interferon-α and ribavirin; QD, once daily; RVR, rapid virologic response.

[a] Data for 1 patient missing at week 12 and not counted in eRVR but had RNA <10 IU/mL at weeks 4 and 16.

Table 3
Inhibitors of HCV NS5A in clinical development

Compound	Sponsor	EC_{50} Genotype 1a (nM)	EC_{50} Genotype 1b (nM)	Other Genotypes	Current Status
A-831	Arrow Therapeutics	550	270	Not disclosed	On hold
AZ-689 (AZD-7295)	Arrow/AstraZeneca	1240	7	Not disclosed	Phase 1[49]
BMS-824393	Bristol-Myers Squibb	Not disclosed	Not disclosed	Not disclosed	Phase 1[50]
PPI-461	Presidio Pharmaceuticals	0.20	0.01	2a: 0.6; 3a: 9.3; 4a: 0.1; 5a: 0.1; 6a: 6.1; 7a: 0.6 (transient transfections)	Phase 1[51,52]
PPI-1301	Presidio Pharmaceuticals	Not disclosed	Not disclosed	Not disclosed	Preclinical
GS-5885	Gilead	0.041	0.005	2a: 0.6; 3a: 9.3; 4a: 0.1; 5a: 0.1; 6a: 6.1; 7a: 0.6 (transient transfections) Chimeric replicons: 2a: 20.8 nM; 3a: 10.1 nM; 4a: 7 pM	Phase 1[53]
EDP-239	Enanta Pharmaceuticals	0.034	0.004	Not disclosed	Preclinical[54]
ACH-2928	Achillion Pharmaceuticals	0.013	0.002	Not disclosed	Preclinical[55]

SUMMARY

With the emergence of newer therapies, such as the NS5A replication complex inhibitors, with their picomolar potency, nonoverlapping resistance profiles, prolonged viral suppression, ability to exert an antiviral effect when used in combination with other direct-acting antivirals, and estimated fewer adverse effects, combination therapy with this exciting class of compounds with protease and polymerase inhibitors is clearly one of the next phases in HCV drug development. The probability is increasing that we will have the opportunity to replace interferon-α and ribavirin with double or triple oral therapy using direct-acting antiviral agents, or with quadruple therapy with medications that replace interferon-α, such as interferon-λ or 4 oral agents. The profound reduction in HCV RNA observed in patients treated with the new NS5A replication complex inhibitors and in patients on triple or quadruple therapy (with pegylated interferon-α and ribavirin as optimal therapy and 1 or 2 other direct-acting antiviral agents) offers hope that we may soon be entering a phase of HCV treatment in which the treatment duration of interferon will be markedly shortened or completely abrogated.

ACKNOWLEDGMENTS

The authors would like to thank Steven Schnittman and Min Gao for their assistance during the preparation of the manuscript. Editorial assistance was provided by Andrew Street at Articulate Science and was funded by Bristol-Myers Squibb Company.

REFERENCES

1. Armstrong GL, Wasley A, Simard EP, et al. The prevalence of hepatitis C virus infection in the United States, 1999 through 2002. Ann Intern Med 2006; 144(10):705–14.
2. Gish RG, Afdhal NH, Dieterich DT, et al. Management of hepatitis C virus in special populations: patient and treatment considerations. Clin Gastroenterol Hepatol 2005;3(4):311–8.
3. World Health Organization. Global Alert and Response (GAR) - hepatitis C. Available at: http://www.who.int/csr/disease/hepatitis/whocdscsrlyo2003/en/index4.html. Accessed January 26, 2011.
4. Centers for Disease Control and Prevention. Division of viral hepatitis. The ABCs of Hepatitis. Available at: http://www.cdc.gov/hepatitis/Resources/Professionals/PDFs/ABCTable.pdf. Accessed January 26, 2011.
5. Perz JF, Armstrong GL, Farrington LA, et al. The contributions of hepatitis B virus and hepatitis C virus infections to cirrhosis and primary liver cancer worldwide. J Hepatol 2006;45(4):529–38.
6. Rumi MG, Aghemo A, Prati GM, et al. Randomized study of peginterferon-alpha2a plus ribavirin vs peginterferon-alpha2b plus ribavirin in chronic hepatitis C. Gastroenterology 2010;138(1):108–15.
7. Fried MW, Shiffman ML, Reddy KR, et al. Peginterferon alfa-2a plus ribavirin for chronic hepatitis C virus infection. N Engl J Med 2002;347(13):975–82.
8. Poynard T, Colombo M, Bruix J, et al. Peginterferon alfa-2b and ribavirin: effective in patients with hepatitis C who failed interferon alfa/ribavirin therapy. Gastroenterology 2009;136(5):1618–28.
9. McHutchison JG, Everson GT, Gordon SC, et al. Telaprevir with peginterferon and ribavirin for chronic HCV genotype 1 infection. N Engl J Med 2009;360(18): 1827–38.

10. Hezode C, Forestier N, Dusheiko G, et al. Telaprevir and peginterferon with or without ribavirin for chronic HCV infection. N Engl J Med 2009;360(18):1839–50.
11. Kwo PY, Lawitz EJ, McCone J, et al. Efficacy of boceprevir, an NS3 protease inhibitor, in combination with peginterferon alfa-2b and ribavirin in treatment-naive patients with genotype 1 hepatitis C infection (SPRINT-1): an open-label, randomised, multicentre phase 2 trial. Lancet 2010;376(9742):705–16.
12. Poordad F, McCone J, Bacon BR, et al. Boceprevir (BOC) combined with peginterferon alfa-2b/ribavirin (P/R) for treatment-naïve patients with hepatitis C virus (HCV) genotype (G) 1: SPRINT-2 final results. Hepatology 2010;52(Suppl S1): 402A–3A [abstract: LB-4].
13. Sherman KE, Flamm SL, Afdhal NH, et al. Telaprevir in combination with peginterferon alfa2a and ribavirin for 24 or 48 weeks in treatment-naïve genotype 1 HCV patients who achieved an extended rapid viral response: final results of phase 3 ILLUMINATE study. Hepatology 2010;52(Suppl S1):401A–2A [abstract: LB-2].
14. Jacobson IM, McHutchison JG, Dusheiko GM, et al. Telaprevir in combination with peginterferon and ribavirin in genotype 1 HCV treatment-naïve patients: final results of phase 3 ADVANCE study. Hepatology 2010;52(Suppl S1):427A [abstract: 211].
15. Bacon BR, Gordon SC, Lawitz E, et al. HCV RESPOND-2 final results: high sustained virologic response among genotype 1 previous non-responders and relapsers to peginterferon/ribavirin when re-treated with boceprevir plus PEGINTRON (peginterferon alfa 2b)/ribavirin. Hepatology 2010;52(Suppl S1):430A [abstract: 216].
16. Rong L, Dahari H, Ribeiro RM, et al. Rapid emergence of protease inhibitor resistance in hepatitis C virus. Sci Transl Med 2010;2(30):30–2.
17. Berg T, Dieterich DT, Lalezari JP, et al. Virological response and safety of 4 weeks treatment with the protease inhibitor BI 201335 combined with 48 weeks of peginterferon alfa 2a and ribavirin for treatment of HCV GT-1 patients who failed peginterferon/ribavirin. Hepatology 2010;52(Suppl S1):704A [abstract: 804].
18. Fried MW, Buti M, Dore GJ, et al. Efficacy and safety of TMC435 in combination with peginterferon-2a and ribavirin in treatment-naive genotype-1 HCV patients: 24-week interim results from the PILLAR study. Hepatology 2010;52(Suppl S1): 403A–4A [abstract: LB-5].
19. Muir AJ, Lawitz E, Ghalib RH, et al. Pegylated interferon lambda (PEG-IFN-λ) phase 2 dose-ranging, active-controlled study in combination with ribavirin (RBV) for treatment-naïve HCV patients (genotypes 1, 2, 3 or 4): safety, viral response, and impact of IL-28B host genotype through week 12. Hepatology 2010;52(Suppl S1):715A [abstract: 821].
20. De Francesco R, Migliaccio G. Challenges and successes in developing new therapies for hepatitis C. Nature 2005;436(7053):953–60.
21. Bartenschlager R. Hepatitis C virus molecular clones: from cDNA to infectious virus particles in cell culture. Curr Opin Microbiol 2006;9(4):416–22.
22. Guedj J, Rong L, Dahari H, et al. A perspective on modelling hepatitis C virus infection. J Viral Hepat 2010;17(12):825–33.
23. Manns MP, Foster GR, Rockstroh JK, et al. The way forward in HCV treatment–finding the right path. Nat Rev Drug Discov 2007;6(12):991–1000.
24. Koev G, Kati W. The emerging field of HCV drug resistance. Expert Opin Investig Drugs 2008;17(3):303–19.
25. Gelman MA, Glenn JS. Mixing the right hepatitis C inhibitor cocktail. Trends Mol Med 2011;17(3):34–46.
26. Lange CM, Sarrazin C, Zeuzem S. Review article: specifically targeted anti-viral therapy for hepatitis C - a new era in therapy. Aliment Pharmacol Ther 2010; 32(1):14–28.

27. Green N, Ott RD, Isaacs RJ, et al. Cell-based assays to identify inhibitors of viral disease. Expert Opin Drug Discov 2008;3(6):671–6.
28. O'Boyle DR 2nd, Nower PT, Lemm JA, et al. Development of a cell-based high-throughput specificity screen using a hepatitis C virus-bovine viral diarrhea virus dual replicon assay. Antimicrob Agents Chemother 2005;49(4):1346–53.
29. Lemm JA, O'Boyle D 2nd, Liu M, et al. Identification of hepatitis C virus NS5A inhibitors. J Virol 2010;84(1):482–91.
30. Romine JL, St Laurent DR, Leet JE, et al. Inhibitors of HCV NS5A: from iminothiazolidinones to symmetrical stilbenes. ACS Med Chem Lett 2011;12(3):224–9.
31. Gao M, Nettles RE, Belema M, et al. Chemical genetics strategy identifies an HCV NS5A inhibitor with a potent clinical effect. Nature 2010;465(7294):96–100.
32. Macdonald A, Harris M. Hepatitis C virus NS5A: tales of a promiscuous protein. J Gen Virol 2004;85(9):2485–502.
33. Schmitz U, Tan SL. NS5A–from obscurity to new target for HCV therapy. Recent Pat Antiinfect Drug Discov 2008;3(2):77–92.
34. Huang Y, Staschke K, De Francesco R, et al. Phosphorylation of hepatitis C virus NS5A nonstructural protein: a new paradigm for phosphorylation-dependent viral RNA replication? Virology 2007;364(1):1–9.
35. Tellinghuisen TL, Marcotrigiano J, Rice CM. Structure of the zinc-binding domain of an essential component of the hepatitis C virus replicase. Nature 2005; 435(7040):374–9.
36. Love RA, Brodsky O, Hickey MJ, et al. Crystal structure of a novel dimeric form of NS5A domain I protein from hepatitis C virus. J Virol 2009;83(9):4395–403.
37. Brillet R, Penin F, Hezode C, et al. The nonstructural 5A protein of hepatitis C virus genotype 1b does not contain an interferon sensitivity-determining region. J Infect Dis 2007;195(3):432–41.
38. Flisiak R, Dumont JM, Crabbe R. Cyclophilin inhibitors in hepatitis C viral infection. Expert Opin Investig Drugs 2007;16(9):1345–54.
39. Tellinghuisen TL, Foss KL, Treadaway J. Regulation of hepatitis C virion production via phosphorylation of the NS5A protein. PLoS Pathog 2008;4(3):e1000032.
40. Appel N, Zayas M, Miller S, et al. Essential role of domain III of nonstructural protein 5A for hepatitis C virus infectious particle assembly. PLoS Pathog 2008; 4(3):e1000035.
41. Shirota Y, Luo H, Qin W, et al. Hepatitis C virus (HCV) NS5A binds RNA-dependent RNA polymerase (RdRP) NS5B and modulates RNA-dependent RNA polymerase activity. J Biol Chem 2002;277(13):11149–55.
42. Appel N, Schaller T, Penin F, et al. From structure to function: new insights into hepatitis C virus RNA replication. J Biol Chem 2006;281(15):9833–6.
43. Dimitrova M, Imbert I, Kieny MP, et al. Protein-protein interactions between hepatitis C virus nonstructural proteins. J Virol 2003;77(9):5401–14.
44. Huang L, Hwang J, Sharma SD, et al. Hepatitis C virus nonstructural protein 5A (NS5A) is an RNA-binding protein. J Biol Chem 2005;280(43):36417–28.
45. Foster TL, Belyaeva T, Stonehouse NJ, et al. All three domains of the hepatitis C virus nonstructural NS5A protein contribute to RNA binding. J Virol 2010;84(18):9267–77.
46. Hwang J, Huang L, Cordek DG, et al. Hepatitis C virus nonstructural protein 5A: biochemical characterization of a novel structural class of RNA-binding proteins. J Virol 2010;84(24):12480–91.
47. Pol S, Everson G, Ghalib R, et al. Once-daily NS5A inhibitor (BMS-790052) plus peginterferon-alpha-2A and ribavirin produces high rates of extended rapid virologic response in treatment-naive HCV-genotype 1 subjects: phase 2A trial. J Hepatol 2010;52(Suppl 1):S462 [abstract: 1189].

48. Lok AS, Gardiner DF, Lawitz E, et al. Combination therapy with BMS-790052 and BMS-650032 alone or with pegIFN/RBV results in undetectable HCV RNA through 12 weeks of therapy in HCV genotype 1 null responders. Hepatology 2010; 52(S1):877A [abstract: LB-8].
49. Gane E, Foster GR, Cianciara J, et al. Antiviral activity, pharmacokinetics, and tolerability of AZD7295, a novel NS5A inhibitor, in a placebo-controlled multiple ascending dose study in HCV genotype 1 AND 3 patients. J Hepatol 2010; 52(Suppl 1):S464 [abstract: 2003].
50. Nettles RE, Wang X, Quadri S, et al. BMS-824393 is a potent hepatitis C virus NS5A inhibitor with substantial antiviral activity when given as monotherapy in subjects with chronic G1 HCV infection. Hepatology 2010;52(Suppl S1):1203A [abstract: 1858].
51. Colonno R, Peng E, Bencsik M, et al. Identification and characterization of PPI-461, a potent and selective HCV NS5A inhibitor with activity against all HCV genotypes. J Hepatol 2010;52(Suppl 1):S14–5 [abstract: 33].
52. Brown NA, Vig P, Ruby E, et al. Safety and pharmacokinetics of PPI-461, a potent new hepatitis C virus (HCV) NS5A inhibitor with pan-genotype activity. Hepatology 2010;52(S1):879A–80A [abstract: LB-12].
53. Link JO, Bannister R, Beilke LD, et al. Nonclinical profile and phase I results in healthy volunteers for the novel and potent HCV NS5A inhibitor GS-5885. Hepatology 2010;52(S1):1215A–6A [abstract: 1883].
54. Owens CM, Brasher B, Polemeropoulos AJ, et al. EDP-239 is a novel potent NS5A inhibitor with an excellent preclinical and resistance profile. Hepatology 2010; 52(S1):1206A [abstract: 1863].
55. Achillion Pharmaceuticals I. Achillion Pharmaceuticals announces nomination of NS5A inhibitor as a lead clinical candidate for treatment of HCV. Available at: http://files.shareholder.com/downloads/ACHN/1150849922x0x388696/b82f8182-53f3-4e95-ae4c-8610528f83be/ACHN_News_2010_7_22_General.pdf. Accessed January 26, 2011.

Hepatitis C Therapy: Other Players in the Game

Joseph Ahn, MD, MS[a], Steven L. Flamm, MD[b,*]

KEYWORDS

• Hepatitis C • Cyclophilin inhibitor • Thiazolide
• Therapeutic vaccine • TLR agonist

Hepatitis C virus (HCV) is a serious worldwide cause of chronic liver disease despite ongoing research in drug development to improve the rates of sustained virologic response (SVR) and reduce the rates of significant side effects. The current standard of care with pegylated interferon (IFN) α2a or 2b (PEG) in combination with ribavirin (RBV) yields SVR of less than 50% in patients with HCV genotype 1 (GT 1). Certain populations have lower SVR, including African Americans, Latino people, and patients with HCV–human immunodeficiency virus (HIV) coinfection.

Because the current standard of care has less than desirable SVR and numerous side effects, active research has been ongoing with the goal of increasing SVR, improving tolerability, and decreasing length of therapy. Direct-acting antiviral agents (DAA) that directly target HCV have been developed, and numerous candidates are being investigated for treatment of chronic HCV. The protease inhibitors telaprevir and boceprevir have completed phase 3 trials and are currently undergoing evaluation by the US Food and Drug Administration for regulatory approval. However, although it seems that SVR will increase and that the length of therapy for many patients with HCV GT 1 will decrease, problems with the DAAs remain. At present, PEG and RBV are necessary in combination with the protease inhibitors. Thus, patients with contraindications to PEG or RBV will be ineligible for the initial DAA regimens. Because of this, there has been interest in developing new IFN-like and ribavirin-like products that may have more favorable tolerability profiles. Second, although SVRs are much higher, a substantial number of patients with HCV GT 1 still do not achieve SVR, including a large number of patients with poor IFN responsiveness. Third, initial data suggest

Financial disclosures: the authors have nothing to disclose in regards to the contents of this manuscript.
[a] Loyola University Medical Center, Room 167, Building 54, South First Avenue, Maywood, IL 60153, USA
[b] Northwestern Feinberg School of Medicine, 676 North Saint Clair Street, Chicago, IL 60611, USA
* Corresponding author.
E-mail address: s-flamm@northwestern.edu

Clin Liver Dis 15 (2011) 641–656
doi:10.1016/j.cld.2011.05.008 liver.theclinics.com

that African Americans continue to have less attractive SVR. In addition, the issue of resistance is pertinent because the DAAs are direct HCV enzyme inhibitors and strategic viral mutations can confer resistance. These issues have increased interest in development of host-targeted HCV life cycle agents such as cyclophilin inhibitors, therapeutic vaccines, and immunomodulators.

This article reviews these other players in the game. The focus is generally on compounds that have moved past preclinical and early phase I trials; however, because the research on these products is early, much of the information is in abstract form.

HOST-TARGETED ANTIVIRAL AGENTS

HCV Life Cycle

Because of limited in vitro models of HCV replication, the precise mechanisms of HCV replication are incompletely understood, especially in the later stages of the HCV life cycle of replication, assembly, and release. However, the main steps of the HCV life cycle are known to include entry into the host cell, viral uncoating, translation of structural and nonstructural HCV proteins, replication, followed by assembly of the viral proteins, and subsequent viral release, as shown in **Fig. 1**.[1]

Viral entry into the host cell has been proposed to be mediated by several host cell surface molecules such as CD81 and human scavenger receptor class B type I (SR-BI), as well as more recently identified tight junction proteins such as Claudin 1 and occludin.[2] They are believed to interact with viral ligands such as glycoprotein E1 and E2 to facilitate HCV entry. Once the virus enters the cell, it undergoes uncoating, with subsequent viral genome exposure that uses the host cell machinery to translate viral proteins, including both structural and nonstructural proteins. The nonstructural proteins such as NS5A and NS5B then establish the viral replication machinery in association with intracellular membranes to initiate viral replication. Although the exact interaction of the viral replication complex with these membranes is not clear, it is postulated that these membranes are used as compartments to

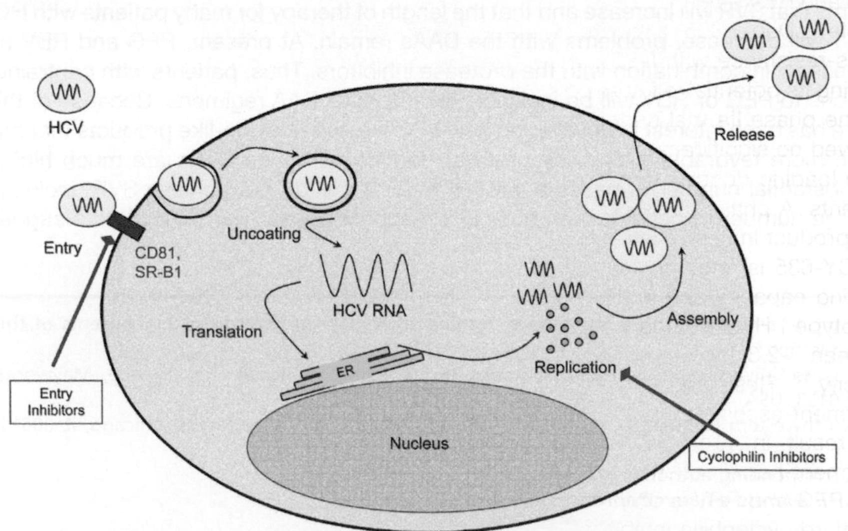

Fig. 1. HCV life cycle, showing 2 potential sites of host-targeted antiviral agents. ER, endoplasmic reticulum.

protect the HCV virus from host defense mechanisms. Subsequently, the virus components are assembled and released into the host circulation.

HCV Entry Inhibitors

HCV entry inhibitors targeting host cell surface molecules are currently being developed, although none have published results of phase 2 clinical treatment trials to date.

Cyclophilins

Cyclophilins are a highly conserved family of human enzymes (peptidyl-prolyl *cis-trans* isomerases) involved in cellular processes associated with protein folding, transport, and secretion as well as mitochondrial function and immune response. However, cyclophilins can be co-opted by the HCV to become a cofactor for viral replication. In the hepatocyte cytoplasm, cyclophilins A and B bind with HCV viral proteins NS5A and NS5B to form a replication complex to mediate the correct folding and trafficking of HCV proteins, thus functioning as a positive modulator for hepatitis C viral replication.[3,4] Via its inhibitory action on cyclophilins, cyclosporine was found to inhibit HCV replication in cell culture replicon models as well as in patients.[4,5] However, cyclosporine has immunosuppressive effects via its inhibition of calcineurin, limiting its usefulness as an anti-HCV product. However, cyclophilin inhibitors without concomitant calcineurin inhibition have been developed.

Debio-025 is a synthetic nonimmunosuppressive form of cyclosporine that has potent activity against a broad range of HCV genotypes[1–4] and HIV in cell culture systems.[6] Phase Ib studies were conducted in 19 HCV/HIV coinfected subjects given 1200 mg twice a day of Debio-025 for 14 days, resulting in a mean HCV RNA reduction of −3.6 log[7] without viral rebound.[8] A phase II dose-ranging trial treated 90 HCV treatment-naive subjects divided into 5 groups for 29 days: PEG with placebo, PEG with 200 mg, 600 mg, or 1000 mg twice daily of Debio-025, and Debio-025 1000 mg twice daily alone.[9] Debio-025 was shown to provide an additive effect in HCV RNA reduction from −2.2 log[7] to −4.75 log[7] with the 1000-mg arm in subjects with HCV GT 1. A follow-up study monitoring these subjects who were administered PEG and RBV after day 29 reported an SVR of 67% without any adverse events attributable to Debio-025.[10] In vitro studies of Debio-025 have reported a lack of significant cross-resistance with NS3 protease inhibitors or various polymerase inhibitors, suggesting its potential in future combination therapy with these agents.[7] The initial report on the phase IIa trial conducted on 50 HCV GT 1 nonresponders to PEG and RBV showed no significant reduction in HCV RNA, leading to questions regarding a need for a loading dose.[11] A mild conjugated hyperbilirubinemia has been noted in some patients. A phase IIb, double-blind, placebo-controlled trial is underway to evaluate this product in combination with PEG and RBV.

SCY-635 is another derivative of cyclosporine shown to have in vitro cyclophilin binding capacity and antifibrogenic activity.[12] A phase I study on 20 subjects with genotype I HCV treated with 300, 600, or 900 mg of SCY-635 for 15 days reported a mean −2.3 log[7] HCV RNA reduction in the 900 mg cohort without significant toxicity.[13] Resistance testing suggested a high barrier to resistance with no treatment-associated mutations in the NS5A protein and mutations in NS5B that did not result in virologic breakthrough.[14] A phase IIa clinical trial in HCV GT 1 treatment-naive patients administered escalating doses of SCY-635 in conjunction with PEG and RBV is ongoing.

A third cyclophilin inhibitor, NIM811, was shown in a phase Ib study in HCV GT 1 relapsers to standard HCV treatment to reduce HCV RNA. Six-hundred milligrams twice a day of NIM811 along with pegylated IFN-α2a led to a −2.78 log[7] reduction compared with −0.58 $\log^7$ with the PEG alone.[15] However, there were significant safety concerns because of development of hyperbilirubinemia and thrombocytopenia. The concern that this may be a potential class-associated adverse effect was ameliorated by a recent report of an in vitro model for assessing the risk of hyperbilirubinemia associated with SCY-635, which showed that SCY-635 was not associated with significant hyperbilirubinemia.[16]

AGENTS AFFECTING THE HOST IMMUNE SYSTEM

Nitazoxanide

Nitazoxanide (NTZ) is an antiprotozoal drug with efficacy against helminths, *Cryptosporidium*, *Giardia*, and *Clostridium difficile*. It was identified incidentally as a potential HCV treatment when patients with HCV and HIV coinfection were noted to have improved alanine aminotransferase (ALT) with long-term NTZ treatment. The postulated mechanism of NTZ is believed to be through selective induction of host-protein kinase R (PKR), which in turn activates eukaryotic initiation factor 2 α (eIF2α) to inhibit HCV RNA translation.[17] In vitro studies have confirmed the ability of NTZ to inhibit HCV in cell culture models.[18] In addition, HCV replicon studies of NTZ resistance did not show susceptibility to cross-resistance with IFN or RBV-associated resistance.[19]

The initial phase II trial was performed in 50 subjects with genotype 4 in Egypt, with NTZ versus placebo monotherapy for 24 weeks, resulting in a 17% SVR in the NTZ group versus 0% in the placebo group.[20] The following trial, STEALTH C-1, was conducted in 120 Egyptian patients with genotype 4, 97 of whom were HCV treatment naive, divided into 3 cohorts. NTZ 500 mg twice daily was given in a 12-week lead-in phase followed by NTZ/PEG double therapy or NTZ/PEG/ RBV triple therapy for 36 weeks compared with PEG/RBV control for 48 weeks. SVR was 79% in the triple therapy group, 61% in the double therapy group, and 50% in the control group. However, in treatment-experienced patients, SVR was only 25% in the triple therapy group and 8% in the double therapy group, raising doubt about the efficacy of NTZ in patients with treatment failure.[21] A follow-up, open-label pilot study of 44 subjects using the STEALTH C-1 PEG+RBV cohort as a historical control group showed that the 12-week lead-in period could be reduced to 4 weeks.[22]

STEALTH C-2, a follow-up phase II study in the United States, was performed in 10 centers on 64 nonresponders to PEG/RBV with HCV GT 1. The population enrolled had difficult-to-treat characteristics, including 7% African American, 40% with stage 3 or 4 fibrosis, 60% with history of null response to PEG/RBV, and 20% with history of partial response. Subjects were assigned to 4 weeks of NTZ lead-in followed by 48 weeks of triple therapy with PEG/RBV/NTZ versus PEG/RBV/placebo. There was no significant change in the HCV RNA during the 4 week NTZ lead-in. The SVR was only 7% in the NTZ group versus 0% in the placebo group, suggesting that NTZ was not effective in treatment of HCV nonresponders.[23]

STEALTH C-3 was performed on treatment-naive patients with HCV GT 1 in the United States with the same treatment arms. One-hundred and twelve subjects were enrolled in 13 centers. SVR was 44% in the NTZ group and 32% in the placebo group. The NTZ group had higher response rates at 12 weeks, but not at 4 weeks. Subgroup analysis showed a higher SVR in difficult-to-treat populations including those with a high viral load and African Americans. NTZ was well tolerated, with similar rates of adverse events compared with the placebo group.[24] A phase III trial with a controlled-release tablet is planned, and NTZ will be assessed with a shorter, 24-week duration of therapy in combination with PEG, RBV, and DAAs.[25]

Therapeutic Vaccines

Preventive vaccination is the commonly recognized form of vaccinations, administered to prevent an infection before initial exposure. Therapeutic vaccination is inoculation after infection, with the goal of clearance of the infections through vaccine-mediated augmentation of the host immune response. No vaccines are yet available for HCV despite the acknowledgment of the importance and potential impact of both preventive and therapeutic vaccination.

It has been difficult to develop a vaccine for HCV because of the extensive sequence diversity among the 7 different known types and numerous subtypes. More importantly, because of the high replication and mutation rate of HCV and the lack of proofreading function in the HCV RNA-dependent RNA polymerase, numerous HCV quasispecies are formed daily, which increases the potential for rapid selection of viral escape mutants for which vaccination may be ineffective.[26] In addition, HCV also directly suppresses the early, innate host immune response by inhibiting the induction of type I IFN, inhibiting natural killer cell activity, and inducing interfering antibodies that cannot resolve or neutralize HCV infection, but interfere with protective antibodies that develop.[27] These factors may also affect the efficacy of therapeutic vaccination.

Patients infected with HCV who progress from acute to chronic infection generate HCV-specific antibodies that are ineffective for clearance of HCV. However, 15% to 20% of patients with acute HCV spontaneously eradicate the virus within 6 months, which highlights the potential of host innate immunity for HCV eradication. Induction of a robust host immune response by vaccine-mediated generation of broad and multispecific T cells with production of cross-genotype neutralizing antibodies may lead to successful HCV prevention and treatment.[26,27] The goal of future vaccine development is the generation of multifunctional CD4+ T cells that are reactive toward a broad spectrum of viral targets to stimulate the host to generate directed and functional CD8+ T cells to eliminate HCV. There are 4 major potential approaches to therapeutic vaccination, including the use of recombinant proteins, DNA, peptide epitopes, or vectors.

Recombinant protein-based therapeutic vaccines use Tarmogens (whole, heat-killed recombinant *Saccharomyces cerevisiae* yeast) that are genetically modified to express protein targets to stimulate the immune system. In particular, natural killer cells are stimulated and subsequently locate and eliminate infected cells expressing these target proteins.

GI-5005 uses Tarmogens targeting HCV NS3 and core antigens to attack HCV-infected cells.[28,29] A phase I study in 66 HCV subjects administered 5 weekly doses of GI-5005 followed by 2 monthly injections at escalating doses versus placebo showed safety and targeted immune response. Immune response was noted in 33% of the GI-5005 group compared with 0% in the placebo group. ALT improvement was observed in 29% of the treatment group versus 17% in the placebo group.[30]

In a phase IIb study, HCV GT 1 treatment-naive and nonresponder subjects were treated with a GI-5005 lead-in for 5 weekly injections followed by 2 monthly doses for 12 weeks followed by triple therapy of monthly GI-5005 in combination with PEG-2a and RBV. Treatment duration was 48 weeks in treatment-naive subjects and 72 weeks in nonresponders, compared with PEG and RBV control (48 weeks in treatment-naive and 72 weeks in nonresponder populations). SVR of 58% was reported in treatment-naive subjects versus 48% in the controls (intention to treat [ITT]). There were no differences in discontinuation rates or adverse events between the groups.[31,32] In the nonresponder population, an SVR of 17% in the treatment group was observed versus 5% in the control group (ITT).[33] In the study arm, T cell responses improved tenfold compared with the control group in the difficult-to-treat IL28B T/T genotype. Therefore, the study was expanded to include an additional 40 patients.[34,35]

DNA-based therapeutic vaccines are also being developed in which naked protein is introduced by DNA electroporation. DNA electroporation is a procedure involving a syringe with the DNA vaccine and needle electrodes inserted into surrounding muscle tissue. The DNA is injected followed by application of controlled pulses of electrical current with the electrodes. The currents create an electrical field that creates openings in the cell membrane, facilitating entrance of the DNA to enter the cells.

ChronVac-C is a DNA-based vaccine with DNA encoding HCV NS3/4A. Inoculated muscle tissue expresses HCV NS3/4A protein and leads to an immune response against these HCV proteins. A phase I study was conducted in 12 HCV GT 1, treatment-naive patients with low HCV RNA levels (<800,000 IU/mL). ChronVac-C was administered monthly for 4 months. No significant, severe adverse effects were noted and modest viral load reductions were noted, especially in the higher dose groups.[36] Further studies are awaited.

Initial studies targeting HCV structure protein E1 in vaccine development were unsatisfactory.[37] However, several new peptide vaccines are being developed. IC41 is a therapeutic vaccine based on a synthetic peptide that contains 7 HCV T cell epitopes including NS3 and NS4. It was found to be safe and effective in inducing HCV-specific T cells in healthy subjects.[38] Further testing in 60 HCV nonresponder subjects resulted in 67% of subjects producing a specific T cell response, 33% with an IFN-γ–secreting CD4+ T cell response. However, only 3 subjects had a decline of HCV RNA levels of more than 1 log.[7,39] In another study, 35 subjects were vaccinated with IC41 during the 28 to 48 weeks of standard PEG/RBV therapy. Although IC41 did not prevent HCV relapse, lower relapse rates than expected were noted and HCV-specific T cell responses were observed.[40] Based on these early results, a combination trial of NTZ, IC41 in combination with PEG, and RBV was announced in October 2010 with a plan to enroll 60 treatment-naive subjects with HCV GT 1 in Europe.

TG4040 is a vector-based vaccine based on a modified Ankara virus, a highly attenuated vaccinia poxvirus strain, expressing NS3, NS4, and NS5B. An open-label, dose-escalation, phase I trial in 15 HCV treatment-naive subjects revealed HCV RNA reduction between 0.5 and 1.4 log[7] in 6 out of 15 subjects and it was well tolerated.[41] The study was extended to include 27 patients in 3 additional cohorts to evaluate the timing of a booster dose and safety in subjects with more advanced liver disease.

Multiple other vaccine candidates are being evaluated, as shown in **Table 1**.[42–47] Further data are awaited.

Antibody Therapy

Polyclonal and monoclonal antibodies directed toward HCV are being evaluated. Hepatitis C immunoglobulin (HCIG) is being assessed in the liver transplant setting. Initial pilot studies revealed that HCIG failed to prevent HCV recurrence after liver transplantation.[48] Nevertheless, a recent phase II trial was conducted with HCIG on liver transplant recipients with the goal of prevention of HCV recurrence after transplantation. Eighteen patients in 4 centers were administered 75 mg/kg or 200 mg/kg of HCIG versus placebo for 17 infusions. All experienced a transfusion-related reaction with myalgias, nausea, headache, and/or vomiting. Six serious adverse events occurred in 3 subjects, including hypotension, coagulopathy, and severe transfusion reaction. The HCIG treatment groups had a higher level of antibody than the control

Table 1
Vaccines

Drug	Vaccine Basis	# Subjects	Trial Phase	References
GI-5005	Recombinant protein	133	II	28–35
ChronVac-C	DNA	12	II	36
IC41	Peptide	95	II	38–40
TG4040	Vector	15	I	41
ISA-51	Peptide	38	I	42,43
ISCOMATRIX	Peptide	30	I	44
CIGB-230	Recombinant protein	15	I	45
MF59+gpE1/2	Peptide	60	I	46
MBL-HCV1	Peptide	31	I	47

group, and all subjects had an expected decrease in HCV antibody levels over time. More importantly, HCV RNA levels did not decline, and there was no impact on hepatic inflammation identified on liver biopsy. The failure of HCIG to prevent HCV recurrence was attributed to limitations of dosing and the inability of the HCIG to neutralize HCV RNA.[49]

Bavituximab is a chimeric monoclonal antibody that targets phosphatidylserine, a specific phospholipid component of cell membranes that become exposed on the outer membrane of cells infected with HCV. Bavituximab helps direct the host immune system to destroy infected cells exhibiting the target phospholipids. It is believed to be less susceptible to the development of viral resistance because the antibody is directed against host-specific proteins rather than viral targets. A phase I study was performed in which 6 patients with HCV who failed or relapsed after standard PEG and RBV treatment were treated with variable doses of bavituximab and followed for 12 weeks. Adverse events were mild and limited to injection site pain, nausea, and headache. A decrease in HCV RNA was noted in the first 24 hours and on day 4, coinciding with the expected upregulation of the host immune response to HCV.[50] A phase II, open-label trial involving 66 HCV GT 1, treatment-naive subjects is underway.

Among antibody therapies that have been stalled in development, those meriting mention include HCV-AbXTL68, a human monoclonal antibody against HCV envelope protein E2, HuMax-HepC, and Hepavaxx C.[51,52]

Immunomodulators

Toll-like receptors (TLR) recognize pathogens and lead to activation of the innate immune system through an increase in nuclear factor KB, activator protein-1, and IFN regulatory factors. TLRs are expressed on cell surfaces and play an important role in the host immune response against viruses such as HCV by sensing viral proteins. Chronic HCV is associated with disruption of TLR signals by HCV-associated viral products that dampen TLR-activated immune responses.[53]

TLR ligands are in development based on the premise that they can enhance the host immune system, and increase the HCV antiviral response by increasing endogenous IFN production. IMO-125 is a TLR9 agonist that has been shown to induce high levels of IFN-α and other T cell–associated cytokines. Phase I data in 41 patients showed excellent tolerability, with flulike symptoms and injection site pruritus as the major complaints.[54] Multiple other TLR agonists such as ANA245, ANA773, and

SD-101 are in early phase studies with preliminary reports of ability to induce endogenous IFN-α.[55–57] Additional data are awaited.

Thymalfasin is a synthetic version of thymosin α1, which is an immunomodulatory peptide found in human circulation. There is a large body of literature indicating a possible adjunctive role in treatment of HCV. However, clinical trials have failed to support the efficacy of thymalfasin. A phase III randomized, controlled trial of HCV nonresponders showed no improvement in SVR, although it was associated with diminished relapse rates among those who completed therapy.[58] Other immunomodulators include CYT107, a recombinant IL-7, which is a multifunctional cytokine associated with an increase of T cells, T cell functional enhancement, and endogenous IFN-α.

Miscellaneous

Other agents that are being evaluated include anti-inflammatory agents such as mitoquinone, a potent antioxidant that has been shown to reduce serum aminotransferases in patients with HCV.[59]

Silybinin, a flavonoid compound found in the milk thistle extract silymarin, is also being studied. It has long been popular as an adjunctive therapy in patients with HCV, despite a paucity of data supporting its efficacy. It is postulated to be a direct inhibitor of HCV RNA-dependent RNA polymerase and a blocker of virus entry and transmission through the target host cell.[60,61] Silybinin was recently successfully used as a rescue treatment of patients on PEG and RBV therapy who had persistent minimal levels of HCV RNA.[62] An NIH-sponsored, randomized, controlled trial involving silymarin as an adjunct to PEG and RBV therapy is ongoing.

α-Glucosidase inhibitors that lead to misfolding of the HCV envelope protein, thereby blocking viral assembly and release, have also been evaluated. However, the most promising candidate, MX-3235, was found to be ineffective.[63]

NEW IFNS

Although there were initial hopes that PEG would be unnecessary with the advent of DAAs, the initial DAA regimens continue to require IFN. PEG is associated with numerous side effects that contraindicate the medication for many and cause substantial morbidity for those who do take it. This problem has provided the impetus to develop new IFNs, particularly ones that have fewer side effects and possibly are administered less frequently.

Albinterferon α-2b (albIFN), a fusion protein of human albumin and IFN-α2b, with the potential for a prolonged half-life and reduced side effects, held promise in the last several years. An initial phase 2 study reported comparable SVR between albIFN 900 μg and 1200 μg every 2 weeks (SVR 58.5%, 55.5%) compared with PEGα-2a 180 μg every week (SVR 57.9%).[64] Two follow-up phase 3 trials were recently published in patients with genotype 1 and genotype 2/3. ACHIEVE-1 enrolled 1331 patients with genotype 1 to 3 open-label 48-week treatment groups comparing albIFN 900 μg every 2 weeks, albIFN 1200 μg every 2 weeks, and PEGα-2a 180 μg every week, all with weight-based ribavirin at 1000 to 1200 mg daily. There were 2 cases of progressive interstitial lung disease, with 1 associated fatality in the albIFN 1200-μg group, as well as a higher rate of discontinuation caused by respiratory adverse events. During the study, the monitoring committee recommended dose reduction for all subjects in the albIFN 1200-μg group to 900 μg. SVR rates were 51% for the PEGα-2a group, 48.2% for the albIFN 900-μg group, and 47.3% for the albIFN 1200-μg group, with demonstration of noninferiority ($P<.05$).[65] ACHIEVE 2/3 enrolled 933 subjects with genotype 2 or 3, with randomization into 1 of 3 groups, similar to the ACHIEVE 1 study. SVR rates were 84.8% for the PEGα-2a group, 79.8% for the albIFN 900-μg group, and 80% for the albIFN 1200-μg group. Dose reductions were instituted during the study in the albIFN 1200-μg group to 900 μg based on the adverse events noted earlier in the ACHIEVE 1 study. As with the ACHIEVE 1 study, more patients in the albIFN groups reported a cough (38%–41%) than in the PEGα-2a group (29%). However, there were no differences in the rates of severe or serious respiratory adverse events or interstitial lung disease between the groups.[66] Although these 2 phase 3 trials showed noninferiority of albIFN compared with PEGα-2a, further development was suspended after regulatory authorities in the United States and Europe expressed concerns regarding the potential risk/benefit ratio.

Pegylated IFN λ (PEG-λ) is a type-III IFN that induces an intracellular antiviral response and inhibits HCV, purportedly with less hematopoietic side effects than PEG. This is because of limited IFN λ receptor expression in hematopoietic cells.[67] Phase IIa trial reports on 57 subjects treated with 4 doses of PEG-λ versus standard PEG showed an equivalent or improved HCV RNA decline without a significant increase in adverse effects.[68,69] A phase IIb study (EMERGE) is ongoing with a plan to enroll 600 patients in 3 PEG-λ and RBV treatment arms compared with a PEG and RBV control arm. Further data on this promising IFN is awaited.

BLX-883, a long-acting, controlled-release formulation of recombinant IFN-α-2b, was shown recently in phase II studies to be safe and well tolerated, with a lower risk of flulike symptoms, and associated with a greater antiviral efficacy than standard PEG.[70,71] Other IFNs in early development include ω IFN, maxy-αIFN, belerofon, infradure, and glycoferon, although data are limited.

RIBAVIRIN-LIKE MOLECULES

There was hope that, with the development of the DAAs, ribavirin would also be unnecessary. However, phase 2 trials with telaprevir and boceprevir have revealed that elimination of ribavirin, or even dose reduction of ribavirin, is associated with lower SVR, increased relapse rates, and increase in resistance-associated variants. Therefore, ribavirin also will remain in the treatment regimens with the DAAs. Ribavirin has many side effects. Most importantly, ribavirin causes hemolytic anemia that can be severe. Therefore, ribavirin-like molecules have been sought that have less hemolysis and equal efficacy compared with ribavirin.

Taribavirin (formerly viramidine), a prodrug of RBV, was compared with RBV in 2 phase 3 trials. The ViSER 1 study enrolled 972 treatment-naive subjects, of whom 68.4% were genotype 1. Subjects were randomized to 600 mg twice daily of taribavirin versus weight-based RBV (1000 or 1200 mg daily), given with PEG α2b dosed at 1.5 μg/kg/wk. SVR rate was significantly lower at 37.7% in the taribavirin group compared with 52.3% in the RBV group, failing to show noninferiority. However, the rates of anemia were approximately 4 times lower with taribavirin than RBV, at 5% versus 24%, respectively.[72] ViSER 2 was a similar study comparing taribavirin versus RBV in conjunction with PEG α2a dosed at 180 μg weekly. Nine-hundred and sixty-two patients were enrolled, including 66% genotype 1. Subjects were randomized to taribavirin 600 mg twice daily versus RBV at 1000 mg or 1200 mg daily, each with PEG α2a. SVR rate was 40% in taribavirin-treated patients and 55% in the RBV-treated patients, again failing to show noninferiority. Anemia rates were lower in the taribavirin group, at 54.3% versus 80.2% in the RBV group.[73]

Although anemia rates were lower in both studies, taribavirin failed to meet noninferiority comparisons with RBV, dampening enthusiasm for further taribavirin development. However, because taribavirin was administered at a flat dose and retrospective

Box 1
HCV drugs in development

- Cyclophilin inhibitors
  - Debio-025
  - SCY-635
- Thiazolides
  - Nitazoxanide
- Antibody therapy
  - HCV immunoglobulin
  - Bavituximab
  - HCV-ABXTL68
  - HuMax-HepC
  - Hepavaxx C
- Toll-like receptor agonists
  - ANA245
  - ANA773
  - ANA975
  - IMO-2125
  - SD-101
- Immunomodulators
  - Thymalfasin
  - Oglufanide disodium
  - NOV-205
  - CYT107
- α-Glucosidase inhibitor
  - MX-3235
- Anti-inflammatory, antifibrotic
  - CTS-1027 matrix metalloproteinase inhibitor
  - PF-03,491,390 (formerly IDN-6556)
  - JKB-122
  - PYN17
- Thrombopoietin receptor agonist
  - LGD-4665
- MicroRNA
  - SPC3649
- RNA interference
  - ALN-VSP
- Anti–liver cancer
  - Sorafenib
  - PI-88

- ZIO-101
- CF102
- Entry inhibitor
  - IDX320
  - IDX375
  - REP9C
- Silybinin
- IFN
  - Locteron
  - Pegylated IFN λ
  - ω IFN
  - Maxy-αIFN
  - Belerofon
  - Infradure
  - Glycoferon
  - Albuferon
- Ribavirin variants
  - Taribavirin

analysis suggested that heavier patients had a lower SVR, an open label, phase IIb trial was conducted using PEG and weight-based taribavirin compared with PEG and weight-based RBV. Although similar SVR rates were noted in the treatment and control groups and anemia rates were lower with taribavirin in the 20 to 25 mg/kg groups at 13% to 16% versus 33% for RBV, overall SVR were all approximately 28%, including the control group. Fewer dose reductions were required in the taribavirin group compared with RBV.[74] Based on these studies, and in light of ongoing development of newer therapies with potentially lower rates of anemia, the future of taribavirin is not promising.

SUMMARY

Box 1 is a summary of some of the current other players in HCV treatment that are in development. This list is in constant flux given the rapid development of new technologies and techniques. At this time, most of the drugs in development still require combination with PEG and RBV. However, the hope is that host-targeted therapies and immune system–mediated approaches, in combination with DAAs, will permit PEG-free and RBV-free regimens for successful eradication of HCV. Although research with these other players in the game is in its infancy, many of the agents are promising.

REFERENCES

1. Sklan EH, Charuworn P, Pang PS, et al. Mechanisms of HCV survival in the host. Nat Rev Gastroenterol Hepatol 2009;6(4):217–27.

2. Chevaliez S, Pawlotsky JM. HCV genome and life cycle. In: Tan SL, editor. Hepatitis C viruses: genomes and molecular biology. Norfolk (UK): Horizon Bioscience; 2006. p. 1–43.
3. Liu Z, Yang F, Robotham JM, et al. Critical role of cyclophilin A and its prolyl-peptidyl isomerase activity in the structure and function of the hepatitis C virus replication complex. J Virol 2009;83:6554–65.
4. Watashi K, Ishii N, Hijikata M, et al. Cyclophilin B is a functional regulator of hepatitis C virus RNA polymerase. Mol Cell 2005;19:111–22.
5. Inoue K, Sekiyama K, Yamada M, et al. Combined interferon alpha 2b and cyclosporine A in the treatment of chronic hepatitis C: controlled trial. J Gastroenterol 2003;38:567–72.
6. Paeshuyse J, Kaul A, De Clercq E, et al. The non-immunosuppressive cyclosporin DEBIO-025 is a potent inhibitor of hepatitis C virus replication in vitro. Hepatology 2006;43:761–70.
7. Coelmont L, Kaptein S, Paeshuyse J, et al. Debio 025, a cyclophilin binding molecule, is highly efficient in clearing hepatitis C virus (HCV) replicon-containing cells when used alone or in combination with specifically targeted antiviral therapy for HCV (STAT-C) inhibitors. Antimicrob Agents Chemother 2009;53:967–76.
8. Flisiak R, Horban A, Gallay P, et al. The cyclophilin inhibitor Debio-025 shows potent anti-hepatitis C effect in patients coinfected with hepatitis C and human immunodeficiency virus. Hepatology 2008;47:817–26.
9. Flisiak R, Feinman SV, Jablkowski M, et al. The cyclophilin inhibitor Debio 025 combined with PEG IFN alpha2a significantly reduces viral load in treatment-naïve hepatitis C patients. Hepatology 2009;49(5):1460–8.
10. Flisiak R, Woynarowski M, Jablkowski M, et al. Efficacy of standard of care therapy following experimental DEBIO 025 treatment in patients with chronic hepatitis C. J Hepatol 2010;52:S291.
11. Nelson DR, Ghalib RH, Sulkowski M, et al. Efficacy and safety of the cyclophilin inhibitor Debio 025 in combination with pegylated interferon alpha-2a and ribavirin in previously null-responder genotype 1 HCV patients. J Hepatol 2009;50:S40.
12. Hopkins S, Scorneaux B, Huang Z, et al. SCY-635, a novel nonimmunosuppressive analog of cyclosporine that exhibits potent inhibition of hepatitis C virus RNA replication in vitro. Antimicrob Agents Chemother 2010;54:660–72.
13. Hopkins S, Heuman D, Gavis E, et al. Safety, plasma pharmacokinetics and antiviral activity of SCY-635 in adult patients with chronic hepatitis C virus infection. J Hepatol 2009;50:S36.
14. Hopkins S, Mosier S, Harris R, et al. Resistance selection following 15 days of monotherapy with SCY-635 a non-immunosuppressive cyclophilin inhibitor with potent anti-HCV activity. J Hepatol 2010;52:S15.
15. Lawitz E, Rouzier R, Nguyen T, et al. Safety and antiviral efficacy of 14 days of the cyclophilin inhibitor NIM811 in combination with pegylated interferon alpha 2a in relapsed genotype I HCV infected patients. J Hepatol 2009;50:S379.
16. Wring S, Wille K, Rewerts C, et al. In vitro models for assessing the relative risk of hyperbilirubinemia associated with cyclophilin inhibitor therapy. J Hepatol 2010; 52(S1):S263.
17. Elazar M, Liu M, McKenna SA, et al. The anti-hepatitis C agent nitazoxanide induces phosphorylation of eukaryotic initiation factor 2a via protein kinase activated by double-stranded RNA activation. Gastroenterology 2009;137:1827–35.
18. Korba BE, Montero AB, Farrar K, et al. Nitazoxanide, tizoxanide and other thiazolides are potent inhibitors of hepatitis B virus and hepatitis C virus replication. Antiviral Res 2008;77:56–63.

19. Korba BE, Elazar M, Lui P, et al. Potential for hepatitis C virus resistance to nitazoxanide or tizoxanide. Antimicrob Agents Chemother 2008;52:4069–71.
20. Rossignol JF, Kabil SM, El-Gohary Y, et al. Clinical trial: randomized, double-blind, placebo-controlled study of nitazoxanide monotherapy for the treatment of patients with chronic hepatitis C genotype 4. Aliment Pharmacol Ther 2008; 28:574.
21. Rossignol JF, Elfert A, El-Gohary Y, et al. Improved virologic response in chronic hepatitis C genotype 4 treated with nitazoxanide, peginterferon, and ribavirin. Gastroenterology 2009;136:856–62.
22. Rossignol J, Elfert A, Keeffe EB. Treatment of chronic hepatitis C using a 4-week lead-in with nitazoxanide before peginterferon plus nitazoxanide. J Clin Gastroenterol 2010;44:504–9.
23. Shiffman ML, Ahmed A, Jacobson IM, et al. Phase 2 randomized, double-blind, placebo-controlled study of nitazoxanide with peginterferon alfa-2a and ribavirin in nonresponders (NR) with chronic hepatitis C genotype 1: final report. J Hepatol 2010;52:S461.
24. Bacon BR, Shiffman ML, Lim JK, et al. Phase 2 randomized, double-blind, placebo-controlled study of nitazoxanide plus peginterferon and ribavirin in HCV genotype 1 naïve patients: week 12 sustained virologic response rate. J Hepatol 2010;52:S463.
25. Korba B, Elazar M, Liu P, et al. Potential role for nitazoxanide in combination with STAT-C agents for the inhibition of HCV replication without the development of resistance. Hepatology 2008;48:356A.
26. Houghton M. Prospects for prophylactic and therapeutic vaccines against the hepatitis C viruses. Immunol Rev 2011;239:99–108.
27. Yu CI, Chiang BL. A new insight into hepatitis C vaccine development. J Biomed Biotechnol 2010;1–12.
28. Haller AA, Lauer GM, King TH, et al. Whole recombinant yeast-based immunotherapy induces potent T cell responses targeting HCV NS3 and Core proteins. Vaccine 2007;25(8):1452–63.
29. Habersetzer F, Baumert TF, Soll-Keller F. GI-5005, a yeast vector vaccine expressing an NS3-core fusion protein for chronic HCV infection. Curr Opin Mol Ther 2009;11:456–62.
30. Schiff E, Everson G, Tsai N, et al. HCV-specific cellular immunity, RNA reductions, and normalization of ALT in chronic HCV subjects after treatment with GI-5005, a yeast-based immunotherapy targeting NS3 and core: a randomized, double blind, placebo controlled phase 1B study. Hepatology 2007;46:816A.
31. Jacobson IM, McHutchison JG, Boyer TD, et al. GI-5005 therapeutic vaccine plus peg-IFN/ribavirin significantly improves virologic response and ALT normalization at end-of-treatment and improves SVR24 compared to peg-IFN/ribavirin in genotype-1 chronic HCV patients. J Hepatol 2010;52:S465–6.
32. McHutchison JG, Goodman ZD, Everson GT, et al. GI-5005 therapeutic vaccine plus peg-IFN/ribavirin improves biopsy necro-inflammatory scores and ALT normalization at 48 weeks versus peg-IFN/ribavirin in genotype 1 chronic HCV patients. J Hepatol 2010;52:S116.
33. Pockros P, Jacobson IM, Boyer TD, et al. GI-5005 Therapeutic vaccine plus Peg-IFN/Ribavirin improves sustained virologic response versus Peg-IFN/Ribavirin in prior non-responders with genotype 1 chronic HCV infection. Hepatology 2010; 50(4):LB-6.
34. McHutchison JG, Thompson AJ, Jacobson IM, et al. Pharmacogenomic analysis reveals improved virologic response in all IL-28b genotypes in naive genotype 1

chronic HCV patients treated with GI-5005 therapeutic vaccine plus peg-IFN/ribavirin. J Hepatol 2010;52:S457.

35. Vierling JM, McHutchison JG, Jacobson IM, et al. GI-5005 therapeutic vaccine improves deficit in cellular immunity in IL28B genotype T/T, treatment-naive patients with chronic hepatitis C genotype 1 when added to standard of care (SOC) Peg-IFN-alfa-2A/Ribavirin. Hepatology 2010;52(4):A1973.
36. Sallberg M, Frelin L, Diepolder H, et al. A first clinical trial of therapeutic vaccination using naked DNA delivered by in vivo electroporation shows antiviral effects in patients with chronic hepatitis C. J Hepatol 2009;50(S1):S18–9.
37. Leroux-Roels G, Batens AH, Desombere I, et al. Immunogenicity and tolerability of intradermal administration of an HCV E1-based vaccine candidate in healthy volunteers and patients with resolved or ongoing chronic HCV infection. Hum Vaccin 2005;1(2):61–5.
38. Firbas C, Jilma B, Tauber E, et al. Immunogenicity and safety of a novel therapeutic hepatitis C virus (HCV) peptide vaccine: a randomized, placebo controlled trial for dose optimization in 128 healthy subjects. Vaccine 2006;24:4343–53.
39. Klade CS, Wedemeyer H, Berg T, et al. Therapeutic vaccination of chronic hepatitis C nonresponder patients with peptide vaccine IC41. Gastroenterology 2008;134:1385–95.
40. Wedemeyer H, Schuller E, Schlaphoff V, et al. Therapeutic vaccine IC41 as late add-onto standard treatment in patients with chronic hepatitis C. Vaccine 2009;27:5142–51.
41. Habersetzer F, Zarski JP, Leroy V, et al. A novel vectorized HCV therapeutic vaccine (Tg4040): results of a phase I study in naive patients chronically infected by HCV. J Hepatol 2009;50:S18.
42. Yutani S, Yamada A, Yoshida K, et al. Phase I clinical study of a personalized peptide vaccination for patients infected with hepatitis C virus (HCV) 1b who failed to response to interferon-based therapy. Vaccine 2007;25(42):7429–35.
43. Yutani S, Komatsu N, Shichijo S, et al. Phase I clinical study of a peptide vaccination for hepatitis C virus-infected patients with different human leukocyte antigen-class I-A alleles. Cancer Sci 2009;100(10):1935–42.
44. Drane D, Maraskovsky E, Gibson R, et al. Priming of CD4+ and CD8+ T cell responses using a HCV core ISCOMATRIX vaccine: a phase I study in healthy volunteers. Hum Vaccin 2009;5(3):151–7.
45. Alvarez-Lajonchere L, Shoukry NH, Gra B, et al. Immunogenicity of CIGB-230, a therapeutic DNA vaccine preparation, in HCV-chronically infected individuals in a phase I clinical trial. J Viral Hepat 2009;16(3):156–67.
46. Frey SE, Houghton M, Coates S, et al. Safety and immunogenicity of HCV E1E2 vaccine adjuvanted with MF59 administered to healthy adults. Vaccine 2010;28:6367–73.
47. Leav BA, Sloan S, Blair BM, et al. Safety and pharmacokinetics of a novel human monoclonal antibody directed against the E2 glycoprotein of hepatitis C virus (MBL-HCV1) in healthy volunteers. J Hepatol 2010;52:S118.
48. Willems J, Ede M, Marotta P, et al. Anti-HCV human immunoglobulins for the prevention of graft infection in HCV-related liver transplantation, a pilot study. J Hepatol 2002;36:S32.
49. Davis GL, Nelson DR, Terrault N, et al. A randomized, open-label study to evaluate the safety and pharmacokinetics of human hepatitis C immune globulin (Civacir) in liver transplant recipients. Liver Transpl 2005;11:941–9.

50. Godofsky E, Shan J. Phase I single dose study of bavituximab, a chimeric anti-phosphatidylserine monoclonal antibody, in subjects with chronic hepatitis C. Hepatology 2006;44:236A.
51. Galun E, Terrault NA, Eren R, et al. Clinical evaluation (phase I) of a human monoclonal antibody against hepatitis C virus: safety and antiviral activity. J Hepatol 2007;46:37–44.
52. Schiano TD, Charlton M, Younossi Z, et al. Monoclonal antibody HCV-AbXTL68 in patients undergoing liver transplantation for HCV: results of a phase 2 randomized study. Liver Transpl 2006;12:1381–9.
53. Seki E, Brenner DA. Toll-like receptors and adaptor molecules in liver disease: update. Hepatology 2008;48:322–35.
54. Muir A, Ghalib R, Lawitz E, et al. A phase 1, multi-center, randomized, placebo-controlled, dose-escalation study of IMO-2125, a TLR9 agonist, in hepatitis C nonresponders. J Hepatol 2010;52:S14.
55. Horsmans Y, Berg T, Desager JP, et al. Isatoribine, an agonist of TLR7, reduces plasma virus concentration in chronic hepatitis C infection. Hepatology 2005;42:724–31.
56. Xiang AX, Webber SE, Kerr BM, et al. Discovery of ANA975: an oral prodrug of the TLR-7 agonist isatoribine. Nucleosides Nucleotides Nucleic Acids 2007;26:635–40.
57. Cianciara J, Martin JT, Spellman MC. Phase 1B dose-escalation study of SD-101, a novel therapeutic TLR-9 agonist, in treatment-naïve chronic hepatitis C patients. J Hepatol 2010;52:S126.
58. Ciancio A, Rizzetto M. Thymalfasin in the treatment of hepatitis B and C. Ann N Y Acad Sci 2010;1194:141–6.
59. Gane EJ, Orr DW, Weilert F, et al. Phase II study of the mitochondrial antioxidant mitoquinone for hepatitis C. J Hepatol 2008;48:S318.
60. Ahmed-Belkacem A, Ahnou N, Barbotte L, et al. Silibinin and related compounds are direct inhibitors of hepatitis C virus RNA-dependent RNA polymerase. Gastroenterology 2010;138:1112–22.
61. Polyak SJ, Morishima C, Shuhart MC, et al. Inhibition of T-cell inflammatory cytokines, hepatocyte NF-kappaB signaling, and HCV infection by standardized Silymarin. Gastroenterology 2007;132:1925.
62. Biermer M, Stoehr L, Schlosser B, et al. Silibinin as a rescue treatment for HCV-infected patients showing suboptimal virologic response to standard combination therapy. J Hepatol 2010;52:S16.
63. Durantel D. Celgosivir, an alpha-glucosidase I inhibitor for the potential treatment of HCV infection. Curr Opin Investig Drugs 2009;10:860–70.
64. Zeuzem S, Yoshida EM, Benhamou Y, et al. Albinterferon alfa-2b dosed every two or four weeks in interferon-naive patients with genotype 1 chronic hepatitis C. Hepatology 2008;48:407–17.
65. Zeuzem S, Sulkowski MS, Lawitz EJ, et al. Randomized trial of albinterferon alfa-2b for the treatment of patients with chronic hepatitis C virus genotype 1. Gastroenterology 2010;139:1257–66.
66. Nelson DR, Benhamou Y, Chuang WL, et al. Randomized trial of albinterferon alfa-2b for the treatment of patients with chronic hepatitis C virus genotype 2 or 3. Gastroenterology 2010;139:1267–76.
67. Brand S, Zitzmann K, Dambacher J, et al. SOCS-1 inhibits expression of the antiviral proteins 2',5'-OAS and MxA induced by the novel interferon-lambdas IL28A and IL-29. Biochem Biophys Res Commun 2005;331:543–8.
68. Freeman JA, Gray TE, Fontana DJ, et al. The effect of treatment group, HCV genotype, and IL28B genotype on early HCV viral kinetics in a phase 2a study

of PEG-interferon lambda (pegIFNλ) in hepatitis C patients. Hepatology 2010; 50(4):A831.
69. Muir AJ, Lawitz E, Ghalib RH, et al. Pegylated interferon lambda (pegIFNλ) Phase 2 dose-ranging, active-controlled study in combination with ribavirin (RBV) for treatment-naïve HCV patients (genotypes 1,2,3, or 4): safety, viral response, and impact of IL28B host genotype through week 12. Hepatology 2010;50(4):A821.
70. Dzyublyk I, Yegorova T, Moroz L, et al. Phase 2a study to evaluate the safety and tolerability and anti-viral of 4 doses of a novel, controlled-release interferon alfa-2b (Locteron) given every 2 weeks for 12 weeks in treatment-naive patients with chronic hepatitis C (genotype 1). Hepatology 2007;46:863A.
71. Long WA, Takov D, Tchernev K, et al. Q2week controlled-release-interferon alpha2b+ribavirin reduces flu-like symptoms >50% and provides equivalent efficacy in comparison to weekly pegylated-interferon-alpha2b+ribavirin in treatment-naïve genotype-1-chronic-hepatitis C: results from EMPOWER, a randomized-open-label-12-week-comparison in 133 patients. J Hepatol 2010;52:S467.
72. Benhamou Y, Afdhal NH, Nelson DR, et al. A phase III study of the safety and efficacy of viramidine vs ribavirin in treatment-naïve patients with chronic hepatitis C: VISER 1 results. Hepatology 2009;50:717–26.
73. Marcellin P, Gish RG, Gitlin N, et al. Safety and efficacy of viramidine versus ribavirin in ViSER2: randomized, double-blind study in therapy-naïve hepatitis C patients. J Hepatol 2010;52:32–8.
74. Poordad F, Lawitz E, Shiffman ML, et al. Virologic rates of weight-based taribavirin versus ribavirin in treatment-naïve patients with genotype 1 chronic hepatitis C. Hepatology 2010;52(4):1208–15.

Mixing and Matching Drugs: What Makes Sense?

Tania M. Welzel, MD, Stefan Zeuzem, MD*

KEYWORDS

- Hepatitis C • Directly acting antiviral combination agents
- Interferon free treatment

The recent advances in the development of directly acting antiviral agents (DAAs), that is, drugs that target and inhibit specific steps in hepatitis C virus (HCV) replication, has revolutionized the treatment of patients with chronic HCV (CHC) infection. The coadministration of the first-generation NS3/4A protease inhibitors telaprevir (VX-950) and boceprevir (SCH-503034) with the current standard of care (SOC), a combination of pegylated interferon-α (PegIFN-α) and weight-based ribavirin (PegIFN/RBV), has been shown to substantially improve sustained virologic response (SVR) rates in patients with HCV genotype 1 infection.[1–4] In regard to the recent approval of the Food and Drug Administration's (FDA's) new drug applications for both protease inhibitors, the interferon-based triple therapy will soon herald a new era in HCV treatment. A comprehensive review on telaprevir and boceprevir as well as other DAAs in the pipeline, including second-generation NS3/4A protease inhibitors, nucleoside and nonnucleoside NS5B polymerase inhibitors, NS5A inhibitors, as well as drugs targeting host cell structures (eg, cyclophilin inhibitors), is provided in previous articles.

DAA COMBINATION STUDIES: THE RATIONALE

Most trials assessed virologic responses of DAA/PegIFN/RBV combinations in comparison with the SOC. Interferon-related adverse effects, however, are challenging for patients undergoing antiviral therapy and frequently affect the treatment adherence. In addition, drug contraindications limit the applicability of interferon-based therapies for a relevant proportion of HCV-infected persons in need for antiviral treatment, such as patients with advanced liver disease, including those awaiting liver

---

Disclosure: Stefan Zeuzem-Consultancies for Abbott, Achillion, Anadys, Boehringer, BMS, Gilead, iTherX, Janssen, Merck, Novartis, Nycomed, Pfizer, Pharmasset, Roche, Santaris, Tibotec, and Vertex.

Department of Medicine 1, JW Goethe University Hospital, Theodor-Stern-Kai 7, 60590 Frankfurt a.M., Germany
* Corresponding author.
E-mail address: zeuzem@em.uni-frankfurt.de

Clin Liver Dis 15 (2011) 657–664
doi:10.1016/j.cld.2011.05.012 **liver.theclinics.com**
1089-3261/11/$ – see front matter

transplantation. For this reason, the development of novel HCV treatment strategies is of major interest. This need was recently acknowledged by the US FDA by encouraging the accelerated design and implementation of DAA combination trials with and without PegIFN-α and/or ribavirin (RBV), aiming for shorter treatment durations of PegIFN-containing regimens and to attain the ultimate goal of a PegIFN-free HCV therapy with a better tolerability.[5]

GENOTYPE DEPENDENCY, EFFICACY, AND RESISTANCE OF DAAs USED FOR COMBINATION

For the successful and durable eradication of HCV using DAA combination approaches, several factors have to be considered. These factors include the drug's genotype sensitivity, the need for a critical level of antiviral efficacy, and the detailed characterization of mutational patterns to avoid cross-resistance between the drugs.

Because most DAAs in clinical development strongly inhibit HCV genotype 1 but exhibit different activities against other HCV genotypes (**Table 1**), the selection of appropriate drugs has particular implications for the design of HCV non–genotype 1 DAA combination trials.

To achieve a rapid and complete viral suppression, individual DAAs should exhibit a strong antiviral activity (see **Table 1**).[6] Results from 3- to 14-day phase 1b monotherapy trials in HCV genotype 1–infected patients indicate high antiviral activities for NS3/4A protease inhibitors and for the first NS5A inhibitor BMS-790052 (up to 4.6 $\log_{10}$ IU/mL and 3.6 $\log_{10}$ IU/mL HCV RNA declines, respectively) and low to medium antiviral activities for nonnucleoside NS5B polymerase inhibitors (0.6–3.7 $\log_{10}$ HCV RNA IU/mL decline). A low antiviral efficacy (0.7–2.7 $\log_{10}$ HCV RNA IU/mL decline) was also shown for earlier nucleoside analogue NS5B polymerase inhibitors. An antiviral efficacy of up to 5.23 $\log_{10}$ HCV RNA IU/mL decline (14-day monotherapy) has been reported recently for the nucleotide analogue PSI-938.[7] The antiviral activity of DAA combinations should at least be additive.

Despite the promising antiviral efficacy of individual DAAs, the high-level replication and high mutation rate turn HCV into a moving target, challenging the successful viral clearance through the emergence of drug-resistant variants. Because of the lack of a proofreading activity of the HCV RNA–dependent RNA polymerase NS5B, numerous variants (quasi-species) are generated during HCV replication. In response to the selection pressures in the host environment (eg, immune escape), a wild-type strain is typically dominant within the viral quasi-species, along with mutant strains that replicate with lower efficacy.[8] Selection pressures to the virus population are also imposed by drug therapy, and, depending on a drug's genetic barrier to resistance (see **Table 1**), viral variants with preexistent resistance mutations may gain a fitness advantage favoring viral breakthrough.[6] In fact, viral resistance was rapidly observed in

Table 1
Characteristics of DAAs used for combination

	Genotype Dependency	Antiviral Efficacy	Barrier to Resistance
NS3A (Protease Inhibitors)	+	+++	+ to ++
NS5A	+ to ++	+++	+ to ++
NS5B (Nucleosides)	+++	+ to ++	+++
NS5B (Nonnucleosides)	+	+ to ++	+

Abbreviations: +, low; ++, moderate; +++, strong.

patients treated with the protease inhibitors telaprevir and boceprevir, indicating a low genetic barrier of resistance. Because of the linear conformation of the NS3/4A binding site, single amino acid substitutions may compromise or inhibit the binding of these drugs. To date, several and partly overlapping resistance mutations have been described for linear and macrocyclic NS3/4A protease inhibitors. The emergence of resistance to telaprevir and boceprevir, as well as several macrocyclic protease inhibitors (RG7227 [danoprevir], BI 201335), differs between patients infected with HCV subtype 1a and subtype 1b.

For the most frequent telaprevir-associated amino acid substitution R155K, this observation can be explained by the different number of nucleotide changes required for the amino acid change (1 nucleotide change in patients infected by HCV subtype 1a and 2 nucleotide changes in those infected by HCV subtype 1b). For NS5B polymerase inhibitors, the genetic barrier to resistance substantially differs between non-nucleoside NS5B inhibitors and nucleoside analogue NS5B inhibitors. This occurrence can be explained by characteristics of the specific binding sites of these drugs. Non-nucleoside inhibitors bind to the allosteric site of the enzyme where numerous amino acid changes can occur without affecting the viral replication; not surprisingly, different resistance patterns were observed for HCV subtypes 1a and 1b. In contrast, mutations at the highly conserved active site of the NS5B polymerase rapidly result in a drastically reduced viral fitness, and no resistance variants or subtype differences are yet clinically reported for the more potent nucleoside polymerase inhibitors. The NS5A inhibitors seem to have a genetic barrier to resistance that is comparable to that of protease inhibitors. Overall, data on the genetic barrier and on possible subtype differences are currently sparse for NS5A inhibitors. The differences in resistance patterns indicate that a combination of 2 or more DAAs with different mechanism of action, nonoverlapping resistance profiles, and a high genetic barrier to resistance are required to achieve strong and durable HCV treatment responses.

DAA COMBINATION STUDIES

The first evidence that combination therapies, including a protease and polymerase inhibitor, may be successfully used for HCV therapy was obtained from in vitro replicon studies and from studies in chimpanzees.[9]

Combination of an NS3/4A Protease Inhibitor and a Nucleoside Analogue NS5B Polymerase Inhibitor

The first clinical study that investigated the safety and efficacy of an oral interferon-free DAA combination regimen was the INterferon-Free regimen for the management of HCV-1 trial.[10] This phase 1, multicenter, randomized, double-blind, placebo-controlled, dose-escalation trial assessed the mean changes in HCV RNA levels after 13 days of oral combination therapy with RG7227 (danoprevir), a macrocyclic HCV NS3/4A protease inhibitor, and RG7128, a nucleoside analogue NS5B polymerase inhibitor. The study population included treatment-naive and treatment-experienced patients with HCV genotype 1 infection who were randomized to 1 of 9 treatment arms of 7 sequentially treated cohorts (A–G, n = 74) or to placebo (n = 14). Cohort A subjects were treated with 4 days of monotherapy with danoprevir (100 mg every 8 hours) or RG7128 (500 mg twice daily) followed by 3 days of combination therapy with RG7128 (500 mg twice daily) or danoprevir (100 mg every 8 hours), respectively. Cohorts B to G received 13 days of treatment with different doses of danoprevir (100 mg or 200 mg every 8 hours or 600 mg or 900 mg twice daily) in combination with RG7128 (500 mg or 1000 mg twice daily), followed by PegIFN and RBV for 46 weeks.

The primary outcome was analyzed for 55 patients who completed 13 days of combination treatment with the study drugs. Compared with an increase of 0.1 log_{10} IU/mL in the placebo group, the median changes in HCV RNA from baseline to day 14 ranged from −3.7 to −5.2 log_{10} IU/mL in cohorts B to G. The strongest antiviral activity was observed in treatment-naive patients who received a combination of 900 mg of danoprevir and 1000 mg of RG7128 twice daily (−5.1 log_{10} IU/mL; interquartile range [IQR] −5.6 to −4.7), and, at this high-dose level, favorable responses were also observed in null responders with previous SOC (−4.9 log_{10} IU/mL; IQR −5.2 to −4.5). Viral rebound was described in 1 patient who experienced an increase of HCV RNA level of 1.4 log_{10} above the nadir on day 13. Although the danoprevir-associated resistance mutation F43S could be identified by clonal sequencing, further phenotypic characterization confirmed the clinical susceptibility to both study drugs. No treatment-related severe or serious adverse events, no grade 3 or 4 changes in laboratory parameters, and no treatment discontinuations were observed.

Combination of an NS3/4A Protease Inhibitor and Nonnucleoside NS5B Polymerase Inhibitor

The results of 2 phase 1b studies investigating the antiviral efficacy of a combination with an NS3/4A protease inhibitor and a nonnucleoside NS5B polymerase inhibitor were presented recently. The SOUND-C1 trial, a randomized open-label trial, investigated rapid virologic response (RVR) rates defined as HCV RNA concentration less than 25 IU/mL at week 4 in all 32 therapy-naive patients with HCV genotype 1 infection.[11] Patients were randomized 1:1 to a 4-week oral therapy with BI 201335, a potent and specific HCV NS3/4A protease inhibitor (120 mg once daily), and BI 207127, a reversible nonnucleoside thumb pocket 1 HCV NS5B polymerase inhibitor (400 or 600 mg 3 times per day), plus weight-based RBV (1000/1200 mg daily in 2 doses). On day 29, all patients were switched to treatment with BI 201335 and PegIFN/RBV. Randomization was stratified by viral load (<800,000 IU/mL and >800,000 IU/mL) and HCV subtype (1a, 1b). The RVR rate at 400 mg of BI 207127 three times a day was 73% at day 29, with higher rates for patients infected with HCV genotype 1b than those infected with genotype 1a. At 600 mg for 3 times a days, the corresponding RVR rate was 100%, and no subtype difference could be detected. One virological breakthrough was observed in the 400-mg BI 207127 group on day 10 that was explained by an R155K amino acid change in NS3A and a P495L in NS5B indicating the selection of double mutants.

In the second study, RVR rates were compared among treatment-naive patients with HCV genotype 1 infection randomized to one of three 4-week regimen with the protease inhibitor GS-9256 and the nonnucleoside NS5B polymerase inhibitor tegobuvir (GS-9190), followed by PegIFN/RBV until week 48.[12] Forty-six patients were randomized to GS-9256 and tegobuvir (n = 16), GS-9256 and tegobuvir plus RBV (n = 15), or GS-9256 and tegobuvir plus PegIFN/RBV (n = 15). GS-9256 was dosed 75 mg twice daily, tegobuvir was dosed 40 mg twice daily, and PegIFN alfa-2a and RBV were given at standard doses. Despite a good antiviral efficacy in all groups with median maximal viral load changes from baseline of −4.1 (range, −5.1 to −1.6), −5.1 (range, −5.6 to −4.1), and −5.7 (range, −6.5 to −3.6) for groups 1, 2, and 3, respectively, RVR rates differed notably between the treatment groups. Compared with a 100% RVR rate in the 4-drug arm, only 38% of the patients in the triple therapy arm and 7% of patients who received the combination of GS-9256 plus tegobuvir alone achieved an RVR. In group 3, HCV RNA rebounded after an initial decline, which was related to the emergence of double resistance mutations in most patients allocated to this regimen. The emergence of double mutants was reduced by the addition of RBV, highlighting its role in the prevention of virologic breakthrough. Treatment with GS-9190 and GS-9256 was well tolerated, and no grade 3 or 4 adverse events or laboratory abnormalities were reported. Further studies combining NS3/4A protease inhibitors with nonnucleoside polymerase inhibitors are ongoing.[13,14]

Combination of an NS3/4A Protease Inhibitor and an NS5A Inhibitor

The results of a 12-week interim analysis of the first study investigating a combination therapy with an NS3/4A protease inhibitor (BMS-650032) and an NS5A inhibitor (BMS-790052) were reported recently.[15] In this randomized, open-label, phase 2a study, 21 HCV genotype 1 treatment-experienced null responders were randomized to 2 treatment groups (A: n = 11 and B: n = 10), receiving an oral combination of BMS-650032 and BMS-790052 (600 mg twice daily and 60 mg once daily), alone or in combination with PegIFN/RBV for 24 weeks. In both groups, a strong median HCV RNA level decline could be observed at week 2 ($-5.1 \log_{10}$ and $-5.3 \log_{10}$). RVR rates were similar in both groups (group A, 63.6%; group B, 60%). However, viral breakthrough by week 12 was frequent in group A subjects (6/11, 54.5%) and occurred exclusively in patients infected with HCV genotype 1a (6/9). In contrast, no viral breakthrough was observed by week 12 in group B receiving both DAAs in combination with the SOC. During the analysis period, treatment was well tolerated and no discontinuations due to adverse events were recorded.

Combination of a Nucleotide Analogue Polymerase Inhibitor and RBV, with and without PegIFN

Only recently, an exploratory phase 2 trial was initiated that investigates the combination of PSI-7977, a nucleotide analogue polymerase inhibitor, and RBV, with 0, 4, 8, or 12 weeks of PegIFN alfa-2a, in treatment-naive patients infected with HCV genotype 2 or 3.[16] HCV RNA response data are currently not yet available.

Combination of a Nucleotide Analogue NS5B Polymerase Inhibitor and a NS5A Inhibitor with and without RBV

This first pharmaceutical cross-collaboration starting in the first half of 2011 will assess the safety and pharmacokinetics of an oral combination therapy with the nucleotide analogue polymerase inhibitor PSI-7977 and the NS5A inhibitor BMS-790052 with and without RBV in treatment-naive patients with CHC genotypes 1, 2, and 3 infection.[17]

Combination of a Purine and a Pyrimidine Nucleotide Analogue NS5B Polymerase Inhibitor

The first study investigating the combination of a purine (PSI-938) and a pyrimidine (PSI-7977) nucleotide analogue polymerase inhibitor has been initiated. In a subsequent phase 2b study, SVR rates will be assessed using different dosing durations of the DAAs, with and without RBV.[18]

Combination of DAAs with Cyclophilin A Inhibitors

Other promising approaches include the combination of DAAs targeting different steps in the viral life cycle with agents directed against host structures, which are involved in the viral replication process. Among those, cyclophilin A inhibitors that block HCV replication in vitro have shown promising results for the treatment of HCV infection in early clinical trials and, furthermore, seem to exhibit a high genetic barrier to resistance. For alisporivir (previously Debio 025), potent antiviral activities were reported in patients infected with HCV genotypes 1, 2, 3, and 4 during monotherapy and in combination with PegIFN, and no viral breakthrough was observed.[19,20] In vitro studies conducted on HCV replicon–containing cell lines indicated an additive antiviral activity of alisporivir with RBV and different DAAs (ie, protease and NS5B polymerase inhibitors).[21] Alisporivir was also shown to delay the selection of resistant strains, turning it into a promising candidate for future in vivo combination trials.

ROLE OF RBV

As an integral part of the current SOC, the role of RBV in future (interferon free) DAA combination therapies has to be further defined. Although the exact mechanism of action of RBV remains incompletely understood, it was shown to substantially improve antiviral responses to PegIFN.[22] Proposed mechanisms of action include the enhancement of the interferon-stimulated gene expression and the alteration of immune responses. Furthermore, RBV may exhibit direct antiviral responses by acting as an RNA mutagen. In fact, several studies provided evidence that RBV favors HCV lethal mutagenesis through genomic incorporation and induction of nonsense mutations that may result in an error catastrophe by exceeding the naturally occurring HCV replication error rate.[23] At this point, data obtained from trials involving novel DAAs and DAA combinations suggest a superiority of antiviral regimens, including RBV in regard to HCV RNA suppression and SVR rates. For example, SVR rates in patients treated for 3 months with telaprevir/PegIFN/RBV were significantly higher compared with SVR rates in those treated for 3 months with telaprevir/PegIFN alone (60% vs 36%), which was attributable to a higher rate of viral relapse in the RBV-free treatment arm (48% vs 30%).[24] The results of PegIFN/RBV-free DAA combination trial as reviewed earlier also highlight the role of RBV in the prevention of resistance.[12]

SUMMARY AND OUTLOOK

The introduction and ongoing development of new substances, including DAAs and drugs targeting host cell structures, will dramatically change the management of patients with CHC infection. The concomitant use of the protease inhibitors telaprevir or boceprevir with SOC will represent the new medical standard for the treatment of HCV genotype 1 infection. Beyond this, the availability of numerous substances belonging to different drug classes opens up new vistas for DAA combination trials with and without PegIFN/RBV to further optimize therapeutic approaches and to develop an all-oral PegIFN-sparing DAA combination therapy. Collaborations among companies may further expand the number of possible drug combinations, and, to date, the optimal number of DAAs used for combinations has to be further defined. The additional emergence of a new generation of nonresponders to triple therapy further highlights the need for the ongoing development and assessment of therapeutic alternatives. As reviewed herein, different combinations of DAAs have been investigated so far. Although these studies provided evidence for a good antiviral activity of the individual DAA combinations with the production of early and steep declines in HCV RNA levels, the reported rates of viral breakthrough through emergence of drug-resistant viruses remains concerning (with the exception of studies including nucleoside polymerase inhibitors and cyclophilin inhibitors). This highlights the need for a better understanding and characterization of the underlying mechanism of resistance (ie, gain of a fitness advantage of preexisting viral quasi-species and/or induction of de novo mutations, number of mutations needed to confer resistance) and the functional results (viral fitness and level of resistance). In this regard, the combination of DAAs with drugs targeting host cell structures represents a promising strategy;

however, further in vivo studies are needed to investigate whether these substances may replace PegIFN and/or RBV. In regard to the genotype dependency of most DAAs, the development of pan-genotypic approaches is of interest, to also meet the therapeutic needs in regions with a predominance of HCV genotypes other than 1. Well-designed pivotal studies are necessary to get answers to these questions, and, as many are underway, some clarity may already be gained in 2012.

REFERENCES

1. Sherman KE, Flamm SL, Afdhal NH, et al. Telaprevir in combination with peginterferon alfa2a and ribavirin for 24 or 48 weeks in treatment naïve genotype 1 HCV patients who achieved an extended rapid viral response: final results of phase 3 ILLUMINATE Study. AASLD 2010 [abstract: LB-2].
2. Bronowicki J, McCone J, Bacon BR, et al. Response-guided therapy (RGT) with boceprevir (BOC) + peginterferon alfa-2b/ribavirin (P/R) for treatment-naïve patients with hepatitis C virus (HCV) genotype (G) 1 was similar to a 48-wk fixed-duration regimen with BOC+P/R in SPRINT-2. AASLD 2010 [abstract: LB-15].
3. Poordad F, McCone J Jr, Bacon BR, et al. Boceprevir with peginterferon/ribavirin for untreated chronic hepatitis C. N Engl J Med 2011;54:1195–206.
4. Bacon BR, Gordon SC, Lawitz E, et al. Boceprevir for treatment of chronic hepatitis C genotype 1 nonresponders. N Engl J Med 2011;54:1207–17.
5. Guidance for industry: chronic hepatitis C virus infection: developing direct-acting antiviral agents for treatment. Draft guidance. Rockville (MD): U.S. Department of Health and Human Services, Food and Drug Administration, Center for Drug Evaluation and Research (CDER); 2010. p. 1–27. Available at: http://www.fda.gov/downloads/Drugs/GuidanceComplianceRegulatoryInformation/Guidances/UCM225333.pdf. Accessed May 19, 2011.
6. Sarrazin C, Zeuzem S. Resistance to direct antiviral agents in patients with hepatitis C virus infection. Gastroenterology 2010;138:447–62.
7. Available at: http://www.pharmasset.com/pipeline. Accessed February 21, 2011.
8. Lauring AS, Andino R. Quasispecies theory and the behavior of RNA viruses. PLoS Pathog 2010;6:e1001005.
9. Olsen DB, Carroll SS, Handt L, et al. HCV antiviral activity and resistance analysis in chronically infected chimpanzees treated with NS3/4A protease and NS513 polymerase inhibitors. J Hepatol 2007;46:S298.
10. Gane EJ, Roberts SK, Stedman CA, et al. Oral combination therapy with a nucleoside polymerase inhibitor (RG7128) and danoprevir for chronic hepatitis C genotype 1 infection (INFORM-1): a randomised, double-blind, placebo-controlled, dose-escalation trial. Lancet 2010;376:1467–75.
11. Zeuzem S, Asselah T, Angus P, et al. Strong antiviral activity and safety of IFN-sparing treatment with the protease inhibitor BI 201335, the HCV polymerase inhibitor BI 207127, and ribavirin, in patients with chronic hepatitis C: the SOUND-C1 trial. AASLD 2010 [abstract: LB-7].
12. Zeuzem S, Buggisch P, Agarwal K, et al. Dual, triple, and quadruple combination treatment with a protease inhibitor (GS-9256) and a polymerase inhibitor (GS-9190) alone and in combination with ribavirin (RBV) or PegIFN/RBV for up to 28 days in treatment naïve, genotype 1 HCV subjects. AASLD 2010 [abstract: LB-1].
13. Available at: http://www.vrtx.com/current-projects/drug-candidates/vx-222.html. Accessed February 21, 2011.
14. Available at: http://www.abbott.com/global/url/pressRelease/en_US/Press_Release_0824.htm. Accessed February 21, 2011.

15. Lok A, Gardiner DF, Lawitz E, et al. Combination therapy with BMS-790052 and BMS-650032 alone or with pegIFN/RBV results in undetectable HCV RNA through 12 weeks of therapy in HCV genotype 1 null responders. AASLD 2010 [abstract: LB-8].
16. Available at: http://www.pharmasset.com/pipeline/psi_7851.aspx. Accessed February 21, 2011.
17. Available at: http://www.natap.org/2010/HCV/011111_01.htm. Accessed February 21, 2011.
18. Available at: http://www.pharmasset.com/pipeline/psi_938_psi_879.aspx. Accessed February 21, 2011.
19. Flisiak R, Feinman SV, Jablkowski M, et al. The cyclophilin inhibitor Debio 025 combined with PEG IFNalpha2a significantly reduces viral load in treatment-naïve hepatitis C patients. Hepatology 2009;49:1460–8.
20. Flisiak R, Horban A, Gallay P, et al. The cyclophilin inhibitor Debio-025 shows potent anti-hepatitis C effect in patients coinfected with hepatitis C and human immunodeficiency virus. Hepatology 2008;47:817–26.
21. Coelmont L, Kaptein S, Paeshuyse J, et al. Debio 025, a cyclophilin binding molecule, is highly efficient in clearing hepatitis C virus (HCV) replicon-containing cells when used alone or in combination with specifically targeted antiviral therapy for HCV (STAT-C) inhibitors. Antimicrob Agents Chemother 2009;53:967–76.
22. Hofmann WP, Herrmann E, Sarrazin C, et al. Ribavirin mode of action in chronic hepatitis C: from clinical use back to molecular mechanisms. Liver Int 2008;28: 1332–43.
23. Dixit NM, Layden-Almer JE, Layden TJ, et al. Modelling how ribavirin improves interferon response rates in hepatitis C virus infection. Nature 2004;432:922–4.
24. Hézode C, Forestier N, Dusheiko G, et al. Telaprevir and peginterferon with or without ribavirin for chronic HCV infection. N Engl J Med 2009;360:1839–50.

Interferon-Free Regimens: The Near Future, the Likely and the Not So Likely

Mitchell L. Shiffman, MD

KEYWORDS

- Chronic hepatitis C virus • Peginterferon
- Sustained virologic response • Protease inhibitors
- Polymerase inhibitors • IL28B genotype

Remarkable progress has been achieved in the treatment of chronic hepatitis C virus (HCV) since interferon was first used to treat this pathogen more than 20 years ago.[1] Standard interferon administered three times weekly for 6 to 12 months was associated with a sustained virologic response (SVR) in only 6% to 12% of patients.[2] Peginterferon was developed approximately a decade ago, and this long-acting form of interferon improved SVR rates 30% to 50%, even in patients with cirrhosis.[3–5] The addition of ribavirin to interferon or peginterferon improved SVR rates to 33% and 40%, respectively, for patients with HCV genotype 1 who received 48 weeks of treatment.[2,6–9] In patients with HCV genotypes 2 or 3, SVR rates of 75% to 85% were achieved with 24 weeks of treatment using either standard or peginterferon and ribavirin.[2,6,7,10]

Within the past several years numerous antiviral agents that directly inhibit the HCV protease or polymerase have been developed by several pharmaceutical companies. Protease inhibitors are highly potent inhibitors of HCV replication, but are typically specific for HCV genotype 1 and associated with the rapid emergence of antiviral resistance when used as monotherapy.[11,12] Polymerase inhibitors tend to be somewhat less potent inhibitors of HCV replication, tend to be active against many different genotypes of HCV, and have lower rates of resistance.[13] As a result, direct-acting antiviral agents for HCV have been used with peginterferon and ribavirin.

Conflicts of Interest: Dr Shiffman has been a consultant to and received fees from Conatus, Exalenz, Human Genome Sciences, Roche/Genentech, and Romark. He has participated in advisor meetings with Bayer, Bristol-Myers Squibb, Gilead, Merck, Novartis, Pfizer, Roche/Genentech, Salix, and Vertex. He has received grant support to conduct clinical trials from Abbott, Anadys, Bristol-Myers Squibb, Conatus, Gilead, Globeimmune, Roche/Genentech, and Zymogenetics. He has been a member of a Data Safety Monitoring Committee for Abbott and Anadys. He is a speaker for Bayer, Bristol-Myers Squibb, Gilead, Merck, Roche/Genentech, Salix, and Vertex.
Liver Institute of Virginia, Bon Secours Health System, 12720 McManus Boulevard, Suite 313, Newport News, VA 23602, USA
E-mail address: mitchell_shiffman@bshsi.org

Clin Liver Dis 15 (2011) 665–675
doi:10.1016/j.cld.2011.05.004 liver.theclinics.com
1089-3261/11/$ – see front matter

Two protease inhibitors, telaprevir and boceprevir, are approved by the US Food and Drug Administration (FDA). Numerous other protease, nucleoside, and nonnucleoside polymerase inhibitors are currently in phase II clinical trials. Many of these agents have been reviewed in this issue. When either boceprevir or telaprevir are used in combination with peginterferon and ribavirin to treat patients with HCV genotype 1, infection SVR rates of 69% to 75% have been achieved.[14,15] Thus, SVR rates in patients with chronic HCV genotype 1, the most common type of this virus in most countries,[16] have increased from only 6% to 75%; a 12-fold increase in just 2 decades.

Numerous highly potent direct-acting antiviral agents that suppress HCV at different sites are currently being evaluated in phase II clinical trials. The availability of these agents provides an opportunity to treat HCV with an all oral formulation. Several studies have been initiated within the past year.[17–19] These data strongly suggest that viral suppression to undetectable levels can be achieved. However, whether a significant percentage of patients can achieve a SVR and be “cured” of chronic HCV without interferon remains to be seen. This manuscript reviews the mechanisms through which interferon is believed to suppress HCV and lead to SVR. These observations are used to speculate as to whether an all-oral antiviral cocktail could “cure” HCV in the near future.

INTERFERONS AND THEIR MECHANISM OF ACTION

Interferons are a diverse group of glycoproteins that are produced by numerous cell types when bacteria, viruses, and other pathogens enter the body.[20] The interferons are divided into three classes based on the location of their genes, the cells they are produced by, the cell surface receptor they bind to, and their mechanism of action. The type I interferons include α, β, Ω. The genes for these interferons are located on chromosome 9. Type I interferons are produced by numerous cells. All type I interferons bind to a common cell surface receptor complex that is located on numerous cells throughout the body.

The type II interferon, interferon-γ, is produced by only a limited number of cells, including natural killer, CD4, and CD8 cytotoxic suppressor cells. The gene for interferon-γ is located on chromosome 12; its cell surface receptor is distinct from the type I interferon receptor complex.

Type III interferons consist of several types of interferon-λ, formerly known as interleukins (ILs)-28 and -29.[21] The genes that code for interferon-λ are located on chromosome 19. Interferon-λ is produced by the same cell types and in response to the same stimuli as type I and II interferons. Interferon-λ also has its own unique cell surface receptor complex. The main difference between interferon-λ and interferon types I and II is that its receptor complex is limited to cells of epithelial origin, including hepatocytes.

The interferon system is intimately involved in the resolution of viral infection. Removing interferon genes or blocking the effects of interferon in experimental animals leads to severe, persistent, and often fatal viral infection.[22,23] Interferons resolve viral infection through two mechanisms: (1) initiating a sequence of intracellular events that suppress viral replication, and (2) modulating the immune response against cells that harbor viral pathogens. Although the various types of interferons bind to cells through different receptor complexes, they all initiate the transcription of numerous interferon-stimulated genes and activate the same basic intracellular antiviral pathways.

The best characterized proteins involved in these events are protein kinase R (PKR), 2’,5’-oligoadenylate synthetase (OAS), and MX. PKR phosphorylates the α subunit of eukaryotic initiation factor, which in turn inhibits the translation of viral proteins[24]; OAS activates intracellular RNase L, which in turn breaks down viral and host RNA[25]; and MX protein blocks the replication of negative-stranded RNA viruses.[26] Collectively, these and other downstream effects inhibit viral replication and are responsible for the indirect antiviral properties of interferon. The immune modulatory effects of interferon include enhanced expression of viral proteins and human leukocyte antigen (HLA) class I and II proteins on the surface of cells infected with virus, enhanced synthesis of ILs and tumor necrosis factor, and stimulation of natural killer cells, cytotoxic T cells, and macrophages.[27,28] As a result, interferon can be considered an indirect antiviral agent that inhibits HCV RNA through these indirect mechanisms, as opposed to directly inhibiting the HCV proteins.

Two forms of interferon-α, 2a and 2b, are currently used to treat chronic HCV. Interferons-β and -γ have also been shown to inhibit HCV but are only used in clinical practice to treat multiple sclerosis and chronic granulomatous disease, and osteopetrosis, respectively.[29,30] Interferon-λ was recently shown to be highly effective in suppressing HCV, and the limited receptor distribution for type III interferon seems to be associated with fewer flu-like symptoms, less bone marrow suppression, and fewer psychiatric side events.[31]

The administration of interferon to patients with chronic HCV leads to a biphasic decline in serum HCV RNA.[32] The first phase occurs within the first 1 to 4 days of initiating treatment and is characterized by a rapid decline in serum HCV RNA. This effect is thought to be secondary to the production of PKR, OAS, and MX, which interfere with HCV replication. The second phase of HCV decline occurs over several weeks to months and is thought to be from the immune response, which leads to apoptosis of HCV-infected hepatocytes and prevents HCV from entering new cells. Both phases of HCV RNA decline are responsible for the global response to interferon, as illustrated in **Fig. 1**. If this global antiviral response is satisfactory, the patient becomes HCV RNA–undetectable and could experience an SVR (see **Fig. 1**A–C). In contrast, if the global HCV RNA response is unsatisfactory the patient will not become HCV RNA–undetectable (see **Fig. 1**D).

Not all patients with chronic HCV experience response to peginterferon and ribavirin in the same way. Rather, a spectrum of virologic responses is influenced by several host genetic, host phenotypic, and virologic factors. These factors include age, sex, race, ethnicity, body weight, insulin resistance, the degree of hepatic fibrosis, the viral genotype, and the serum level of HCV RNA.[6–10,33–37] Each of these factors could potentially affect both the first and second phase responses. However, the major impact of many of these factors seems to be on the slope of the second phase decline (see **Fig. 1**). This phase is most dependent on the immune response to HCV and is primarily responsible for when patients become HCV RNA–undetectable during treatment. The single most important factor affecting the slope of the phase two decline during treatment with peginterferon seems to be the host gene IL-28B.[38]

THE ROLE OF IL-28B IN MODULATING THE RESPONSE TO INTERFERON

Studies from three different laboratories and countries have conclusively shown that at least two single nucleotide polymorphisms (SNP) near the gene that codes for IL-28B, one of the interferon λ genes, affects the patients ability to respond to peginterferon and experience an SVR.[39] A commercial test for the SNP at position rs12979860 is now available in the United States and many other countries. Patients who have the CC genotype at this position in this gene have a twofold higher likelihood of experiencing an SVR compared with patients with either the CT or TT haplotype, regardless of race or

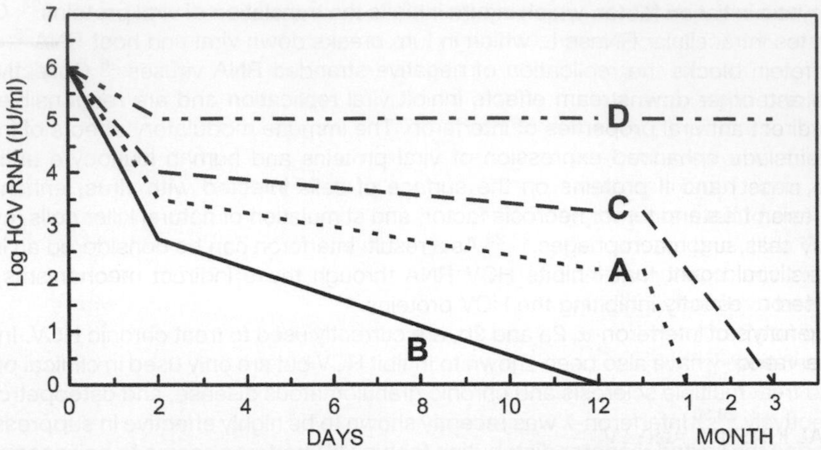

Fig. 1. Various patterns of phase one and two decline in HCV RNA during treatment with peginterferon and ribavirin. (A) Phase one and rapid phase two decline leading to HCV RNA clearance within 4 weeks. This pattern is seen in patients with rapid virologic response to peginterferon and ribavirin therapy. (B) Rapid phase one and two decline in HCV RNA leading to HCV RNA clearance within 2 weeks. This pattern is seen in patients with rapid virologic response to telaprevir, peginterferon, and ribavirin. (C) Phase one and slower phase two decline in HCV RNA leading to HCV RNA clearance within 12 weeks. This pattern is seen in patients with complete early virologic response. (D) Slow phase one and very slow phase two decline in HCV RNA. This pattern is seen in patients with null response.

ethnicity. The higher rates of SVR observed in patients of Asian descent and the lower rates of SVR observed in African Americans compared with Caucasians is directly related to the frequency of the IL-28B CC genotype in these racial and ethic populations.[38] Most patients with spontaneous resolution of HCV after acute infection have also been shown to have the IL-28B CC genotype.[40] This finding suggests that these patients are also highly responsive to endogenous interferon, can mount an appropriate immune response, and can experience HCV resolution after the acute infection.

The genotype of IL-28B modulates interferon responsiveness through affecting the phase two decline in HCV RNA during treatment. Patients with the CC genotype have a more rapid decline in HCV RNA during phase two than patients with either the CT or the TT genotypes.[41] Therefore, most patients with the CC genotype become HCV RNA–undetectable within the first 12 weeks after peginterferon and ribavirin therapy is initiated. In Caucasians with chronic HCV, 94% become HCV RNA–undetectable during treatment compared with only 56% and 51% of those with the CT or TT genotypes, respectively. Fifty percent of African American patients with the CC genotype become HCV RNA–undetectable within 12 weeks compared with only 26% of patients with a non–IL-28B CC genotype. The IL-28B gene also affects the immune response against chronic hepatitis B virus (HBV). In patients with e antigen–positive chronic HBV, a higher percentage of patients with IL-28B CC genotype experience seroconversion after treatment with peginterferon compared with patients with non-CC genotypes.[42] Seroconversion from e antigen–positive to anti–e antigen in patients with chronic HBV is known to be influenced by the immune response. This recent observation further supports the data suggesting that IL-28B modulates the immune-mediated interferon response.

Because the phase two decline in HCV RNA during treatment with peginterferon and ribavirin is thought to be secondary to the interferon immune response against cells harboring HCV, it is highly likely that the low rates of SVR observed in patients with IL-28B CT and TT are secondary to downregulation of the immune response to interferon treatment. It is unlikely that this defect could be overcome simply through administering exogenous interferon, and that is why treating HCV with higher doses (more) of interferon does not lead to significant increases in SVR.[43] If this is correct, patients who have the least response to interferon, those likely to have the TT genotype, might require an alternative therapy that restores immune responsiveness before interferon treatment is initiated. This hypothesis is supported by a recent preliminary study that suggested that administration of the NS5A vaccine GI5005 for several weeks could restore the blunted immune response against HCV proteins, improve interferon responsiveness, and produce higher SVR rates in patients with the IL-28B TT genotype.[44] Additional studies of this HCV vaccine are warranted to confirm this observation.

VIRAL KINETICS AND SVR

Although IL-28B genotype is an important predictor of SVR after interferon therapy, the time to experience a virologic response and become HCV RNA–undetectable is the single most important determinant of SVR.[41] The time to virologic response has been conveniently divided into three categories: rapid virologic response (RVR; becoming HCV RNA–undetectable within 4 weeks after initiating interferon and ribavirin treatment), complete early virologic response (cEVR; becoming HCV RNA–undetectable after week 4 and by week 12), and slow to respond (STR; becoming HCV RNA–undetectable after week 12 and by week 24).[45] These virologic response patterns depend on both phase one and two viral kinetics. Patients with an RVR have rapid rates of viral decline during both phase one and two (see **Fig. 1**A). In contrast, patients with a cEVR have much lower rates of viral decline during phase one and two (see **Fig. 1**C). Patients who do not experience a response to interferon generally have a phase one response but no significant decline in HCV RNA during phase two (see **Fig. 1**D).

SVR rates for RVR, cEVR, and STR range from 85% to 95%, 60% to 70%, and 33% to 45% respectively. Patients with an RVR have exceptionally high SVR rates regardless of HCV genotype.[46] Both retrospective and prospective studies have now shown that treatment could be shortened from 48 to 24 weeks in patients with genotype 1 who experience an RVR.[47–49] These concepts form the basis of response-guided therapy.[50] Patients with an RVR also have exceptionally high rates of SVR regardless of their IL-28B genotype.[41] Most patients who experience an RVR have the IL-28B CC genotype. However, patients with the IL-28B CT or TT genotype who experience an RVR also have SVR rates that approach 90%.[41] This finding strongly suggests that the IL-28B genotype is not the only factor affecting phase one and two viral decline. Rather, other undefined host genetic factors, host phenotypic factors, and viral factors also affect the response to peginterferon and contribute to viral clearance.

Two direct-acting antiviral agents, telaprevir and boceprevir, have completed phase III clinical trials, and their approval by the FDA is anticipated during the summer of 2011. The addition of either of these two protease inhibitors to peginterferon and ribavirin has been shown to markedly enhance phase one and two viral decline and lead to RVR in 80% to 85% of patients, as illustrated in **Fig. 1**B.[14,15] Virtually all patients with the IL-28B CC genotype and most with the IL-28B CT gentoype experience an RVR when treated with these protease inhibitors. In contrast, the largest group of patients who did not achieve an RVR after treatment with triple combination therapy were IL-28B TT and experienced poor response to interferon on a genetic basis.[51,52]

IMPACT OF HCV ON THE IMMUNE RESPONSE AND THE IMPACT OF ANTIVIRAL SUPPRESSION

One of the primary reasons that HCV persists after an acute infection is that it directly inhibits the immune response. Once this RNA virus enters cells, it translates a polyprotein that is subsequently cleaved into several structural and nonstructural proteins. At least two of these proteins, the envelope protein E2 and the nonstructural protein NS5A, directly inhibit PKR and other steps in the interferon cascade.[53,54] This function blunts the interferon-mediated antiviral response against HCV and allows HCV to replicate and persist even in the presence of an immune response. One possible explanation as to why patients with the IL-28B CC genotype have such a high rate of spontaneous resolution after acute infection is that their immune response to endogenous interferon is sufficient to overcome the antiviral effects of these HCV proteins.[40]

Inhibiting HCV replication reduces the production of the viral proteins that inhibit the intracellular response to interferon. Investigators currently hypothesize that this effect enhances the intracellular effects of interferon therapy and, together with interferon's effect on the immune response, which seems to be modulated by IL-28B, can eradicate HCV and produce an SVR. The addition of a potent antiviral agent to peginterferon and ribavirin is simply much more effective in suppressing HCV replication, leads to a much more rapid decline in HCV proteins, and may therefore enhance the interferon-induced immune response. However, whether suppressing HCV with a combination of potent antiviral agents will trigger an immune response without using exogenous interferon remains to be seen.

The first of the studies to evaluate interferon-free therapy used a protease and polymerase inhibitor for 14 days.[17] All patients had a marked decline in serum HCV RNA and 25% became HCV RNA–undetectable. The antiviral agents were then discontinued and treatment with peginterferon and ribavirin was initiated. All patients became HCV RNA–undetectable shortly after peginterferon and ribavirin were initiated, but approximately 25% developed recurrent viremia while still receiving peginterferon and ribavirin. Three additional studies have also used a protease and polymerase inhibitor without interferon.[18,19,55] In each of these studies, more than half of the patients developed a virologic breakthrough several months into treatment.

However, in one study, 5 of 11 patients remained HCV RNA–undetectable throughout the 6-month treatment course, and 4 of 11 remained HCV RNA–undetectable for at least 3 months after stopping the antiviral agents. This finding strongly suggests that the combination of a protease and polymerase inhibitor without interferon could eradicate HCV in a limited number of patients. It is likely that these patients have an intact endogenous interferon response, and either the IL-28B CC genotype or other host genetic or phenotypic factors associated with SVR. If this hypothesis is correct, an interferon-free regimen would be expected to achieve a SVR in only 25% to 33% of patients with chronic HCV.

CAN HCV BE CURED WITHOUT INTERFERON

A major impediment to treating chronic HCV is the adverse effect profile of interferon, which leads to morbidity in virtually all patients but rarely is associated with mortality.[56] These adverse events cause 15% to 20% of patients to prematurely discontinue therapy. Some patients cannot receive interferon because it may stimulate or exacerbate a coexistent immune or psychiatric disorder. Most patients with chronic HCV defer treatment because they simply do not wish to receive weekly injections or because they fear developing adverse events. Shortening the duration that interferon is used or replacing interferon entirely with an all oral antiviral regimen would be widely embraced options.

The primary question is whether viral suppression with antiviral agents alone would lead to eradication of HCV or if it would require an immune response. The answer is currently purely speculative. Clinical trials currently underway will undoubtedly answer this question within the coming year. For now, all one can do is compare the various mechanisms through which antiviral agents and peginterferon affect HCV and the immune response. These mechanisms are summarized in **Box 1**.

Patients who experience an RVR when treated with peginterferon and ribavirin have a very low relapse rate and high SVR rate.[45,46] Therefore, these patients may be treated for only 24 weeks.[47–49] The use of a single potent antiviral agent along with peginterferon and ribavirin increases the percentage of patients who experience an RVR from 15% to 20% to 50% to 66%.[14,15] Preliminary studies have shown that the addition of a polymerase to this three-drug regimen (four drugs) leads to an RVR in 100% of patients, including those who experienced no prior response.[18,19,55] In the only study that currently provides SVR data, 9 of 10 patients experienced an SVR after 24 weeks of treatment.[55] Reducing the duration of peginterferon and ribavirin to less than 24 weeks in patients with an RVR seems to increase relapse and marginally reduce SVR regardless of HCV genotype.[10,50] However, given the high potency of a four-dug regimen and that most patients become HCV RNA–undetectable within 2 weeks after initiating treatment, the possibility that treatment could be shortened to only 12 weeks and still produce an SVR in nearly all patients is entirely possible and will undoubtedly be evaluated in the future.

Several questions must be considered in developing an all oral treatment for HCV, the most important of which is whether interferon exerts its effects and eradicates HCV through acting as an antiviral agent alone or as both an antiviral and immune-modulating agent. The bulk of the evidence discussed earlier clearly supports both, with the immune effect mediated through the IL-28B gene and other host genetic and phenotypic factors. If this is the case, then an all-oral regimen is likely to have a limited SVR rate, possibly confined to those patients with an IL-28B CC genotype and an intact endogenous interferon response.

The second possibility is that simply suppressing HCV long enough with multiple antiviral agents to prevent the emergence of resistant species will ultimately lead to

Box 1
Mechanisms involved in eradicating HCV with antiviral agents versus peginterferon and ribavirin

- Oral antiviral agents
  - Antiviral response mediated by direct suppression of HCV replication at one or more sites.
  - Require multiple antiviral agents that act at different sites and with adequate potency to prevent the emergence of resistant species.
  - Suppress HCV replication to reduce HCV proteins that inhibit the effects of endogenous interferon.
  - Long-term suppression will lead to degradation of existing HCV RNA.
- Peginterferon and ribavirin
  - Antiviral response mediated by stimulating intracellular proteins that interfere with HCV replication.
  - Interferon enhances T-cell immune response against HCV-infected cells.

the degradation and eradication of HCV. A recent study has shown that treatment of patients with HCV with telaprevir monotherapy increased the rate of the phase two HCV RNA decline.[57] Mathematical modeling has suggested that intracellular HCV must be degraded to account for this observation. Additional studies have suggested that at least three antiviral agents would be required to prevent the emergence of antiviral resistance in the absence of interferon.[58] Two studies have shown that the combination of a protease, polymerase, and ribavirin can suppress and maintain HCV RNA at undetectable levels without breakthrough viremia for several months. What percentage of patients will remain HCV RNA–undetectable and experience a SVR when these treatments are stopped remains to be seen. At least two additional studies to evaluate the hypothesis that HCV can be cured by a two- (protease and polymerase) or three- (protease, polymerase, and ribavirin) drug regimen were initiated in early 2011. The final results are anxiously awaited.

Patients with chronic HCV and their physicians should be very optimistic about the future. Within a few short months, 70% to 75% of patients will be cured of chronic HCV when treated with a protease inhibitor, peginterferon, and ribavirin. In the near future, it is likely that four-drug therapy consisting of a protease, polymerase inhibitor, peginterferon, and ribavirin will be administered for a shorter period, possibly 12 weeks, and cure nearly all patients. Although an all-oral cocktail is likely to cure some patients with chronic HCV, it is not so likely that it would be effective in all patients.

REFERENCES

1. Bisceglie AM, Martin P, Kassianides C, et al. Recombinant interferon alfa therapy for chronic hepatitis C. N Engl J Med 1989;321:1506–10.
2. McHutchinson JG, Gordon SC, Schiff ER, et al. Interferon alfa-2b alone or in combination with ribavirin as initial treatment for chronic hepatitis C. N Engl J Med 1998;339:1485–92.
3. Lindsay KL, Trepo C, Heintges T, et al. A randomized, double-blind trial comparing peginterferon alfa-2b to interferon alfa-2b as initial treatment for chronic hepatitis C. Hepatology 2001;34:395–403.
4. Reddy KR, Wright TL, Pockros PJ, et al. Efficacy and safety of pegylated (40-KD) interferon α-2a compared with interferon α-2a in non-cirrhotic patients with chronic hepatitis C. Hepatology 2001;33:433–8.
5. Heathcote EJ, Shiffman ML, Cooksley WG, et al. Peginterferon alfa-2a in patients with chronic hepatitis C and cirrhosis. N Engl J Med 2000;343:1673–80.
6. Manns MP, McHutchinson JG, Gordon SC, et al. Peginterferon-alfa-2b plus ribavirin compared with interferon alfa-2b plus ribavirin for initial treatment of chronic hepatitis C: a randomized trial. Lancet 2001;358:958–65.
7. Fried MW, Shiffman ML, Reddy KR, et al. Combination of peginterferon alfa-2a (40 kd) plus ribavirin in patients with chronic hepatitis C virus infection. N Engl J Med 2002;347:975–82.
8. Hadziyannis SJ, Sette H Jr, Morgan TR, et al. Peginterferon-alfa 2a and ribavirin combination therapy in chronic hepatitis C: a randomized study of treatment duration and ribavirin dose. Ann Intern Med 2004;140:346–55.
9. McHutchison JG, Lawitz EJ, Shiffman ML, et al. Peginterferon alfa-2b or alfa-2a with ribavirin for treatment of hepatitis C infection. N Engl J Med 2009;361:580–93.
10. Shiffman ML, Suter F, Bacon BR, et al. Peginterferon alfa-2a and ribavirin for 16 or 24 weeks in HCV genotype 2 or 3. N Engl J Med 2007;357:124–34.
11. Weisberg IS, Jacobson IM. Telaprevir: hope on the horizon, getting closer. Clin Liver Dis 2009;13:441–52.

12. Berman K, Kwo PY. Boceprevir, an NS3 protease inhibitor of HCV. Clin Liver Dis 2009;13:429–39.
13. Burton JR Jr, Everson GT. HCV NS5B polymerase inhibitors. Clin Liver Dis 2009; 13:453–65.
14. Poordad F, McCone J Jr, Bacon BR, et al. Boceprevir for untreated chronic HCV genotype 1 infection. N Engl J Med 2011;364:1195–11206.
15. Jacobson IM, McHutchison JG, Dusheiko GM, et al. Telaprevir in combination with peginterferon and ribavirin in genotype 1 HCV treatment naïve patients: final results of phase 3 Advance study. Hepatology 2010;52(Suppl):427A.
16. Lavanchy D. The global burden of hepatitis C. Liver Int 2009;29(Suppl 1):74–81.
17. Gane EJ, Roberts SK, Stedman CA, et al. Oral combination therapy with a nucleoside polymerase inhibitor (RG7128) and danoprevir for chronic hepatitis C genotype 1 infection (INFORM-1): a randomised, double-blind, placebo-controlled, dose-escalation trial. Lancet 2010;376:1467–75.
18. Zeuzem S, Buggisch P, Agarwal K, et al. Dual, triple and quadruple combination treatment with a protease inhibitor (GS-9256) and a polymerase inhibitor (GS-9190) alone and in combination with ribavirin or Peginterferon/ribavirin for up to 28 days in treatment naïve, genotype 1 HCV subjects. Hepatology 2010; 52(Suppl):400A.
19. Di Bisceglie AM, Nelson DR, Gane E, et al. VX-222 with telaprevir alone or in combination with peginterferon alfa-2a and ribavirin in treatment-naïve patients with chronic hepatitis C: Zenith study interim results. J Hepatol 2011;54(Suppl):S540.
20. Samuel CE. Antiviral actions of interferons. Clin Microbiol Rev 2001;14:778–809.
21. Donnelly RP, Kotenko SV. Interferon-lambda: a new addition to an old family. J Interferon Cytokine Res 2010;30:555–64.
22. Vilcek J, Zinkernagel RM, Aguet M. Immune response in mice that lack the interferon-gamma receptor. Science 1993;259:1742–5.
23. Hwang SY, Hertzog PJ, Holland KA, et al. A null mutation in the gene encoding a type I interferon receptor component eliminates antiproliferative and antiviral responses to interferons alpha and beta and alters macrophage responses. Proc Natl Acad Sci U S A 1995;92:11284–8.
24. Samuel CE, Kuhen KL, George CX, et al. The PKR protein kinase—an interferon-inducible regulator of cell growth and differentiation. Int J Hematol 1997;65:227–37.
25. Witt PL, Marie I, Robert N, et al. Isoforms p69 and p100 of 2′,5′-oligoadenylate synthetase induced differentially by interferons in vivo and in vitro. J Interferon Res 1993;13:17–23.
26. Staeheli P, Pitossi F, Pavlovic J. Mx proteins: GTPases with antiviral activity. Trends Cell Biol 1993;3:268–72.
27. Rehermann B. Chronic infections with hepatotropic viruses: mechanisms of impairment of cellular immune responses. Semin Liver Dis 2007;27:152–60.
28. Seo YJ, Hahm B. Type I interferon modulates the battle of host immune system against viruses. Adv Appl Microbiol 2010;73:83–101.
29. Frese M, Schwarzle V, Barth K, et al. Interferon-γ inhibits replication of subgenomic and genomic hepatitis C virus RNAs. Hepatology 2002;35:694–703.
30. Chan HL, Ren H, Chow WC, et al. Randomized trial of interferon beta-1a with or without ribavirin in Asian patients with chronic hepatitis C. Hepatology 2007;46:315–23.
31. Muir AJ, Shiffman ML, Zaman A, et al. Phase 1b study of pegylated interferon lambda 1 with or without ribavirin in patients with chronic genotype 1 hepatitis C virus infection. Hepatology 2010;52:822–32.
32. Herrmann E, Neumann AU, Schmidt JM, et al. Hepatitis C virus kinetics. Antivir Ther 2000;5:85–90.

33. Conjeevaram HS, Fried MW, Jeffers LJ, et al. Peginterferon and ribavirin treatment in African American and Caucasian American patients with hepatitis C genotype 1. Gastroenterology 2006;131:470–7.
34. Muir AJ, Bornstein JD, Killenberg PG. Peginterferon alfa-2b and ribavirin for the treatment of chronic hepatitis C in blacks and non-Hispanic whites. N Engl J Med 2004;350:2265–71.
35. Shiffman ML, Mihas AA, Millwala F, et al. Treatment of chronic hepatitis C virus in African Americans with genotypes 2 and 3. Am J Gastroenterol 2007;102:1–6.
36. Rodriguez-Torres M, Jeffers LJ, Sheikh MY, et al. Peginterferon alfa-2a and ribavirin in Latino and non-Latino whites with hepatitis C. N Engl J Med 2009;360:257–67.
37. Romero-Gomez M, Del Mar Viloria M, Andrade RJ, et al. Insulin resistance impairs sustained response rate to peginterferon plus ribavirin in chronic hepatitis C patients. Gastroenterology 2005;128:636–41.
38. Ge D, Fellay J, Thompson AJ, et al. Genetic variation in IL28B predicts hepatitis C treatment-induced viral clearance. Nature 2009;461:399–401.
39. Afdhal NH, McHutchison JG, Zeuzem S, et al. Hepatitis C pharmacogenetics: state of the art in 2010. Hepatology 2011;53:336–45.
40. Thomas DL, Thio CL, Martin MP, et al. Genetic variation in IL28B and spontaneous clearance of hepatitis C virus. Nature 2009;461:798–801.
41. Thompson AJ, Muir AJ, Sulkowski MS, et al. IL28B polymorphism improves viral kinetics and is the strongest pre-treatment predictor of SVR in HCV-1 patients. Gastroenterology 2010;139:120–9.
42. Sonneveld MJ, Wong VWS, Woltman AM, et al. Polymorphisms at RS12979860 and RS 12980275 near IL28B predict serological response to INF/Peginterferon in HBEG-positive chronic hepatitis B. J Hepatol 2011;54(Suppl):S32.
43. Reddy KR, Shiffman ML, Rodriguez-Torres M, et al. Induction pegylated interferon alfa-2a and high dose ribavirin do not increase SVR in heavy patients with HCV genotype 1 and high viral loads. Gastroenterology 2010;139:1972–83.
44. Pockros P, Jacobson I, Boyer TD, et al. GI-5005 therapeutic vaccine plus peginterferon/ribavirin improves sustained virologic response versus peginterferon/ribavirin in prior non-responders with genotype 1 chronic HCV infection. Hepatology 2010;52(Suppl):404A.
45. Shiffman ML. Optimizing the current therapy for chronic hepatitis C virus: peginterferon and ribavirin dosing and the utility of growth factors. Clin Liver Dis 2008; 12:487–505.
46. Fried MW, Hadziyannis SJ, Shiffman ML, et al. Rapid virological response is the most important predictor of sustained virological response across genotypes in patients with chronic hepatitis C virus infection. J Hepatol, in press.
47. Jensen DM, Morgan TR, Marcellin P, et al. Early identification of HCV genotype 1 patients responding to 24 weeks peginterferon alpha-2a (40 kd)/ribavirin therapy. Hepatology 2006;43:954–60.
48. Ferenci P, Laferl H, Scherzer TM, et al. Peginterferon alfa-2a and ribavirin for 24 weeks in hepatitis C type 1 and 4 patients with rapid virological response. Gastroenterology 2008;135:451–8.
49. Lee SS, Sherman M, Ramji A, et al. 36 versus 48 weeks of treatment with peginterferon alfa-2a plus ribavirin for genotype 1/4 patients with undetectable HCV RNA at week 8: final results of a randomized multicenter study. Hepatology 2010;52(Suppl):359A.
50. Shiffman ML. HCV response guided therapy: should treatment length be shortened or extended? Curr Hepat Rep 2011;10:4–10.

51. Jacobson IM, Catlett I, Marcellin P, et al. Telaprevir substantially improved SVR rates across all IL28B genotypes in the advance trial. J Hepatol 2011;54(Suppl):S542.
52. Poordad F, Bronowicki JP, Gordon SC, et al. IL28B polymorphism predicts virologic response in patients with hepatitis C genotype 1 treated with boceprevir combination therapy. J Hepatol 2011;54(Suppl):S6.
53. Gale M, Katze MG. Molecular mechanisms of interferon resistance mediated by viral-directed inhibition of PKR, the interferon induced protein kinase. Pharmacol Ther 1998;78:29–46.
54. Taylor DR, Shi ST, Romano PR, et al. Inhibition of the interferon-inducible protein kinase PKR by HCV E2 protein. Science 1999;285:107–10.
55. Lok A, Gardiner D, Lawitz E, et al. Quadruple therapy with MBS-790052, BMS-650032 and peginterferon/ribavirin for 24 weeks results in 100% SVR12 in HCV genotype 1 null responders. J Hepatol 2011;54(Suppl):S536.
56. Shiffman ML. Side effects of medical therapy for chronic hepatitis C. Ann Hepatol 2004;3:5–10.
57. Guedj J, Perelson AS. Second-phase hepatitis C virus RNA decline during telaprevir-based therapy increases with drug effectiveness: implications for treatment duration. Hepatology 2011;53(6):1801–8.
58. Rong L, Dahari H, Ribeiro RM, et al. Rapid emergence of protease inhibitor resistance in hepatitis C virus. Sci Transl Med 2010;2(30):30ra32.

Index

Note: Page numbers of article titles are in **boldface** type.

Clin Liver Dis 15 (2011) 677–684
doi:10.1016/S1089-3261(11)00079-1 liver.theclinics.com

C

D

E

G

H

R

S

T

Printed and bound by CPI Group (UK) Ltd, Croydon, CR0 4YY
03/10/2024
01040448-0002